1994 Revised EMT-Basic National Standards Review Self-Test

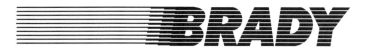

1994 Revised EMT-Basic National Standards Review Self-Test

Charly D. Miller, REMT-P

David White, RN

Based on the
1994 Revision of the
Emergency Medical Technician
National Standard Curriculum
U.S. Department of Transportation,
National Highway Traffic Safety Administration

Keyed to
Brady's *Emergency Care*
7th Edition, © 1995

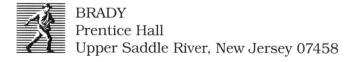

BRADY
Prentice Hall
Upper Saddle River, New Jersey 07458

Library of Congress Cataloging-in-Publication Data

Miller, C. D. (Charly D.), (date)
  1994 revised EMT-basic national standards review self-test/by Charly D. Miller and David White.
    p.   cm.
    "Based on the 1994 revision of the Emergency medical technician national standard curriculum [by] U.S. Department of Transportation, National Highway Traffic Safety Administration".
    "Answers page-keyed to Brady's emergency care, 7th edition, 1994".
    ISBN 0-8359-4948-6
    1. Emergency medicine—Examinations, questions, etc. 2. First aid in illness and injury—Examinations, questions, etc. 3. Emergency medical technicians—Examinations, questions, etc. I. White, David, 1964– . II. Grant, Harvey D., 1934– Brady emergency care, 1995. III. United States. National Highway Traffic Safety Administration. IV. Title.
    RC86.7.G7   1995 Suppl.
    616.02'5—dc20   95-16025
                                                                CIP

Editorial/Production Supervision: *Susan Geraghty*
Page Layout: *DeNee Reiton Skipper*
Publisher: *Susan Katz*
Marketing Manager: *Judy Streger*
Managing Production Editor: *Patrick Walsh*
Production Editor: *Cathy O'Connell*
Director of Manufacturing and Production: *Bruce Johnson*
Manufacturing Buyer: *Ilene Sanford*
Editorial Assistant: *Carol Sobel*
Printer/Binder: *The Banta Company, Harrisonburg*

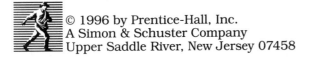

© 1996 by Prentice-Hall, Inc.
A Simon & Schuster Company
Upper Saddle River, New Jersey 07458

All rights reserved. No part of this book may be reproduced in any form or by any means, without permission in writing from the publisher.

Printed in the United States of America
10 9 8 7 6 5 4 3 2 1

ISBN 0-8359-4948-6

PRENTICE-HALL INTERNATIONAL (UK) LIMITED, *London*
PRENTICE-HALL OF AUSTRALIA PTY, LIMITED, *Sydney*
PRENTICE-HALL CANADA INC., *Toronto*
PRENTICE-HALL HISPANOAMERICANA, S.A., *Mexico*
PRENTICE-HALL OF INDIA PRIVATE LIMITED, *New Delhi*
PRENTICE-HALL OF JAPAN, INC., *Tokyo*
SIMON & SCHUSTER ASIA PTE. LTD., *Singapore*
EDITORA PRENTICE-HALL DO BRASIL, LTDA., *Rio De Janeiro*

NOTICE ON CARE PROCEDURES

It is the intent of the authors and publisher that this textbook be used as part of a formal EMT-Basic education program taught by qualified instructors and supervised by a licensed physician. The procedures described in this textbook are based upon consultation with EMT and medical authorities. The authors and publisher have taken care to make certain that these procedures reflect currently accepted clinical practice; however, they cannot be considered absolute recommendations.

The material in this textbook contains the most current information available at the time of publication. However, federal, state, and local guidelines concerning clinical practices, including without limitation, those governing infection control and universal precautions, change rapidly. The reader should note, therefore, that the new regulation may require changes in some procedures.

It is the responsibility of the reader to familiarize himself or herself with the policies and procedures set by federal, state, and local agencies as well as the institution or agency where the reader is employed. The authors and the publisher of this textbook and the supplements written to accompany it disclaim any liability, loss, or risk resulting directly or indirectly from the suggested procedures and theory, from any undetected errors, or from the reader's misunderstanding of the text. It is the reader's responsibility to stay informed of any new changes or recommendations made by any federal, state, and local agency as well as by his or her employing institution or agency.

Contents

Introduction ("Read Me Before You Start!") **ix**

Acknowledgments **xiii**

About the Authors **xv**

Suggestions for Written Examination Preparation and Execution **xvii**

Suggestions for Practical Examination Preparation and Execution **xxv**

TEST SECTION ONE: PREPARATORY **1**

Introduction to Emergency Medical Care; Well-being of the EMT-Basic; Medical, Legal, and Ethical Issues; The Human Body; Baseline Vital Signs and SAMPLE History; Lifting and Moving Patients

TEST SECTION TWO: AIRWAY **57**

Respiration Anatomy Review; Opening the Airway; Techniques of Artificial Ventilation; Airway Adjuncts; Suctioning and Suction Devices; Oxygen Therapy; Special Airway Considerations

TEST SECTION THREE: PATIENT ASSESSMENT **79**

Scene Size-up; The Initial Assessment; The Focused History and Physical Exam of Trauma Patients; The Focused History and Physical Exam of Medical Patients; The Detailed Physical Exam; Ongoing Assessment; Communications; Documentation; Elective Group of Medical Terminology and Abbreviations Questions

TEST SECTION FOUR: MEDICAL/BEHAVIORAL EMERGENCIES AND OBSTETRICS/GYNECOLOGY **123**

General Pharmacology; Respiratory Emergencies; Cardiac Emergencies; Diabetes and Altered Mental Status; Allergies; Poisonings and Overdoses; Environmental Emergencies; Behavioral Emergencies; Obstetrics and Gynecology

TEST SECTION FIVE: TRAUMA **215**

Bleeding and Shock; Soft-tissue Injuries; Musculoskeletal Injuries; Injuries to the Head and Spine

TEST SECTION SIX: INFANTS AND CHILDREN **249**

Age Group Definitions for Infants and Children; Developmental Differences between Age Groups; Pediatric Airway Differences; General Special Assessment Considerations for Infants and Children; General Special Emergency Care Considerations for Infants and Children; Pediatric Seizures, Poisonings, Fevers, and Drownings; Sudden Infant Death Syndrome; Pediatric Trauma, Child Abuse, and Child Neglect

TEST SECTION SEVEN: OPERATIONS **261**

Ambulance Operations; Gaining Access; Hazardous Materials Incident Management; Multiple-Casualty Incident Management

TEST SECTION EIGHT: ADVANCED AIRWAY MANAGEMENT (*ELECTIVE SECTION*) **271**

Airway Anatomy Review (per repeated DOT emphasis); Adult Orotracheal Intubation; Pediatric Orotracheal Intubation; Nasogastric Tube Insertion; Endotracheal Tube Suctioning

TEST SECTION NINE: APPENDIX A (ALS-ASSIST SKILLS) AND APPENDIX B (INFECTIOUS DISEASES) OF BRADY'S *EMERGENCY CARE,* 7th Ed. (*ELECTIVE SECTION*) **293**

Assisting with Endotracheal Intubation; Assisting with ECG Application and Use; Pulse Oximeter Use; Assisting with IV Therapy; Infectious Diseases

NATIONAL REGISTRY OF EMERGENCY MEDICAL TECHNICIANS SKILLS SHEETS **313**

TEST SECTION ANSWER SHEETS **331**

SECTION ONE ANSWER KEY **347**

SECTION TWO ANSWER KEY **353**

SECTION THREE ANSWER KEY **356**

SECTION FOUR ANSWER KEY **361**

SECTION FIVE ANSWER KEY **369**

SECTION SIX ANSWER KEY **373**

SECTION SEVEN ANSWER KEY **375**

SECTION EIGHT ANSWER KEY **376**

SECTION NINE ANSWER KEY **379**

GUIDE TO COMMON MEDICAL ABBREVIATIONS AND SYMBOLS **383**

Introduction
("Read Me Before You Start!")

Dear Reader,

This text was written **by** EMTs **for** EMTs. Our test questions are based primarily on the 1994 revised EMT-Basic National Standard Curriculum as set forth by the National Highway Traffic Safety Administration's Department of Transportation (DOT). This text is designed to assist you in your preparation for **any** written examination (local, county, state, and/or National Registry). Its self-test format is designed to challenge you, to pinpoint the subjects in which you require additional study, and to test your skill at reading and responding to test questions.

The answer keys for each section are accompanied by reference page numbers that correspond to Brady's **Emergency Care**, 7th ed. They also are accompanied by the question's subject title. Thus, if you don't have Brady's **Emergency Care** text (and cannot purchase it), you can use the index of the text you do have to seek information on the subjects you had difficulty with. Each section has questions on medical terminology. The answer key for some of these questions will direct you to reference your text glossary or a medical dictionary.

Be sure to read the sections we have included that provide tips on mental and physical preparation for taking written **and** practical exams. All too frequently, students fail tests **not** because they don't know the material but because they **don't read the questions carefully** or because they are **ill-prepared to**

successfully perform in the testing environment. By purchasing and using this text, you already are on the road to successful written test performance. But your preparation must also include consideration of your practical test performance.

SPECIAL NOTES REGARDING SOME TEST SECTIONS

Long Test Sections: Because our test sections follow the divisions set by the DOT curriculum modules (and the ***Emergency Care*** text modules), some sections are ***quite long*** (specifically, Test Sections One, Three, and Four). We suggest that you determine how much time you have to spend during each study session and plan to accomplish ***one question per minute*** of that study time. Place a pencil mark in the text (and on the answer sheet) at the point where you have set your time limit. In this way, you will begin to acquaint yourself with the normal test's question time allotment.

Question Difficulty: Our test sections are more complete and contain more difficult questions than any "average" test will. We require absolutely perfect knowledge of each DOT-listed EMS subject. Our goal is to help you pinpoint subjects that represent your potential "weaknesses." This gives you the opportunity to study these specific subjects and to feel comfortable with the information you already have mastered. Thus, if you can pass ***our*** tests with a 90 percent score (or better), you should be able to achieve a significantly higher score on ***any*** written exam that you may face.

Repeated Test Questions: As you progress through the test sections, you may notice that ***some questions are repeated*** (or very similar questions are asked). This repeat emphasis on certain subjects directly corresponds with repeat emphasis in the DOT guidelines. Since these subjects are so often repeated in the DOT, it is our opinion that they will be ***the most likely subjects to be covered*** in every actual written test. Thus, they represent information that is critically important to your test-taking preparation.

Seemingly Obvious Answers: Some DOT guidelines stipulate knowledge of fairly "silly" or simple information. Unfortunately, this "silly" information may be the straw that breaks your test score. Our inclusion of questions with answers that seem obvious to you is our way of ensuring that we help you to obtain the highest test score possible!

Elective Questions: In some test sections (for example, the last 59 questions of Test Section Three and the last 8 questions of Test Section Four), we have included "elective questions." Usually, these are medical terminology questions that represent subject matter not specifically required by the DOT but that may appear on your local, county, or state tests. If you want to skip them, you certainly may! However, you may enjoy testing yourself on these terms and subjects. Excellence in EMS includes more than simply mastering the minimum DOT requirements.

Questions with Long and Involved Answers: Most actual tests do not have questions with long and involved answers. Our "place the following in the correct order of performance" question/answers represent our desire to ensure that you have a mastery of all DOT-required orders of specific skill performance steps. Usually, you will be tested on these kinds of skill steps during a practical skills examination. It *is* possible, however, that an actual written test may include this sort of question. We will warn you to stop timing your performance when you are about to encounter one of our long and involved questions. You may stop timing and/or take a break and/or skip these questions altogether. Remember, though, that these questions are designed to help you prepare for *all* aspects of EMS testing. Thus, you may want to complete them.

Author's Tips on Questions with Long and Involved Answers: Rather than try to sort through all the steps provided (sometimes as many as 19!), just read through them first. Then, on lined paper, write out the correct sequence of step performance, as you remember it. Write one performance activity on each line, leaving a margin on the left side of your paper. After that, look at the steps provided in the text's question options. Find the step that most closely corresponds to each of your listed performance activities, and put that step's number in the margin to the left of each line. When you are done, compare the left margin numbered sequence of your performance activities to the available answers.

While using this text, if none of your selections match the available answers, you should "flag" that question for study and review.

On an actual test, try this technique: Find a step that you know is absolutely ***not*** a correct selection. Any available answer containing that step's number is NOT THE CORRECT ANSWER. Find another incorrect selection and check the remaining answers to rule out more available answers. Continue this process until (it is hoped) only one answer is left.

No Options to Summon ALS Backup: Written tests rarely reflect "reality." Get used to it! Although summoning ALS backup is a real solution in many EMS situations, it is **not** a solution in the testing situation. For the vast majority of testing situations, the EMT-Basic is on her/his own!

"Elective" Test Sections: Test Sections Eight and Nine are "elective" sections, containing information that would be present only on exams that include coverage of Advanced Airway Techniques, ALS-Assist Skills, or Infectious Diseases. Yet these sections are included in the 1994 EMT-Basic DOT guidelines. Thus, they contain information that may be tested on **any** written examination. It probably is to your advantage to test yourself on these skills prior to taking any written or practical EMT-Basic examination.

We sincerely hope that our text will assist you to excel in your examination. We do not wish you good luck, because luck is not a factor. Only your dedicated preparation and review will help you to achieve high scores and excellent performance on your upcoming examination. We do, however, wish you the best of performances!

Sincerely yours,

Charly D. Miller   David M. White

Charly D. Miller and David M. White

Acknowledgments

The authors wish to express their gratitude and appreciation to Susan B. Katz, our extraordinary editor.

Lastly, the authors enjoy saying "Hi, Mom! Hi, Dad!" (Raymond and Carol Miller, James and Carolyn White).

About the Authors

Charly D. Miller is a field paramedic, currently employed by Denver General Hospital's Paramedic Division. She has been involved in EMS since 1983, when she received her EMT-Basic certificate in the state of Nebraska. In addition to "working the streets," she has been an in-hospital Psychiatric Technician-EMT and a helicopter medic for the Army National Guard. She is also a nationally recognized EMS educator and author of EMS texts and journal articles. She received her paramedic training at Creighton University in Omaha, Nebraska, and has been a Nationally Registered EMT-Paramedic since 1986. Her first Brady book, **Home Meds; A Paramedic's Pocket Guide to Prescription Medications,** was published in the fall of 1991.

David White is a Registered Nurse who began his EMS career in 1985 as a firefighter EMT in Sheridan, Colorado. In 1986 he was certified at the EMT/IV level and began working for a private ambulance service in Cheyenne, Wyoming. He received his paramedic training in 1989 and completed his registered nursing program in Denver, Colorado, in 1994. With Charly, he is also the coauthor of Brady's **EMT-Basic National Standards Review Self-Test,** 2nd Edition; he also has coauthored EMS journal articles.

Suggestions for Practical Examination Preparation and Execution

Throughout your entire EMS career you will periodically be subjected to the dreaded practical skills examination stations. They accompany all levels of EMS courses, certification exams, recertification exams, and National Registry examinations. More and more often, practical stations also accompany continuing education workshops (such as Critical Trauma Care or Prehospital Trauma Life Support). Even the most veteran of EMS providers tremble in their boots when faced with the ordeal of performing in the situational exam station environment.

Why?

Skills and performance, knowledge and physical abilities are placed under the strictest scrutiny. It is unnerving to be so acutely observed and evaluated, especially when your livelihood is threatened should you fail. Even the best simulations contain components that must be recognized and remembered without actually seeing, feeling, hearing, or smelling them. You frequently are either alone or paired with people you have never worked with before. The equipment you are given is rarely in the configuration that you are accustomed to. Consequently, you may fumble around, hunting for instruments that your hands would normally, in a "real" situation, find on their own. Often, when you do find the equipment, it is of a different brand, make, or model and is unfamiliar to you. Additionally, the evaluators themselves may appear to be "out to get you." In their effort to remain unbiased and objective, even the friendliest evaluators often appear cold and perhaps hostile.

What can you do about these dilemmas?

Of course, regardless of the volume of calls you actually respond to, it is imperative that you remain skilled at operating all EMS equipment and that you frequently refresh yourself regarding patient assessment and treatment protocols. Periodic practice and review are essential. In the last section of this text, you will find copies of the skills station score sheet used by the National Registry of EMTs. Prior to the practical exam, get together with a small group of peers and use these score sheets to practice the practical skills. Volunteering your time for the testing of others (spending time as "the patient") is also helpful in developing an awareness of common performance mistakes. But the biggest improvement between past and present performances can be made by changing your approach to the situational or practical exam station itself.

When appearing for a written exam, you bring your own pencil and eraser, do you not? A similar rule applies to any practical skills exam station. At the very least, wear your own equipment holster. This puts vital items like scissors, penlight, pens, and the like at your fingertips, just where you are accustomed to finding them. Your own stethoscope ought to be draped, bundled, or strapped in its usual position. Actually changing into your uniform before going through the stations is ideal. This may appear "gung-ho" to others, but these others are not grading your performance. Indeed, if you have your own emergency care kit, **bring it**. Your goal should be to clothe and equip yourself in a manner that makes you feel comfortable and makes your surroundings as familiar as possible.

The previous suggestions are easily applied to any practical skills exam station. The "assessment" or "situation" stations present a greater challenge, however. Here, the most difficult and most vital improvement you can make is in your performance style itself.

RULES FOR SITUATIONAL PRACTICAL SKILLS STATIONS

1. ***Fix your eyes and your attention on the evaluator.*** As you enter this station, do not preoccupy yourself with eyeing the patient or the scene to get a head start on the situation. Fix your eyes and your attention on the evaluator. Concentrate on the instructions and information she/he is providing.

2. ***If you are offered time to examine the equipment, do so.*** Look at the equipment carefully, especially if it differs from the equipment you are accustomed to using. If possible, arrange it in a manner that is familiar to you. Do not leave it in a messy pile beside the patient.

3. ***When the evaluator describes the scenario, be alert for indications of the mechanism of injury or descriptions of the scene that cannot be simulated.*** If you are told that the steering wheel is bent, or the windshield fractured, or the furniture broken, **it means something**. Take time to consider the information these clues provide.

   If this type of information is not offered, **you must ask for it**. What is the condition of her apartment? Is it tidy? Messy? What does it smell like? What does the car look like? Where was the point of impact, and where was the patient sitting? Did the patient wear her/his seat belt? Is there compartmental intrusion involving the patient's space? Is the steering wheel bent/broken? Is there glass damage from patient contact?

4. ***As you are directed to begin your performance, no matter what the situation, the first words you should utter are "Is the scene safe?"*** In real life, you usually can detect potential dangers on approach. You can see smoke, smell a gas leak, hear a domestic altercation, or observe that the police have not yet arrived. Situational exams are usually unable to simulate signs of these dangers, however. So, for situational exams, the first words out of your mouth must be "Is the scene safe?"

5. ***From this moment on, there is no longer any reason for you to look at the evaluator.*** This is very important. Looking back and forth between the evaluator and the patient is distracting. It will interrupt your concentration

and continuity. Focus your eyes and attention on the scene and the patient. Your eyes and hands should never leave the patient (except to obtain equipment). The evaluator doesn't need to see your face. She/he is listening to what you say and watching your skills performance as much as possible.

6. **Never stop talking.** Whether you are questioning the evaluator, questioning the patient, or describing your actions, you should never stop talking. Frequently, evaluators miss actions/skills performed by the testing party while they are making notes on a skills performance sheet. Verbalize every single thing you are doing, everything you are **thinking**.

7. **Don't forget to talk to your patient.** This may sound difficult, but it can be easily incorporated with the previous suggestion. Since you should be addressing your attention to the patient, but verbalizing all your thoughts and actions for the evaluator, **tell the patient what you are thinking and doing**. As often as you are able, address all your questions and explanations to the patient.

8. **If the patient doesn't have the answers, ask the evaluator, but do not remove your eye contact from the patient.** The evaluator is in the same room. She/he can hear you without your needing to look at her/him.

What follows is a written example of what a situational practical skills station should **sound like**:

EVALUATOR: You may begin.

PERFORMER: Is the scene safe?

EVALUATOR: The scene is safe.

PERFORMER: Then I am observing the scene as I approach. Is the mechanism of injury apparent?

I can see that my patient has some blood on his left thigh. Is the blood spurting as though it is an arterial bleed? It's not? Okay.

First, I place my hand on his head and assess his level of consciousness.

Sir? Sir? Can you hear me?

Hi. My name is Mork. I'm an Emergency Medical Technician and I'm here to help you. I need you to keep very still and not move your head.

What's your name?

Okay, Endor, any pain in your neck as I run my fingers down it?

My invisible partner, Mindy, is going to hold your head to help you keep it absolutely still while I examine you. She will not stop holding your head until we have secured you to a long backboard.

First I'd like to check your airway. I'm going to look inside and make sure it's clear. Anything loose in there, Endor?

Good. Are you having any difficulty breathing?

When I listen to his chest with this stethoscope, can I hear any unusual noises when he breathes?

Does your chest hurt at all when I compress it?

It feels even in excursion and I don't feel any crepitus or see any wounds or deformities.

My invisible partner, Mindy, will observe your airway and respiratory effort as she continues to maintain immobilization of your C-spine, and she will alert me to any changes while I examine you further.

I'm going to check his pulses now. Do I feel his radial pulse?

What quality and rate do I feel?

Is he sweaty?

What is his skin color?

Temperature?

Endor, I'm going to give you some oxygen to help you feel better. This is a nasal cannula and may tickle your nose a bit, but I'll run it at four liters per minute and it will help you feel much better.

Yes, an evaluator could be scoring this performance over the telephone!

A continuous narration of your thoughts and activities assists your score in a number of ways. It keeps you focused on your patient and your task, ensuring that you proceed without forgetting things. This extra degree of attention also helps to calm you down, improving your physical and mental concentration. Perhaps most important, verbalizing everything you do and think will make it nearly impossible for the evaluator to miss what you have done. Without this technique, the evaluator may miss your sweeping check of the patient's clothing for gross bleeding because she/he was making notes on the skills performance sheet, or the like.

GROUP APPROACHES TO THE SITUATIONAL EXAM STATION

All the previous suggestions apply here as well. However, now you are working with other participants who probably were total strangers only moments ago. The old adage "Too many cooks spoil the broth" applies here in quadruplicate. Few things are as debilitating and disastrous as having two, three, or four EMTs crawling all over each other, trying to treat a patient at the same time.

The secret is **organization and assignment of tasks**. Each group member must have an assigned task, with an assigned group leader in charge—**before the group enters the examination station**. As each new station is approached, the tasks should be clearly reassigned to allow each participant an opportunity to rotate through each different task performance.

Groups of two are easy. For trauma situational exam stations, one partner is Group Leader and the other is the C-spine/Airway Monitor. The Group Leader introduces self and partner, directing partner to maintain immobilization of the C-spine continuously and to monitor for changes in airway status after the initial examination. The Group Leader examines the patient and performs all other necessary treatments.

The C-spine/Airway Monitor maintains spinal immobilization and observes airway/respiratory status no matter how tempted she/he is to help with other treatment. While doing so, however, she/he may **verbally** assist whenever the Group Leader seems to have forgotten something.

For groups of two in the **medical** situational exam stations, the C-spine/Airway Monitor becomes an Equipment Operator. The Equipment Operator manages oxygen equipment and delivery, takes vital signs, applies the EKG monitor (if available), positions the backboard and/or gurney, and so on. The Group Leader is still responsible for the patient examination. But when an Equipment Operator is present, the Group Leader may direct application of treatments.

Groups of three responders are broken down into assignments of the Group Leader, the C-spine/Airway Monitor, and the Equipment Operator.

Groups of four responders may be broken down into assignments of the Group Leader, the C-spine Immobilizer, the Airway Monitor, and the Equipment Operator. If active airway maintenance is not required, the Airway Monitor becomes a secondary Equipment Operator, and the C-spine Immobilizer resumes observation of the airway.

If you have the misfortune of operating in a five-member or more team, send the fifth or more members to direct traffic!

The most important key to group performance, no matter how you designate the tasks, is that the assignments are clearly understood by each member.

IN SUMMARY:

1. Wear your own equipment holster and stethoscope. Bring your own kit if you have one, and wear your uniform. Make the testing environment as comfortable and familiar as possible.

2. As you first enter the station, fix your eyes and attention on the evaluator. Don't "jump the gun." Listen to the clues that the evaluator provides. Take time to consider the clues and to check the equipment provided. Ask for scene or situation information if it is not offered.

3. Ask, "Is the scene safe?"

4. After beginning your performance, never let your eyes or hands leave the patient.

5. Never stop talking. Talk to the patient, ask questions, and describe everything you are thinking and doing. Don't look away from the patient to ask questions of the evaluator; she/he does not need to see your face to answer you.

6. Clearly assign specific tasks to group members and take turns with task performance.

7. Do not physically deviate from your assigned task. However, you may **verbally** remind partners of business if they appear to have forgotten something.

8. Above all, enjoy yourself! Take pride in the performance level you have worked so hard to achieve, and have confidence in your abilities.

Suggestions for Written Examination Preparation and Execution

Written examinations are generally as delightful as a visit to the dentist. Nonetheless, anesthesia is not an appropriate solution.

Test preparation should start well before the exam day. Use this text to determine your strengths and weaknesses and to practice your test-taking skills.

First, read each question carefully. Many written examinations are failed by knowledgeable and experienced EMTs **simply because they don't read the questions well**. Don't read more into the question than what is presented. Is the question asking you to identify a correct answer (a true answer), an incorrect answer (a false answer), or the "best" answer? Read each answer carefully. After making your selection, go back and reread the question, inserting that answer. Does it still seem correct?

In an exam situation, a guess is better than leaving the answer completely blank (a blank answer is an error). When taking the self-tests, however, **do not guess** at the answers. If you cannot answer a question with confidence, you ought to review that particular subject. If you **do** guess, you may answer correctly by pure accident. There is no guarantee that you will guess in the same (accidentally correct) manner when faced with a similar question on your actual exam. Skip that question, circle its number on your answer sheet, and move on.

When you have completed the self-test section, compare your answers to the key provided. Highlight or write down the subject and/or reference page number for each incorrect or skipped answer. Then refer to your text and study that material.

After you have studied, retake the self-test. If you again have difficulty with some subjects, return to your text and repeat your review. The more often you are able to repeat this process, the better you will fare on your examination.

As you are taking the self-tests, begin to practice timing yourself. Most examinations allow one minute per question: 60 questions, one-hour time limit; 150 questions, 2½-hour time limit; and so on. Timed practice sessions will actually help you to increase your test-taking speed. This will afford you extra time for those questions that require extra thought.

Learn not to let yourself become "bogged down" on a difficult or confusing question. You can skip it and come back. When you do skip a question, however, make sure you also skip the corresponding answer sheet entry! Although everyone will warn you about making "unnecessary stray marks or erasures" on an answer sheet, it is better to **lightly** circle the number of a skipped question than to cause all your subsequent questions to be incorrectly answered. But make darn sure that you erase all extra marks before turning in your answer sheet.

If you have coworkers or friends who will be taking the same exam, get together with them and do group study and practice sessions during the week or two before the test. (This is especially helpful in preparation for **practical skills** examinations.) "Teaching" others is often the best way to study for a written or practical skills examination.

Okay. You've done all that "good student" stuff. You've done your homework and practiced your skills, but you're still apprehensive and uncertain about taking this stupid test. What **more** can you do? You can **relax**!

Often people respond to that kind of encouragement with the reply, "I'm trying!" Well, there is no need to "try!" There is no effort involved in letting yourself relax and feel confident in your abilities. If you have studied and prepared, **congratulate yourself** with the certainty of success.

Be sure to get a good night's sleep before the test. If you stay up all night studying, you'll certainly do more harm than good. If you've delayed your review and cannot avoid last-minute studying, you **still** should go to bed early! But then get up early and study the morning of the test, ideally over a good breakfast.

If you are one of those "night shift" people who feel they don't think well in the early hours of the morning, you will need to arrange for a good sleep the previous afternoon and evening.

Now let's discuss the definition of a "good breakfast." Guess what? Contrary to popular EMT behavior (of **all** levels), a good breakfast does not consist of coffee and doughnuts. Whether or not you adopt good nutrition in your normal day-to-day living, it will be to your great advantage to do so on the morning of an event as stressful as a written and/or practical skills examination.

First, the sugar contained in the doughnuts will quickly peak, producing lethargy, while the caffeine in the coffee will provide artificial stimulation. Do you truly want to approach any exam situation **sideways**?

A breakfast high in complex carbohydrates, along with some protein, is the key to the sustained energy levels you'll need during a high-stress situation. Lean meats, eggs, and milk products (such as yogurt, cheeses, and low-fat milk) are good sources of protein. Carbohydrates are found in fresh fruits and juices, whole-grain breads, pancakes, and rice products.

A truly good breakfast will fuel your body **and** your brain. It will produce energy slowly and efficiently and help you to perform at your best. An important point to remember, however, is that the largest shunting of blood supply to the stomach (instead of to the brain) is **immediately after** ingestion of food. So allow yourself a couple of hours between your good breakfast and your test-taking. In this way, your body will be sending energy and nutrients to your brain during the time you sit for the test.

Structured review, sleep, and efficient nutrition will give you an undeniable "edge" and improve your performance in any testing situation.

Test Section One

This test section covers the following subjects:

* Introduction to Emergency Medical Care
* Well-being of the EMT-Basic
* Medical, Legal, and Ethical Issues
* The Human Body
* Baseline Vital Signs and SAMPLE History
* Lifting and Moving Patients

1994 Revised EMT-Basic National Standards Review Self-Test

1. The EMT's roles and responsibilities include assessing patients, providing patient care based on assessment findings, lifting and moving, transporting patients or transferring patient care, acting as a patient advocate, and ensuring

    (a) personal safety.
    (b) safety of the crew and patient.
    (c) safety of bystanders.
    (d) Answers (a) and (b) only.
    (e) Answers (a), (b), and (c).

2. Professional attributes of an EMT include a neat and clean appearance; knowledge of local, state, and national EMS issues; and

    (a) a positive attitude.
    (b) putting the patient's needs ahead of personal safety.
    (c) attending continuing education and refresher courses.
    (d) Both answers (a) and (c).
    (e) Both answers (b) and (c).

3. The definition of _____ is: A system of internal/external reviews and audits of all aspects of an EMS system designed to identify those areas needing improvement to ensure that the public receives the highest quality prehospital care.

    (a) quality improvement
    (b) medical direction
    (c) patient advocacy
    (d) Any of the above.
    (e) None of the above.

4. The definition of a _____ is: A physician responsible for the clinical and patient care aspects of an EMS system. Every ambulance service or rescue squad must have one.

    (a) quality improvement officer
    (b) medical director
    (c) patient advocate
    (d) Any of the above.
    (e) None of the above.

5. Quality improvement requires that an EMT attend continuing education and skills maintenance refresher courses, gather feedback from patients and hospital staff, attend run reviews and audits, and
    (a) document patient contacts completely and legibly.
    (b) conduct basic maintenance on equipment to assure proper functioning.
    (c) perform patient care without deviating from care protocols unless permission to do so is granted.
    (d) Answers (a) and (c) only.
    (e) Answers (a), (b), and (c).

6. "On-line" medical direction is when care is performed according to
    (a) telephone contact instructions from the medical director or receiving facility during a specific call.
    (b) radio contact instructions from the medical director or receiving facility during a specific call.
    (c) "standing orders" or care protocols previously written by the medical director.
    (d) Answers (a) and (b) only.
    (e) Answers (a), (b), and (c).

7. "Off-line" medical direction is when care is performed according to
    (a) telephone contact instructions from the medical director or receiving facility during a specific call.
    (b) radio contact instructions from the medical director or receiving facility during a specific call.
    (c) "standing orders" or care protocols previously written by the medical director.
    (d) Answers (a) and (b) only.
    (e) None of the above.

8. Which of the following statements regarding EMS stress is false?
    (a) Multiple-casualty incidents (MCIs) are the only stressful events any EMT may ever have to face.
    (b) Pediatric or elderly abuse/neglect incidents often are causes of great stress to the EMT.
    (c) Severe injuries (distortions of the human face from crushing, limb amputations, hangings, and the like) are very stressful for any prehospital provider.
    (d) Any single event may affect any EMT with profound stress, depending upon her/his private history or personal responses.
    (e) Personal life problems combined with stressful EMS incidents may result in a serious stress level for any EMT.

9. Signs and symptoms of stress include irritability, inability to concentrate, indecisiveness, difficulty sleeping, and

  (a) guilt.
  (b) loss of appetite.
  (c) loss of interest in sexual activities.
  (d) Answers (a) and (b) only.
  (e) Answers (a), (b), and (c).

10. All of the following lifestyle or work environment changes can be helpful in dealing with EMS stress, except

  (a) dietary changes, including reducing the intake of sugar, caffeine, alcohol, and fatty foods.
  (b) avoiding the embarrassment of seeking "professional" help.
  (c) requesting a duty assignment to a less busy area.
  (d) requesting work shift changes to allow extra relaxation time with family or friends.
  (e) safely increasing physical exercise and learning relaxation techniques.

11. Which of the following statements regarding Critical Incident Stress Debriefing (CISD) is true?

  (a) A CISD team is composed only of mental health professionals.
  (b) CISD is designed to accelerate the normal recovery process of experiencing a critically stressful incident.
  (c) CISD is reserved for MCIs of 20 or greater casualties.
  (d) CISD is helpful only if it occurs within 12 to 24 hours of the incident.
  (e) CISD is often a helpful method of investigating the incident because all information shared during a CISD meeting is considered "public record."

12. Dealing with death and dying produces specific stages of reactions that are experienced by patients and family members. Which of the following statements regarding death and dying stages is (are) true?

  (a) The stages may occur in any order.
  (b) Some stages may be experienced simultaneously.
  (c) Some people display emotions or attitudes that do not seem to fit any of the stages.
  (d) Only answers (a) and (c) are true.
  (e) Answers (a), (b), and (c) are true.

13. All of the following are considered response stages of death and dying, except the
    (a) bargaining stage ("If I can live, I'll never do such-and-such again."); an attempt to postpone death.
    (b) healing stage ("I'm feeling much better! Really!"); a sudden remission of all signs and symptoms of the patient's illness.
    (c) anger stage ("Why me?!"); the patient focuses anger about her/his impending death upon those around her/him.
    (d) denial stage ("Not me!"); a defense mechanism creating a buffer between the shock of dying and dealing with the illness/injury.
    (e) acceptance stage ("Well, I need to get everything in order now."); the patient accepts the fact of impending death (but not that the patient is happy about dying).

14. Which of the following death and dying stages may pose a risk of personal injury to the responding EMT?
    (a) Bargaining stage ("If I can live, I'll never do such-and-such again.").
    (b) Healing stage ("I'm feeling much better! Really!").
    (c) Anger stage ("Why me?!").
    (d) Denial stage ("Not me!").
    (e) Acceptance stage ("Well, I need to get everything in order now.").

15. Diseases are caused by _____, such as viruses and bacteria.
    (a) halogens
    (b) carcinogens
    (c) pathogens
    (d) biogens
    (e) germogens

16. Infectious diseases may be spread by
    (a) direct contact with infected blood or other body fluids.
    (b) droplet infection from airborne organisms (coughing, sneezing, or breathing).
    (c) indirect contact via handling objects or materials contaminated with infectious secretions.
    (d) Answers (a) and (c) only.
    (e) Answers (a), (b), and (c).

17. Which of the following statements regarding personal protective equipment is false?

(a) Hand washing before and after every patient contact is required only if protective gloves are not worn throughout the entire patient contact.
(b) Protective gloves should be worn for every patient contact, and a separate pair should be used for each separate patient.
(c) Eye protection should be worn whenever airborne droplet (or splashing fluid) contact is anticipated.
(d) Masks should be worn whenever airborne droplet (or splashing fluid) contact is anticipated.
(e) A gown should be worn whenever spilling or splashing of infectious fluid is anticipated.

18. Immunizations are available for EMS personnel against all of the following diseases, except

(a) tetanus.
(b) hepatitis-C.
(c) measles.
(d) chickenpox.
(e) hepatitis-B.

19. Which of the following statements regarding hazardous material incidents is false?

(a) Every ambulance should be equipped with a pair of binoculars and **The Emergency Response Handbook**, published by the U.S. Department of Transportation, so that hazardous material may be identified from a safe distance.
(b) If a patient is in immediate life-threat, untrained EMTs may borrow hazardous material suits and enter the contaminated area to provide emergency patient care.
(c) A self-contained breathing apparatus (SCBA) is required for entering any scene where poisonous gases, dust, or fumes are present or suspected to be present.
(d) EMTs should provide emergency care only after the patient is decontaminated.
(e) Placards with hazardous material symbols, colors, and identification numbers must be displayed on all vehicles (or containers) carrying hazardous materials.

20. Rescue operations often involve potential life threats from hazards such as electricity, fire, explosion, hazardous materials, cave-ins, and the like. Which of the following statements regarding rescue operations is true?

(a) Appropriate protective clothing (such as turnout gear, puncture-proof gloves, or helmets) must be worn by any responder before engaging in a rescue operation.
(b) An EMT's first responsibilities are to ensure personal and public safety, to identify potential dangers or rescue needs, and to call for appropriate rescue teams to be dispatched.
(c) Untrained persons must **never** attempt rescues.
(d) Only answers (a) and (b) are true.
(e) Answers (a), (b), and (c) are true.

21. Scenes involving violence are not uncommon. Crime perpetrators, bystanders, family members, and even patients may present a personal threat to the responding EMT. Which of the following statements regarding violent scenes is true?

(a) The scene should be controlled by law enforcement before an EMT provides care.
(b) EMS crews should have preplanned procedures for dealing with violence that erupts after entering the scene and should never be without radio contact.
(c) An EMT wearing body armor (such as a bulletproof vest) is safe, and her/his first responsibility should be to shield the patient from further harm.
(d) Only answers (a) and (b) are true.
(e) Answers (a), (b), and (c) are true.

22. The EMT has legal, medical, and ethical duties to her/his patient, public, and medical director. Which of the following statements regarding the EMT's **scope of practice** is false?

(a) The scope of practice defines the extent and limits of an EMT's job responsibilities.
(b) The medical skills and interventions that an EMT is allowed to perform are defined by state legislation.
(c) Within the limits set by state legislation, the medical skills and interventions that an EMT is allowed to perform are defined by local protocols (as set forth by the EMT's medical director) and may vary from region to region within the state.
(d) All regions within a state must share the same definition of an EMT's scope of practice, as set forth by state legislation.
(e) Legislation about an EMT's scope of practice, skills, and intervention may vary from state to state.

23. When considered in the context of EMS, the term *battery* may be defined as

   (a) unlawfully touching a patient without her/his consent.
   (b) providing emergency care to a competent patient who does not consent to the treatment.
   (c) providing emergency care to an unconscious patient.
   (d) Answers (a) and (b) only.
   (e) Answers (a), (b), and (c).

24. Which of the following statements regarding *expressed consent* is false?

   (a) The patient must be of legal age and able to make a rational decision.
   (b) The patient must be informed of the procedures' steps and all related risks.
   (c) Expressed consent must be obtained from every conscious, mentally competent adult before rendering treatment or transportation.
   (d) All of the above are false.
   (e) None of the above are false.

25. Which of the following statements regarding *implied consent* is false?

   (a) To be effective, implied consent must be *informed* consent.
   (b) With *any* unconscious patient, the law presumes that the patient would give her/his consent to treatment.
   (c) The law presumes that the unconscious patient would give her/his consent to treatment *only* if there is a significant risk of death if the treatment were withheld.
   (d) Both answers (a) and (b) are false.
   (e) Both answers (a) and (c) are false.

26. Which of the following statements regarding minors (children) and mentally incompetent adults is true?

   (a) Consent for treatment must be obtained from the patient's parent (or legal guardian) if she/he is present.
   (b) Some states consider a married minor, minor parent, or otherwise "emancipated" minor to have rights of consent or refusal of treatment.
   (c) In life-threatening situations, if the parent or legal guardian is unavailable, emergency treatment may be rendered based upon implied consent.
   (d) All of the above are true.
   (e) None of the above are true.

TEST SECTION ONE

27. Which of the following statements regarding refusal of care is false?

   (a) Every patient has a right to refuse treatment and/or transport.
   (b) Refusals are honored only when made by mentally competent adults following the rules of expressed consent.
   (c) Every patient refusing treatment must be informed of all the risks and consequences associated with such refusal and should be able to demonstrate understanding of all the risks and consequences.
   (d) All of the above are false.
   (e) None of the above are false.

28. In cases where the patient is unable to give consent but has life-threatening problems, the EMT may provide care under the law of

   (a) implied consent.
   (b) informed consent.
   (c) actual consent.
   (d) involuntary consent.
   (e) unconscious consent.

29. Which of the following statements regarding refusal of care is false?

   (a) Any unconscious patient who regains consciousness and demonstrates mental competency has a right to refuse further treatment or transportation.
   (b) Once any patient signs a "release from liability" form, the EMT is guaranteed freedom from liability for the patient's refusal of treatment or transportation.
   (c) When in doubt of the patient's competency to refuse treatment and transportation, the EMT should err in favor of providing care.
   (d) All of the above are false.
   (e) None of the above are false.

30. An EMT's best protection from liability when a patient refuses treatment or transportation is

   (a) a good EMS lawyer.
   (b) an accurate, detailed written report, describing all attempts made to obtain the patient's consent to treatment and transportation.
   (c) a more experienced partner.
   (d) stating "I cannot remember," as often as possible.
   (e) a "release from liability" form signed by the patient.

31. Another term for Do Not Resuscitate (DNR) orders is
  (a) death wish directives (DWDs).
  (b) dying wills.
  (c) advanced directives.
  (d) hold-treatment directives (HTDs).
  (e) hospice directives.

32. Which of the following statements regarding DNR orders is true?
  (a) Every mentally competent patient has the right to refuse resuscitative efforts in advance of their actual need.
  (b) DNR orders require a physician's signature and the signature of the patient or the patient's legal guardian.
  (c) Some DNR orders stipulate only that intubation, CPR, and chemical resuscitation be withheld.
  (d) When in doubt, or when written orders are not present, the EMT should perform all possible resuscitation efforts.
  (e) All of the above are true.

33. An EMT may be convicted of negligence only if which of the following is proven to have occurred?
  (a) The EMT had a duty to act and provide care for the patient.
  (b) The EMT failed to perform *or* deviated from care measures within her/his scope of practice.
  (c) The patient was injured physically *or* emotionally by the EMT's actions.
  (d) Answers (a) and (b) only.
  (e) Answers (a), (b), and (c).

34. You have transferred a nursing-home resident to the emergency department (ED) for evaluation of a urinary problem. As you arrive, your dispatcher notifies you that a 911 emergency call is waiting for you. All of the ED nurses are busy, but the ED clerk listens to your patient report and assures you that she will inform the nurse. You leave the patient in the care of the clerk. Which of the following statements regarding this situation is true?
  (a) In every state in the United States, this is viewed as abandonment.
  (b) Only some states view this as abandonment.
  (c) Emergency calls take precedence over transfers; therefore, this is not abandonment.
  (d) You have completed the transfer to the ED because the patient was received by the ED clerk; therefore, this is not abandonment.
  (e) None of these statements is true.

35. Some states have "Good Samaritan Laws." These laws are intended to grant immunity from negligence prosecution to
    (a) EMTs who operate under a physician's license.
    (b) EMTs who have lawsuits filed against them.
    (c) untrained individuals who volunteer to help an injured person at the scene of an accident.
    (d) All of the above.
    (e) None of the above.

36. Patient confidentiality rules stipulate that information obtained through the interview or examination of a patient may be shared with other persons
    (a) **only** when a written release is signed by the patient or an established legal guardian.
    (b) **only** when a verbal release is made by the patient or an established legal guardian.
    (c) **never**, under **any** circumstances.
    (d) when the patient (or established legal guardian) gives permission **either** in writing or over the telephone.
    (e) **only** after the patient's physician orders the release of information form.

37. The exceptions to patient confidentiality rules involve
    (a) other health care providers who need the information to continue patient care.
    (b) incidents that must be reported as a matter of state law, such as sexual assault and child or elderly abuse/neglect.
    (c) legal subpoenas to disclose the information.
    (d) Answers (a) and (c) only.
    (e) Answers (a), (b), and (c).

38. A medical identification device is designed to provide emergency medical information about a patient. It may list allergies, diabetic conditions, epilepsy, or other pertinent medical information about the patient. A medical identification device may include an information tube kept in the refrigerator or
    (a) a bracelet on the patient.
    (b) a necklace on the patient.
    (c) a card in the patient's wallet, pocket, or purse.
    (d) Answers (a) and (b) only.
    (e) Answers (a), (b), and (c).

39. Which of the following statements regarding crime scenes and evidence preservation is false?

    (a) The EMT's first priority is scene and evidence preservation.
    (b) An EMT should not disturb any item at the scene unless emergency care requires it—and then, only after making a mental note about the scene's condition prior to disruption.
    (c) When necessary to cut clothing, an EMT should never cut through holes from gunshot wounds or stabbings.
    (d) An EMT should observe, report, and/or document anything unusual at the scene.
    (e) An EMT should never enter a potential crime scene until the police have secured it.

40. State legislation requires the reporting of special situations, which may vary from state to state. Situations that commonly require reporting include all of the following, except suspected

    (a) child or elderly abuse.
    (b) prostitution.
    (c) sexual assault or injuries resulting from violent crimes.
    (d) infectious disease exposure.
    (e) spousal abuse.

41. Anatomy is the study of

    (a) body structure.
    (b) body function.
    (c) body strength.
    (d) All of the above.
    (e) None of the above.

42. Physiology is the study of

    (a) body structure.
    (b) body function.
    (c) body strength.
    (d) All of the above.
    (e) None of the above.

43. The ***anatomical position*** refers to the human body in which of the following positions?

    (a) Standing upright with arms outstretched above the head.
    (b) Lying prone with arms along the side of the body.
    (c) Lying supine with arms along the side of the body.
    (d) All of the above.
    (e) None of the above.

44. In the anatomical position, the thumb is on the _____ side of the hand.

    (a) superior
    (b) medial
    (c) midline
    (d) inferior
    (e) lateral

45. The umbilicus is considered to be in the _____ area of the abdomen.

    (a) superior
    (b) circumflex
    (c) midline
    (d) inferior
    (e) lateral

46. The small toe is on the _____ side of the foot

    (a) superior
    (b) medial
    (c) midline
    (d) inferior
    (e) lateral

47. A finding noted on only one side of the body (or body region) may be called a(n) _____ finding.

    (a) unilateral
    (b) bilateral
    (c) trilateral
    (d) quadrilateral
    (e) unusual

48. A finding noted on both sides of the body (or body region) may be called a(n) _____ finding.

    (a) unilateral
    (b) bilateral
    (c) trilateral
    (d) quadrilateral
    (e) unusual

49. Which of the following best defines *lateral rotation*?

    (a) Standing in an upright position.
    (b) To straighten a joint.
    (c) To bend a joint.
    (d) To turn a joint or limb away from the body's midline.
    (e) To turn a joint or limb toward the body's midline.

50. Which of the following best defines *extension*?

(a) Standing in an upright position.
(b) To straighten a joint.
(c) To bend a joint.
(d) To turn a joint or limb away from the body's midline.
(e) To turn a joint or limb toward the body's midline.

51. Which of the following best defines *medial rotation*?

(a) Standing in an upright position.
(b) To straighten a joint.
(c) To bend a joint.
(d) To turn a joint or limb away from the body's midline.
(e) To turn a joint or limb toward the body's midline.

52. Which of the following best defines *flexion*?

(a) Standing in an upright position.
(b) To straighten a joint.
(c) To bend a joint.
(d) To turn a joint or limb away from the body's midline.
(e) To turn a joint or limb toward the body's midline.

53. The best definition of the *mid-clavicular line* is an imaginary line drawn from the middle of either clavicle down to the

(a) great toe.
(b) lower chest margin.
(c) umbilicus.
(d) Answers (a) or (b).
(e) Answers (a) or (c).

54. The best definition of the *mid-axillary line* is an imaginary line drawn

(a) horizontally, from armpit to armpit.
(b) diagonally, from an armpit to the opposite hip.
(c) vertically, from the middle of an armpit to the middle of the lateral ankle.
(d) horizontally, from hip to hip.
(e) vertically, from the chin to the pubic bone.

55. The *apex* of an organ is best defined as the organ's

(a) pointed portion.
(b) superior portion.
(c) inferior portion.
(d) flat portion.
(e) largest (usually rounded) portion.

56. The tibia is _____ to the femur.
- (a) superior
- (b) medial
- (c) midline
- (d) inferior
- (e) lateral

57. The cranium is _____ to the spine.
- (a) superior
- (b) medial
- (c) midline
- (d) inferior
- (e) lateral

58. The great toe is on the _____ side of the foot.
- (a) superior
- (b) medial
- (c) midline
- (d) inferior
- (e) lateral

59. In the anatomical position, the ulna is _____ to the humerus.
- (a) proximal
- (b) anterior
- (c) superior
- (d) posterior
- (e) distal

60. The sternum is _____ to the thoracic spine.
- (a) proximal
- (b) anterior
- (c) superior
- (d) posterior
- (e) distal

61. The tarsals are _____ to the metatarsals.
- (a) proximal
- (b) anterior
- (c) superior
- (d) posterior
- (e) distal

62. The cervical spine is _____ to the esophagus.

    (a) proximal
    (b) anterior
    (c) superior
    (d) posterior
    (e) distal

63. In the anatomical position, the palm of the hand is considered to be the _____ surface.

    (a) proximal
    (b) superior
    (c) anterior
    (d) inferior
    (e) posterior

64. A person in the **supine** position is lying

    (a) on her/his stomach.
    (b) on her/his side.
    (c) on the floor.
    (d) on a bed with her/his head elevated 40 degrees.
    (e) on her/his back.

65. A person in the **prone** position is lying

    (a) on her/his stomach.
    (b) on her/his side.
    (c) on the floor.
    (d) on a bed with her/his head elevated 40 degrees.
    (e) on her/his back.

66. A person in the **lateral recumbent** position is lying

    (a) on her/his stomach.
    (b) on her/his side.
    (c) on the floor.
    (d) on a bed with her/his head elevated 40 degrees.
    (e) on her/his back.

67. In the medical sense, **abduction** refers to

    (a) movement toward the body.
    (b) movement toward the head.
    (c) movement away from the body.
    (d) movement toward the feet.
    (e) movement toward the back.

68. **Adduction** refers to
    - (a) movement toward the body.
    - (b) movement toward the head.
    - (c) movement away from the body.
    - (d) movement toward the feet.
    - (e) movement toward the back.

69. Another term for the **posterior** surface of the body is the _____ surface.
    - (a) dorsal
    - (b) ventral
    - (c) plantar
    - (d) palmar
    - (e) inguinal

70. Another term for the **anterior** surface of the body is the _____ surface.
    - (a) dorsal
    - (b) ventral
    - (c) plantar
    - (d) palmar
    - (e) inguinal

71. Another term for the **anterior** surface of the hand is the _____ surface.
    - (a) dorsal
    - (b) ventral
    - (c) plantar
    - (d) palmar
    - (e) inguinal

72. Another term for the **inferior** surface of the foot is the _____ surface.
    - (a) dorsal
    - (b) ventral
    - (c) plantar
    - (d) palmar
    - (e) inguinal

73. In addition to producing red blood cells (within bone marrow), the musculoskeletal system functions to
    - (a) give the body shape.
    - (b) protect vital internal organs.
    - (c) provide for body movement.
    - (d) Answers (a) and (b) only.
    - (e) Answers (a), (b), and (c).

74. The skull consists of

    (a) the cranium (which contains the brain) only.
    (b) the cranium (which contains the brain) and the face.
    (c) the cranium (which contains the brain), the face, and the first vertebra of the spine.
    (d) the cranium (which contains the brain), the face, and the first two vertebrae of the spine.
    (e) None of the above.

75. The bony facial structure that surrounds each eye is called the

    (a) mandible.
    (b) orbit.
    (c) nasal bone.
    (d) maxilla.
    (e) zygoma (zygomatic bone).

76. The bony facial structure that provides shape to the nose is called the

    (a) mandible.
    (b) orbit.
    (c) nasal bone.
    (d) maxilla.
    (e) zygoma (zygomatic bone).

77. The bony facial structure that is the upper jaw is called the

    (a) mandible.
    (b) orbit.
    (c) nasal bone.
    (d) maxilla.
    (e) zygoma (zygomatic bone).

78. The bony facial structure that is also called the cheekbone is the

    (a) mandible.
    (b) orbit.
    (c) nasal bone.
    (d) maxilla.
    (e) zygoma (zygomatic bone).

79. The bony facial structure that is the lower jaw is called the

    (a) mandible.
    (b) orbit.
    (c) nasal bone.
    (d) maxilla.
    (e) zygoma (zygomatic bone).

80. Which of the following statements regarding the spinal column is false?

(a) The spinal column encloses the spinal cord.
(b) The spinal cord connects with the brain through an opening at the base of the skull.
(c) The spinal column consists of 33 bones, known as *vertebrae*.
(d) The spine is divided into five sections.
(e) The coccyx does not enclose any portion of the spinal cord and therefore is not considered a part of the spine.

81. The sacral section of the spine (the sacrum) is located

(a) in the upper back, having ribs attached to it.
(b) immediately inferior to the lower back, forming the posterior wall of the pelvis.
(c) in the lower back and does not have attached ribs.
(d) in the neck.
(e) at the very end of the spine.

82. The thoracic section of the spine is located

(a) in the upper back, having ribs attached to it.
(b) immediately inferior to the lower back, forming the back wall of the pelvis.
(c) in the lower back and does not have attached ribs.
(d) in the neck.
(e) at the very end of the spine.

83. The cervical section of the spine is located

(a) in the upper back, having ribs attached to it.
(b) immediately inferior to the lower back, forming the back wall of the pelvis.
(c) in the lower back and does not have attached ribs.
(d) in the neck.
(e) at the very end of the spine.

84. The coccygeal section of the spine (the coccyx) is located

(a) in the upper back, having ribs attached to it.
(b) immediately inferior to the lower back, forming the back wall of the pelvis.
(c) in the lower back and does not have attached ribs.
(d) in the neck.
(e) at the very end of the spine.

85. The lumbar section of the spine is located

- (a) in the upper back, having ribs attached to it.
- (b) immediately inferior to the lower back, forming the back wall of the pelvis.
- (c) in the lower back and does not have attached ribs.
- (d) in the neck.
- (e) at the very end of the spine.

86. The chest is also sometimes called the

- (a) cervical cavity (cervix).
- (b) lumbar cavity.
- (c) thoracic cavity (thorax).
- (d) sacral cavity (sacrum).
- (e) coccygeal cavity (coccyx).

87. The cervical spine consists of ____ vertebrae.

- (a) 12
- (b) 10
- (c) 7
- (d) 5
- (e) 4

88. The thoracic spine consists of ____ vertebrae.

- (a) 12
- (b) 10
- (c) 7
- (d) 5
- (e) 4

89. The lumbar spine consists of ____ vertebrae.

- (a) 12
- (b) 10
- (c) 7
- (d) 5
- (e) 4

90. The sacral spine (sacrum) consists of ____ fused vertebrae.

- (a) 12
- (b) 10
- (c) 7
- (d) 5
- (e) 4

91. The coccyx consists of _____ fused vertebrae.
    (a) 12
    (b) 10
    (c) 7
    (d) 5
    (e) 4

92. The chest consists of ___ pairs of ribs.
    (a) 11
    (b) 12
    (c) 8
    (d) 7
    (e) 14

93. Almost all of the pairs of ribs are attached posteriorly to vertebrae and anteriorly to the breastbone. ___ pair(s) are attached only to the vertebrae and are called "floating" ribs.
    (a) 1
    (b) 2
    (c) 3
    (d) 4
    (e) 5

94. Another term for the entire breastbone is the
    (a) xiphoid process.
    (b) ilium.
    (c) sternum.
    (d) manubrium.
    (e) acetabular process.

95. Another term for the superior section of the breastbone is the
    (a) xiphoid process.
    (b) ilium.
    (c) sternum.
    (d) manubrium.
    (e) acetabular process.

96. Another term for the inferior tip of the breastbone is the
    (a) xiphoid process.
    (b) ilium.
    (c) sternum.
    (d) manubrium.
    (e) acetabular process.

97. The **hip** is defined as

(a) the pelvis.
(b) the joint between the pelvis and the thighbone.
(c) the thighbone.
(d) the joint between the spine and the thighbone.
(e) the joint between the spine and the pelvis.

98. The pelvis consists of several bones fused together. There are two large "wings" of the pelvis—wide bones that form each lateral (and superior) portion of the pelvis. Each of these bones is called the

(a) ilium (also referred to as the iliac crest).
(b) ischium (also referred to as the ischiac crest).
(c) pubis (also referred to as the pubic crest).
(d) Any of the above.
(e) None of the above.

99. The anterior pelvis is formed by a joining of bones, which is called the

(a) ilium.
(b) ischium.
(c) pubis.
(d) Any of the above.
(e) None of the above.

100. The socket portion of the hip is the

(a) tibia.
(b) fibula.
(c) femur.
(d) acetabulum.
(e) patella.

101. The anatomical term for the thighbone is the

(a) tibia.
(b) fibula.
(c) femur.
(d) acetabulum.
(e) patella.

102. The anatomical term for the kneecap is the

(a) tibia.
(b) fibula.
(c) femur.
(d) acetabulum.
(e) patella.

103. The anatomical term for the bone in the anterior lower leg is the

    (a) tibia.
    (b) fibula.
    (c) femur.
    (d) acetabulum.
    (e) patella.

104. The anatomical term for the bone in the posterior lower leg is the

    (a) tibia.
    (b) fibula.
    (c) femur.
    (d) acetabulum.
    (e) patella.

105. The anatomical term for the ankle bone on the great-toe side of the foot is the

    (a) medial malleolus.
    (b) lateral malleolus.
    (c) medial tuberosity.
    (d) lateral tuberosity.
    (e) dorsal tuberosity.

106. The anatomical term for the ankle bone on the small-toe side of the foot is the

    (a) medial malleolus.
    (b) lateral malleolus.
    (c) medial tuberosity.
    (d) lateral tuberosity.
    (e) dorsal tuberosity.

107. The anatomical term for the bones of the toes is the

    (a) tarsals and metatarsals.
    (b) carpals and metacarpals.
    (c) phalanges.
    (d) calcaneus.
    (e) sacrals and metasacrals.

108. The anatomical term for the bones of the foot is the

    (a) tarsals and metatarsals.
    (b) carpals and metacarpals.
    (c) phalanges.
    (d) calcaneus.
    (e) sacrals and metasacrals.

109. The anatomical term for the bone of the heel is the

(a) tarsal or metatarsal.
(b) carpal or metacarpal.
(c) phalanx.
(d) calcaneus.
(e) sacral or metasacral.

110. The anatomical term for the bones of the fingers is the

(a) tarsals and metatarsals.
(b) carpals and metacarpals.
(c) phalanges.
(d) calcaneus.
(e) sacrals and metasacrals.

111. The anatomical term for the bones of the hands is the

(a) tarsals and metatarsals.
(b) carpals and metacarpals.
(c) phalanges.
(d) calcaneus.
(e) sacrals and metasacrals.

112. The shoulder is composed of several bones. The anatomical term for the collarbone is the

(a) ulna.
(b) acromion.
(c) scapula.
(d) clavicle.
(e) olecranon.

113. The anatomical term for the shoulder blade (in the back) is the

(a) ulna.
(b) acromion.
(c) scapula.
(d) clavicle.
(e) olecranon.

114. The very end of the collarbone, where it forms the shoulder joint, is called the

(a) ulna.
(b) acromion.
(c) scapula.
(d) clavicle.
(e) olecranon.

115. The bone of the upper arm is the
    (a) ulna.
    (b) humerus.
    (c) radius.
    (d) carpalus.
    (e) olecranon.

116. The lateral bone of the lower arm is the
    (a) ulna.
    (b) humerus.
    (c) radius.
    (d) carpalus.
    (e) olecranon.

117. The medial bone of the lower arm is the
    (a) ulna.
    (b) humerus.
    (c) radius.
    (d) carpalus.
    (e) olecranon.

118. Joints are where bones connect to bones and accommodate movement. An example of a ball-and-socket joint is the
    (a) elbow.
    (b) hip.
    (c) neck.
    (d) Both answers (a) and (c).
    (e) Both answers (a) and (b).

119. An example of a hinge joint is the
    (a) elbow.
    (b) hip.
    (c) neck.
    (d) Both answers (a) and (c).
    (e) Both answers (a) and (b).

120. Muscles come in three different types. Voluntary muscle is best described as muscle that
    (a) requires no conscious control.
    (b) is consciously controlled.
    (c) has properties of automaticity (able to generate and conduct its own electrical impulses).
    (d) Both answers (a) and (c).
    (e) Both answers (b) and (c).

121. Involuntary muscle is best described as muscle that

    (a) requires no conscious control.
    (b) is consciously controlled.
    (c) has properties of automaticity (able to generate and conduct its own electrical impulses).
    (d) Both answers (a) and (c).
    (e) Both answers (b) and (c).

122. Cardiac muscle is best described as muscle that

    (a) requires no conscious control.
    (b) is consciously controlled.
    (c) has properties of automaticity (able to generate and conduct its own electrical impulses).
    (d) Both answers (a) and (c).
    (e) Both answers (b) and (c).

123. _____ attaches to the bones of the skeleton, forms the major muscle mass of the body, and is controlled by the nervous system and the brain. It also can be contracted and relaxed by the individual's will and is responsible for body movement.

    (a) Involuntary muscle
    (b) Cardiac muscle
    (c) Voluntary muscle
    (d) Any of the above.
    (e) None of the above.

124. _____ is found in the walls of the gastrointestinal tract and urinary system as well as the blood vessels and bronchi. It controls the flow of materials through these structures, carries out the automatic muscular functions of the body, is under no direct control by the individual, and responds to stimuli such as stretching, heat, and cold.

    (a) Involuntary muscle
    (b) Cardiac muscle
    (c) Voluntary muscle
    (d) Any of the above.
    (e) None of the above.

125. _____ is found only in the heart and has its own rich supply of blood. It can tolerate only a very short interruption of blood supply.

    (a) Involuntary muscle
    (b) Cardiac muscle
    (c) Voluntary muscle
    (d) Any of the above.
    (e) None of the above.

126. The respiratory system is responsible for the
    (a) introduction of carbon dioxide to the bloodstream and excretion of oxygen.
    (b) introduction of oxygen to the bloodstream and excretion of carbon dioxide.
    (c) muscular function of inhalation and exhalation only.
    (d) Answers (a) and (c) only.
    (e) Answers (a), (b), and (c).

127. When breathing through the mouth, the first area that air enters is the
    (a) pharynx.
    (b) nasopharynx.
    (c) larynx.
    (d) endopharynx.
    (e) oropharynx.

128. When breathing through the nose, the first area that air enters is the
    (a) pharynx.
    (b) nasopharynx.
    (c) larynx.
    (d) endopharynx.
    (e) oropharynx.

129. A leaf-shaped valve that prevents food and liquid from entering the windpipe is called the
    (a) cricoid cartilage.
    (b) larynx.
    (c) valecula.
    (d) epiglottis.
    (e) trachea.

130. The medical term for the windpipe is the
    (a) cricoid cartilage.
    (b) larynx.
    (c) valecula.
    (d) epiglottis.
    (e) trachea.

131. The firm ring that forms the lower portion of the voice box is the
    (a) cricoid cartilage.
    (b) larynx.
    (c) valecula.
    (d) epiglottis.
    (e) trachea.

132. The medical term for the voice box is the

(a) cricoid cartilage.
(b) larynx.
(c) valecula.
(d) epiglottis.
(e) trachea.

133. The windpipe divides into two large air tubes at a junction called the carina. The medical term for these air tubes is the

(a) right or left rhonchi.
(b) right or left bronchi.
(c) right or left alveoli.
(d) anterior or posterior rhonchi.
(e) anterior or posterior bronchi.

134. At the end of the respiratory "tree" are groups of tiny sacs. These sacs are called the

(a) rhonchi.
(b) bronchi.
(c) alveoli.
(d) petechia.
(e) cilia.

135. When the diaphragm and rib (intercostal) muscles are activated,

(a) the larynx opens and air flows in.
(b) the chest cavity becomes smaller and air flows out.
(c) the larynx opens and air flows out.
(d) the chest cavity enlarges and the lungs fill with air.
(e) None of the above.

136. When the diaphragm and rib (intercostal) muscles relax,

(a) the larynx opens and air flows in.
(b) the chest cavity becomes smaller and air flows out.
(c) the larynx opens and air flows out.
(d) the chest cavity enlarges and the lungs fill with air.
(e) None of the above.

137. The inhalation phase of respiration is considered _____ phase of respiration because it requires energy to accomplish.

(a) an active
(b) a passive
(c) the second
(d) the formal
(e) None of the above.

138. The exhalation phase of respiration is considered _____ phase of respiration because it requires energy to accomplish.

    (a) an active
    (b) a passive
    (c) the first
    (d) an informal
    (e) None of the above.

139. The respiratory gas exchange of oxygen and carbon dioxide occurs

    (a) in the alveoli only.
    (b) in the rhonchi and bronchi only.
    (c) in the cells of the body (via capillaries) only.
    (d) in the alveoli and the cells of the body (via capillaries) only.
    (e) in the rhonchi, bronchi, alveoli, and the cells of the body.

140. For an adult, an adequate rate of respiration at rest is considered to be _____ breaths per minute.

    (a) 10 to 12
    (b) 12 to 20
    (c) 15 to 30
    (d) 25 to 35
    (e) 25 to 50

141. For an infant, an adequate rate of respiration at rest is considered to be _____ breaths per minute.

    (a) 10 to 12
    (b) 12 to 20
    (c) 15 to 30
    (d) 25 to 35
    (e) 25 to 50

142. For a child, an adequate rate of respiration at rest is considered to be _____ breaths per minute.

    (a) 10 to 12
    (b) 12 to 20
    (c) 15 to 30
    (d) 25 to 35
    (e) 25 to 50

143. The complete assessment of respiration includes assessing the rate of breathing, the rhythm of breathing (is it regular or irregular?), and the

   (a) clarity and equality of breath sounds.
   (b) equality and fullness of chest expansion.
   (c) use of accessory muscles.
   (d) Answers (a) and (b) only.
   (e) Answers (a), (b), and (c).

144. Which of the following statements regarding pediatric airway anatomy considerations is false?

   (a) In general, all pediatric airway structures are smaller and more easily obstructed than adult airway structures.
   (b) The trachea is harder and less flexible in children, providing greater protection from direct injury.
   (c) Children's tongues take up proportionally more space in the mouth than adults'.
   (d) All of the above are false.
   (e) None of the above are false.

145. Which of the following statements regarding pediatric airway anatomy considerations is true?

   (a) Children have narrower tracheas that can be obstructed more easily by swelling.
   (b) Like other cartilage in the child, the cricoid cartilage is less developed and less rigid than in the adult.
   (c) The chest wall is softer, and children tend to depend more heavily on the diaphragm for breathing.
   (d) All of the above are true.
   (e) None of the above are true.

146. The heart is the circulatory pump of the body. The right side of the heart pumps _____ blood through the _____ circulation.

   (a) oxygen rich/systemic
   (b) oxygen poor/systemic
   (c) oxygen rich/pulmonary
   (d) oxygen poor/pulmonary
   (e) either oxygenated or deoxygenated/systemic or pulmonary.

147. The _____ receives blood from the veins of the body and the heart.

   (a) left ventricle
   (b) right ventricle
   (c) ventricular septum
   (d) right atrium
   (e) left atrium

148. The _____ receives blood from the lungs (via pulmonary veins).

 (a) left ventricle
 (b) right ventricle
 (c) ventricular septum
 (d) right atrium
 (e) left atrium

149. The _____ pumps blood to the lungs.

 (a) left ventricle
 (b) right ventricle
 (c) ventricular septum
 (d) right atrium
 (e) left atrium

150. The _____ pumps blood to the body.

 (a) left ventricle
 (b) right ventricle
 (c) ventricular septum
 (d) right atrium
 (e) left atrium

151. The cardiac valves

 (a) propel blood from one chamber of the heart to another.
 (b) propel blood from heart chambers into blood vessels.
 (c) prevent back flow of blood.
 (d) Both answers (a) and (b).
 (e) Both answers (a) and (c).

152. All arteries

 (a) carry blood away from the heart.
 (b) carry blood back to the heart.
 (c) carry only oxygenated blood.
 (d) Both answers (a) and (c).
 (e) Both answers (b) and (c).

153. All veins

 (a) carry blood away from the heart.
 (b) carry blood back to the heart.
 (c) carry only deoxygenated blood.
 (d) Both answers (a) and (c).
 (e) Both answers (b) and (c).

154. Pulmonary arteries

(a) carry blood away from the heart.
(b) carry blood back to the heart.
(c) carry only deoxygenated blood.
(d) Both answers (a) and (c).
(e) Both answers (b) and (c).

155. Pulmonary veins

(a) carry blood away from the heart.
(b) carry blood back to the heart.
(c) carry only oxygenated blood.
(d) Both answers (a) and (c).
(e) Both answers (b) and (c).

156. A major blood vessel that originates from the heart, then descends through the thoracic and abdominal cavities (in front of the spine), is the

(a) superior vena cava.
(b) inferior vena cava.
(c) aorta.
(d) Both answers (a) and (b).
(e) Both answers (b) and (c).

157. A major blood vessel that returns blood to the heart is the

(a) superior vena cava.
(b) inferior vena cava.
(c) aorta.
(d) Both answers (a) and (b).
(e) Both answers (b) and (c).

158. The heart muscle is supplied with blood by the _____, which branch off from the aorta.

(a) femoral arteries
(b) radial arteries
(c) carotid arteries
(d) coronary arteries
(e) brachial arteries

159. The head is supplied with blood by the _____, producing a pulse that can be palpated on either side of the neck.

(a) femoral arteries
(b) radial arteries
(c) carotid arteries
(d) coronary arteries
(e) brachial arteries

160. Major arteries of each thigh, the _____ supply the groin and lower extremities with blood. Their pulse can be palpated in the groin area.

    (a) femoral arteries
    (b) radial arteries
    (c) carotid arteries
    (d) coronary arteries
    (e) brachial arteries

161. The _____ produce a pulse that can be palpated between the elbow and the shoulder on the inside of the arm.

    (a) femoral arteries
    (b) radial arteries
    (c) carotid arteries
    (d) coronary arteries
    (e) brachial arteries

162. The _____ produce a pulse that can be palpated on the _____ side of either wrist.

    (a) radial arteries / small-finger (medial)
    (b) radial arteries / thumb (lateral)
    (c) pulsitile arteries / small-finger (lateral)
    (d) brachial arteries / thumb (lateral)
    (e) brachial arteries / small-finger (medial)

163. The pulse produced by the _____ is auscultated when using a sphygmomanometer and stethoscope to determine the blood pressure.

    (a) femoral artery
    (b) radial artery
    (c) carotid artery
    (d) coronary artery
    (e) brachial artery

164. An artery on the posterior surface of the medial malleolus that can be palpated for a pulse is the

    (a) anterior tibial artery.
    (b) posterior tibial artery.
    (c) dorsalis pedis artery.
    (d) superior pedal artery.
    (e) posterior pedal artery.

165. An artery on the anterior surface of the foot that can be palpated for a pulse is the

 (a) anterior tibial artery.
 (b) posterior tibial artery.
 (c) dorsalis pedis artery.
 (d) superior pedal artery.
 (e) posterior pedal artery.

166. Capillaries are found in all parts of the body. They are tiny blood vessels that

 (a) receive blood from the smallest arteries and send it to the smallest veins.
 (b) receive blood from the smallest veins and send it to the smallest arteries.
 (c) are responsible for the exchange of nutrients and waste, oxygen and carbon dioxide, at the cellular level of the body.
 (d) Both answers (a) and (c).
 (e) Both answers (b) and (c).

167. The smallest branch of an artery is called

 (a) a capillary.
 (b) an arteriette.
 (c) an arteriole.
 (d) All of the above.
 (e) None of the above.

168. The smallest branch of a vein is called

 (a) a capillary.
 (b) a veinette.
 (c) a venule.
 (d) Both answers (a) and (b).
 (e) None of the above.

169. Blood is made up of several components. Red blood cells (RBCs, or red corpuscles) carry oxygen to the tissues and carbon dioxide away from the tissues. Another medical term for RBCs is

 (a) leukocytes.
 (b) platelets.
 (c) erythrocytes.
 (d) plasma.
 (e) packed cells.

170. White blood cells (WBCs, or white corpuscles) are the body's immune defense against infections. Another medical term for WBCs is

(a) leukocytes.
(b) platelets.
(c) erythrocytes.
(d) plasma.
(e) packed cells.

171. The formation of blood clots is largely dependent upon the _____ found in blood.

(a) leukocytes
(b) platelets
(c) erythrocytes
(d) plasma
(e) packed cells

172. The fluid that carries the blood cells and nutrients is called

(a) whole blood.
(b) platelets.
(c) erythroliquid.
(d) plasma.
(e) packed cells.

173. A pulse is formed when the _____ contracts, sending a wave of blood through the arteries.

(a) left atrium
(b) right atrium
(c) left ventricle
(d) right ventricle
(e) ventricular septum

174. A pulse can be palpated

(a) only at the neck, inner arm, wrist, groin, and foot.
(b) anywhere an artery simultaneously passes near the skin surface and over a bone.
(c) anywhere a vein simultaneously passes near the skin surface and over a bone.
(d) anywhere a vein or artery simultaneously passes near the skin surface and over thick muscle.
(e) only at the neck, inner arm, wrist, groin, ankle, and foot.

175. ***Peripheral*** pulses include all of the following, except the _____ pulse.

(a) femoral
(b) brachial
(c) radial
(d) dorsalis pedis
(e) posterior tibial

176. ***Central*** pulses consist of the carotid pulse and the _____ pulse.

(a) femoral
(b) brachial
(c) radial
(d) dorsalis pedis
(e) posterior tibial

177. When measuring the blood pressure, the pressure on the walls of the artery when the left ventricle contracts is called the _____ blood pressure.

(a) diastolic
(b) endostolic
(c) systolic
(d) Any of the above.
(e) None of the above.

178. When measuring the blood pressure, the pressure on the walls of the artery when the left ventricle is at rest or relaxed is called the _____ blood pressure.

(a) diastolic
(b) endostolic
(c) systolic
(d) Any of the above.
(e) None of the above.

179. Which of the following statements regarding the nervous system is false?

(a) It controls voluntary and involuntary activities of the body.
(b) It consists of the central nervous system and peripheral nervous system.
(c) It governs sensation, movement, and thought.
(d) All of the above are false.
(e) None of the above are false.

180. The components of the central nervous system include the brain and the

  (a) spinal cord.
  (b) sensory nerves.
  (c) motor nerves.
  (d) Both answers (a) and (b).
  (e) Both answers (a) and (c).

181. Peripheral nervous system components include the

  (a) spinal cord.
  (b) sensory nerves.
  (c) motor nerves.
  (d) Both answers (a) and (c).
  (e) Both answers (b) and (c).

182. The spinal cord is located within the spinal column. It begins at the brain and ends in the

  (a) cervical vertebrae.
  (b) thoracic vertebrae.
  (c) lumbar vertebrae.
  (d) sacrum.
  (e) coccyx.

183. The _____ nerves carry information from the body to the brain.

  (a) motor
  (b) sensory
  (c) antegrade
  (d) Both answers (a) and (b).
  (e) Both answers (b) and (c).

184. The _____ nerves carry information from the brain to the body.

  (a) motor
  (b) sensory
  (c) retrograde
  (d) Both answers (a) and (b).
  (e) Both answers (b) and (c).

185. Involuntary motor functions are controlled by a division of the peripheral nervous system called the

  (a) heterogenic nervous system.
  (b) independent nervous system.
  (c) autonomic nervous system.
  (d) Any of the above.
  (e) None of the above.

186. All of the following functions are performed by the skin, except

(a) protection of the body from the environment and provision of a barrier to keep out bacteria and other organisms.
(b) prevention of body water loss and provision of a barrier to keep out environmental water.
(c) production of WBCs to combat infection.
(d) body temperature regulation.
(e) reception and transmission of environmental information to the brain.

187. The outermost layer of skin that is composed primarily of dead cells that constantly are rubbed or sloughed off and replaced is the

(a) endodermis.
(b) epidermis.
(c) dermis.
(d) subcutaneous layer.
(e) sebaceous layer.

188. The layer of skin containing sweat and sebaceous glands is the

(a) endodermis.
(b) epidermis.
(c) dermis.
(d) subcutaneous layer.
(e) sebaceous layer.

189. The layer of skin containing hair follicles, blood vessels, and nerve endings is the

(a) endodermis.
(b) epidermis.
(c) dermis.
(d) subcutaneous layer.
(e) sebaceous layer.

190. The layer of skin containing fat and soft tissue is largely responsible for temperature insulation and shock absorption (protection from impact injuries to the body organs). This layer is called the

(a) endodermis.
(b) epidermis.
(c) dermis.
(d) subcutaneous layer.
(e) sebaceous layer.

191. The endocrine system of the body is responsible for the secretion of chemicals that regulate body activities and functions (such as insulin and adrenaline). These chemicals are called

    (a) adrenal secretions.
    (b) hormones.
    (c) immunosuppressants.
    (d) Any of the above.
    (e) None of the above.

192. The thoracic and abdominal cavities are separated by the

    (a) duodenum.
    (b) xiphoid process.
    (c) lower rib margin.
    (d) cerebellum.
    (e) diaphragm.

193. If a patient sustained a blunt injury to the right upper quadrant of the abdomen, what organ should you be most concerned about?

    (a) The heart.
    (b) The kidney.
    (c) The liver.
    (d) The spleen.
    (e) The appendix.

194. If a patient sustained a penetrating injury to the left lower quadrant of the abdomen, what organ should you be most concerned about?

    (a) The heart.
    (b) The large intestine.
    (c) The liver.
    (d) The spleen.
    (e) The appendix.

195. If a patient sustained a blunt injury to the lateral aspect of the left upper abdominal quadrant, what organ should you be most concerned about?

    (a) The heart.
    (b) The large intestine.
    (c) The liver.
    (d) The spleen.
    (e) The appendix.

196. If a patient complained of severe pain in the right lower quadrant of the abdomen, what organ should you be most concerned about?

    (a) The heart.
    (b) The kidney.
    (c) The liver.
    (d) The spleen.
    (e) The appendix.

197. The term *vital signs* includes all of the following outward signs of a patient's status, except

    (a) mental status.
    (b) respirations.
    (c) pulse.
    (d) skin condition.
    (e) blood pressure.

198. Which of the following statements regarding measuring the respiratory rate of a patient is false?

    (a) The patient should be told that her/his respiratory rate is being counted so that the patient will cease talking or crying and perform "normal" respiration.
    (b) Respiratory rates are assessed by observing the patient's chest rise and fall.
    (c) The quality of respirations should be determined simultaneously with the rate of respiration.
    (d) All of the above are false.
    (e) None of the above are false.

199. The medical term for a fast respiratory rate is

    (a) normopnea.
    (b) apnea.
    (c) tachypnea.
    (d) bradypnea.
    (e) dyspnea.

200. The medical term for a slow respiratory rate is

    (a) normopnea.
    (b) apnea.
    (c) tachypnea.
    (d) bradypnea.
    (e) dyspnea.

201. The medical term for difficulty breathing is

(a) normopnea.
(b) apnea.
(c) tachypnea.
(d) bradypnea.
(e) dyspnea.

202. The medical term for absence of breathing is

(a) normopnea.
(b) apnea.
(c) tachypnea.
(d) bradypnea.
(e) dyspnea.

203. To obtain an accurate respiratory rate per minute, you should count the number of breaths (each inhalation and exhalation cycle) the patient makes in

(a) 10 seconds, then multiply that number by 6.
(b) 15 seconds, then multiply that number by 4.
(c) 30 seconds, then multiply that number by 2.
(d) a full 60 seconds.
(e) Any of the above.

204. Determining the *quality* of respiratory effort includes assessing all of the following, except

(a) rate of chest movement.
(b) equality of chest wall movement.
(c) depth of chest excursion.
(d) effort of chest excursion (use of accessory muscles).
(e) noisy respirations (snoring, wheezing, gurgling, crowing, or the like).

205. In the adult patient, the assessment of accessory muscle use includes observing any or all of the following, except

(a) pulling in of the shoulder or neck muscles when inhaling (suprasternal retractions).
(b) excessive abdominal movement when inhaling.
(c) pulling in of the skin between the ribs when inhaling (intercostal retractions).
(d) grasping of the neck with both hands while inhaling.
(e) widening of the nostrils (nasal flaring) while inhaling.

206. Noisy breathing can indicate some sort of respiratory obstruction. Snoring respirations generally indicate

(a) the presence of fluid in the upper airway, indicating a need for suction.
(b) obstruction of inhalation in the upper airway, usually relieved with airway-opening maneuvers.
(c) difficulty exhaling past clogged lower airways, a condition that may respond to inhaled medications.
(d) obstruction of inhalation in the upper airway that often will not respond to airway-opening maneuvers or treatments rendered by EMTs.
(e) a normal respiratory manifestation that is not a concern for prehospital care providers.

207. Wheezing respiration generally indicates

(a) the presence of fluid in the upper airway, indicating a need for suction.
(b) obstruction of inhalation in the upper airway, usually relieved with airway-opening maneuvers.
(c) difficulty exhaling past clogged lower airways, a condition that may respond to inhaled medications.
(d) obstruction of inhalation in the upper airway that often will not respond to airway-opening maneuvers or treatments rendered by EMTs.
(e) a normal respiratory manifestation that is not a concern for prehospital care providers.

208. Gurgling respiration generally indicates

(a) the presence of fluid in the upper airway, indicating a need for suction.
(b) obstruction of inhalation in the upper airway, usually relieved with airway-opening maneuvers.
(c) difficulty exhaling past clogged lower airways, a condition that may respond to inhaled medications.
(d) obstruction of inhalation in the upper airway that often will not respond to airway-opening maneuvers or treatments rendered by EMTs.
(e) a normal respiratory manifestation that is not a concern for prehospital care providers.

209. Crowing respiration generally indicates

(a) the presence of fluid in the upper airway, indicating a need for suction.
(b) obstruction of inhalation in the upper airway, usually relieved with airway-opening maneuvers.
(c) difficulty exhaling past clogged lower airways, a condition that may respond to inhaled medications.
(d) obstruction of inhalation in the upper airway that often will not respond to airway-opening maneuvers or treatments rendered by EMTs.
(e) a normal respiratory manifestation that is not a concern for prehospital care providers.

210. Which of the following statements regarding respiratory rhythm is true?

(a) Even and regular respiration is the only respiration considered "normal."
(b) In an unconscious patient, irregular respiration is a cause for concern.
(c) In the conscious patient, irregular respiration is common (and not a cause for concern) because things such as speech, mood, and physical activity normally cause irregular respiratory patterns.
(d) Both answers (a) and (b) are true.
(e) Both answers (b) and (c) are true.

211. To count a pulse rate, the EMT should place her/his

(a) thumb on the pulse site, because the thumb is the most sensitive to touch.
(b) small finger ("pinkie") on the pulse site, because the small finger is the most sensitive to touch.
(c) first two or three fingers on the pulse site, avoiding the use of the thumb because the thumb has its own pulse and may produce an inaccurate patient pulse measurement.
(d) Any of the above.
(e) None of the above.

212. The carotid pulse is located in the patient's

(a) wrist.
(b) groin.
(c) upper arm.
(d) neck.
(e) foot.

213. Which of the following statements regarding assessment of the carotid pulse is false?

   (a) It is important to assess both carotid pulses at the same time, to determine equality of their pulse nature.
   (b) Excessive pressure on the carotid pulse can slow the patient's heart rate.
   (c) If you cannot feel a carotid pulse on one side, immediately attempt assessment of the other side's carotid pulse.
   (d) Both answers (a) and (b) are false.
   (e) Both answers (b) and (c) are false.

214. The radial pulse is located in the patient's

   (a) wrist.
   (b) groin.
   (c) upper arm.
   (d) neck.
   (e) foot.

215. In all patients over the age of 1 year, the radial pulse should be assessed first. Per the DOT EMT guidelines, the initial method of determining a patient's vital sign pulse rate per minute consists of counting the number of pulse beats that can be felt in

   (a) 10 seconds, then multiplying that number by 6.
   (b) 15 seconds, then multiplying that number by 4.
   (c) 30 seconds, then multiplying that number by 2.
   (d) a full 60 seconds.
   (e) Any of the above.

216. While counting the vital sign pulse rate, the **quality** of the pulse also should be assessed. Pulse quality is characterized by whether the pulse is

   (a) strong (normal or "full"), or weak and thin (abnormal or "thready").
   (b) regular in beat rhythm (normal) or irregular in beat rhythm (abnormal).
   (c) fast or slow.
   (d) Answers (a) and (b) only.
   (e) Answers (a) and (c) only.

217. If the patient's pulse rate is noted to be irregular in rhythm, the pulse rate per minute should be obtained by counting the number of pulse beats that can be felt in

   (a) 10 seconds, then multiplying that number by 6.
   (b) 15 seconds, then multiplying that number by 4.
   (c) 30 seconds, then multiplying that number by 2.
   (d) a full 60 seconds.
   (e) Any of the above.

218. If the first attempt at assessing a radial pulse yields a pulse that cannot be felt, the EMT should next assess the

(a) other arm's radial pulse.
(b) dorsalis pedis pulse.
(c) popliteal pulse.
(d) femoral pulse.
(e) carotid pulse.

219. If the second attempt at assessing a radial pulse yields a pulse that cannot be felt, the EMT should next assess the

(a) other arm's radial pulse.
(b) dorsalis pedis pulse.
(c) popliteal pulse.
(d) femoral pulse.
(e) carotid pulse.

220. In an average adult, the "normal" resting pulse rate is between

(a) 20 and 40 beats per minute.
(b) 40 and 60 beats per minute.
(c) 60 and 100 beats per minute.
(d) 80 and 120 beats per minute.
(e) 100 and 150 beats per minute.

221. Adult athletes usually have more developed, stronger heart muscle. Thus, in the adult athlete, the "normal" resting pulse rate may be between

(a) 20 and 40 beats per minute.
(b) 40 and 60 beats per minute.
(c) 60 and 100 beats per minute.
(d) 80 and 120 beats per minute.
(e) 100 and 150 beats per minute.

222. Emergency situations often cause the "normal" adult patient's pulse to be ***temporarily*** between _____. Thus, this finding should not be considered unusual, or a sign of serious injury, unless it is maintained throughout several pulse checks.

(a) 20 and 40 beats per minute
(b) 60 and 80 beats per minute
(c) 80 and 100 beats per minute
(d) 100 and 150 beats per minute
(e) 150 and 200 beats per minute

223. A sign of serious injury or illness is a **maintained** pulse rate that is slower than ___ **or** faster than ___ beats per minute.

    (a) 20/80
    (b) 50/120
    (c) 40/150
    (d) 150/200
    (e) 80/250

224. The medical term for a fast heart rate is

    (a) normocardia.
    (b) cardiomyopathy.
    (c) tachycardia.
    (d) bradycardia.
    (e) endocardia.

225. The medical term for a slow heart rate is

    (a) normocardia.
    (b) cardiomyopathy.
    (c) tachycardia.
    (d) bradycardia.
    (e) endocardia.

226. Infants and children normally have different pulse rate ranges than adult patients. Which of the following general statements regarding infant and child pulse rates is false?

    (a) A maintained pulse rate of greater than 100 in an infant or child is a cause for serious illness or injury concern.
    (b) A maintained pulse rate of lower than 60 in an infant or child is not a cause for serious illness or injury concern.
    (c) In infants and children, maintenance of a faster pulse rate (100 to 120) is a much greater concern than maintenance of a slower pulse rate (40 to 60).
    (d) Only answers (a) and (b) are false.
    (e) All of the above are false.

227. Skin assessment is most important in determining the adequacy of

    (a) hemodynamic perfusion.
    (b) pulse rate.
    (c) respiratory rate.
    (d) mental faculty.
    (e) blood pressure.

228. Pink skin color is normal in light-skinned patients. To determine the normal "pinkness" of dark-skinned patients, the EMT should assess pinkness of the

(a) inner eyelids (conjunctiva).
(b) inner lips or cheeks (oral mucosa).
(c) nail beds.
(d) Answers (a) and (b) only.
(e) Answer (a), (b), or (c).

229. The color of cyanotic skin (cyanosis) is commonly described as being

(a) red.
(b) white.
(c) normal.
(d) blue-gray.
(e) yellow.

230. Cyanosis usually indicates inadequate perfusion (lack of oxygen in the tissues) because of

(a) poor ventilation.
(b) poor circulation.
(c) poor cardiac function.
(d) Answers (a) and/or (b) only.
(e) Answers (a), (b), and/or (c).

231. The color of jaundiced skin is commonly described as being

(a) red.
(b) white.
(c) normal.
(d) blue-gray.
(e) yellow.

232. A patient's jaundiced skin color suggests the possibility of

(a) liver disease.
(b) shock.
(c) high blood pressure.
(d) Any of the above.
(e) None of the above.

233. A patient's red, "flushed" skin color suggests the possibility of

(a) high blood pressure, heat exposure, or emotional excitement.
(b) spinal injury shock.
(c) alcohol overdose.
(d) Answers (a) and/or (b) only.
(e) Answers (a), (b), and/or (c).

234. Pale skin or mucosal membranes may indicate poor perfusion from the constriction of blood vessels because of

    (a) emotional distress.
    (b) blood loss or other types of shock.
    (c) heart attack.
    (d) Answers (b) and/or (c) only.
    (e) Answers (a), (b), and/or (c).

235. The best places for determining a patient's skin color include the nail beds, the inside of the lower eyelids, and the

    (a) mucosa of the inner mouth.
    (b) palms of pediatric patients.
    (c) soles of the feet of pediatric patients.
    (d) Answers (a) and/or (b) only.
    (e) Answers (a), (b), and/or (c).

236. To determine skin temperature, place the back of your hand on the patient's skin, simultaneously noting skin moisture or condition. Skin temperature, moisture, and condition signs of moderate fever or brief exposure to heat include

    (a) cool, moist ("clammy") skin.
    (b) cold, dry skin.
    (c) hot, dry skin.
    (d) hot, moist skin.
    (e) "goose pimples."

237. Skin temperature, moisture, and condition signs of prolonged fever or extreme exposure to heat include

    (a) cool, moist ("clammy") skin.
    (b) cold, dry skin.
    (c) hot, dry skin.
    (d) hot, moist skin.
    (e) "goose pimples."

238. Skin temperature, moisture, and condition signs of poor cellular perfusion include

    (a) cool, moist ("clammy") skin.
    (b) cold, dry skin.
    (c) hot, dry skin.
    (d) hot, moist skin.
    (e) "goose pimples."

239. Skin temperature, moisture, and condition signs of extreme exposure to cold include

    (a) cool, moist ("clammy") skin.
    (b) cold, dry skin.

(c) hot, dry skin.
(d) hot, moist skin.
(e) "goose pimples."

240. Capillary refill should be assessed (only in pediatric patients) by pressing on the patient's skin or nail beds and determining the amount of time for a return of the initial color. Normal capillary refill time in children is

(a) less than 1 second.
(b) less than 2 seconds.
(c) 2 to 3 seconds.
(d) 3 to 4 seconds.
(e) 4 full seconds.

241. When bright light is shone into them, the pupils should react by

(a) constricting, becoming larger.
(b) dilating, becoming larger.
(c) dilating, becoming smaller.
(d) constricting, becoming smaller.
(e) elongating, becoming more oval in shape.

242. When introduced to a dark environment, the pupils should react by

(a) constricting, becoming larger.
(b) dilating, becoming larger.
(c) dilating, becoming smaller.
(d) constricting, becoming smaller.
(e) elongating, becoming more oval in shape.

243. Fright may cause pupils to become

(a) constricted.
(b) dilated.
(c) elongated.
(d) unequal in size or reactivity to light.
(e) Both answers (c) and (d).

244. Stroke or head injury may cause pupils to become

(a) equally constricted.
(b) equally dilated.
(c) unequally elongated in shape.
(d) unequal in size or reactivity to light.
(e) Both answers (c) and (d).

245. The term *auscultation* refers to the process of
- (a) listening to areas of the body with a stethoscope.
- (b) systematically gathering information from the patient.
- (c) touching and feeling the patient to detect injuries or pain.
- (d) watching the patient closely for changes in level of consciousness.
- (e) tapping on the chest or abdomen.

246. The term *palpation* refers to the process of
- (a) listening to areas of the body with a stethoscope.
- (b) systematically gathering information from the patient.
- (c) touching and feeling the patient to detect injuries or pain.
- (d) watching the patient closely for changes in level of consciousness.
- (e) tapping on the chest or abdomen.

247. The medical term for a blood pressure cuff is
- (a) spiromanometer.
- (b) hemomanometer.
- (c) stethomanometer.
- (d) sphygmomanometer.
- (e) None of the above.

248. To obtain a patient's blood pressure by listening with a stethoscope, you should place the diaphragm of the stethoscope over the
- (a) carotid artery.
- (b) brachial artery.
- (c) radial artery.
- (d) femoral artery.
- (e) coronary artery.

249. To obtain a patient's blood pressure by feeling for a return of the patient's pulse, you should find the pulse at the _____ pulse site prior to inflation, maintaining contact during inflation of the blood pressure cuff.
- (a) carotid
- (b) brachial
- (c) radial
- (d) femoral
- (e) coronary

250. To obtain a patient's blood pressure reading by listening with a stethoscope, you should place the diaphragm of the stethoscope on the

   (a) medial side of the antecubital area (anterior to the elbow).
   (b) lateral side of the antecubital area (anterior to the elbow).
   (c) center of the antecubital area (anterior to the elbow).
   (d) medial side of the anterior wrist.
   (e) lateral side of the anterior wrist.

251. To obtain a patient's blood pressure by feeling for a return of the patient's pulse, you should feel the pulse on the

   (a) medial side of the antecubital area (anterior to the elbow).
   (b) lateral side of the antecubital area (anterior to the elbow).
   (c) center of the antecubital area (anterior to the elbow).
   (d) medial side of the anterior wrist.
   (e) lateral side of the anterior wrist.

252. When listening to obtain a blood pressure, the gauge number at which the pulse is *first heard* represents the patient's _____ blood pressure.

   (a) diastolic
   (b) hypostolic
   (c) systolic
   (d) hyperstolic
   (e) None of the above.

253. When listening to obtain a blood pressure, the gauge number at which the pulse is *last heard* represents the patient's _____ blood pressure.

   (a) diastolic
   (b) hypostolic
   (c) systolic
   (d) hyperstolic
   (e) None of the above.

254. When feeling the patient's pulse to obtain a blood pressure, the gauge number at which the return of a pulse is *first felt* represents the patient's _____ blood pressure.

   (a) diastolic
   (b) hypostolic
   (c) systolic
   (d) hyperstolic
   (e) None of the above.

255. When feeling the patient's pulse to obtain a blood pressure, the gauge number at which the pulse is **last felt** represents the patient's _____ blood pressure.

- (a) diastolic
- (b) hypostolic
- (c) systolic
- (d) hyperstolic
- (e) None of the above.

256. The medical term for low blood pressure is

- (a) hypothermia.
- (b) hyperthermia.
- (c) hypotension.
- (d) hypertension.
- (e) hypocardia.

257. A patient should be considered to have seriously low blood pressure when her/his _____ reading is less than _____ mmHg (millimeters of mercury).

- (a) diastolic/150
- (b) hypostolic/120
- (c) hyperstolic/90
- (d) systolic/90
- (e) systolic/120

258. A patient should be considered to have seriously high blood pressure when her/his _____ reading is greater than _____ mmHg (millimeters of mercury).

- (a) systolic/150
- (b) hyperstolic/150
- (c) diastolic/120
- (d) diastolic/150
- (e) hypostolic/120

259. The medical term for high blood pressure is

- (a) hypothermia.
- (b) hyperthermia.
- (c) hypotension.
- (d) hypertension.
- (e) hypercardia.

260. When a patient is stable, vital signs should be assessed

- (a) after every medical intervention.
- (b) every 30 minutes.

(c) every 15 minutes.
(d) Both answers (a) and (b).
(e) Both answers (a) and (c).

261. When a patient is unstable, vital signs should be assessed

   (a) after every medical intervention.
   (b) every 10 minutes.
   (c) every 5 minutes.
   (d) Both answers (a) and (b).
   (e) Both answers (a) and (c).

262. In the phrase **signs and symptoms,** a "sign" is something

   (a) a bystander knows about the patient.
   (b) the patient refuses to explain.
   (c) the care provider is told about the scene.
   (d) the patient feels and tells the care provider.
   (e) the care provider sees, hears, feels, or smells about the patient.

263. In the phrase **signs and symptoms,** a "symptom" is something

   (a) a bystander knows about the patient.
   (b) the patient refuses to explain.
   (c) the care provider is told about the scene.
   (d) the patient feels and tells the care provider.
   (e) the care provider sees, hears, feels, or smells about the patient.

264. To obtain a complete patient history, the EMT may use the mnemonic (a memory aid) SAMPLE to remember what questions to ask. The "S" of a SAMPLE history stands for

   (a) Signs and Symptoms—What is wrong with the patient?
   (b) Size—What is the weight and height of the patient?
   (c) Speech—How well does the patient speak?
   (d) Snoring—Does the patient have an airway?
   (e) Sleeping—Does the patient "pass out" often?

265. The "A" of a SAMPLE history stands for

   (a) Aftereffects—complaints following the incident.
   (b) Allergies—to medications, foods, or environmental substances.
   (c) Altered level of consciousness.
   (d) Affect—What does the patient look like?
   (e) Anxiety—Is the patient upset?

266. The "M" of a SAMPLE history stands for

(a) Major—What are the patient's major complaints?
(b) Minor—What are the patient's minor complaints?
(c) Multiple—number of patient complaints.
(d) Married—Is the patient married, single, divorced, or widowed?
(e) Medications—current and/or recent prescription or non-prescription drugs.

267. The "P" of a SAMPLE history stands for

(a) Plan—your planned course of treatment.
(b) Potential—the suspected diagnosis.
(c) Previous—the treatment already rendered.
(d) pertinent Past medical history—medical, surgical, or trauma.
(e) Pulse—Does the patient have a pulse?

268. The "L" of a SAMPLE history stands for

(a) Likes and dislikes.
(b) Last menstrual period.
(c) Last meal or oral intake—time, quantity, and substance(s).
(d) Looks—What is the patient's appearance?
(e) Late—late developing signs and symptoms.

269. The "E" of a SAMPLE history stands for

(a) Equal—equality of grips, pupils, and movement.
(b) Energy—Is the patient fatigued?
(c) Events leading to the injury or illness.
(d) Extra—What extra things can you think to ask?
(e) Evaluation—the suspected diagnosis.

270. Which of the following statements regarding EMT safety in lifting and moving patients is false?

(a) Do not try to handle too heavy a load. When in doubt, call for help.
(b) Avoid twisting when lifting, lowering, or pulling.
(c) When lifting a heavy patient, keep your legs straight and rely on shoulder and arm muscles.
(d) Avoid bending at the waist.
(e) Communicate clearly and frequently with your partner.

271. Which of the following statements regarding EMT safety when pushing or pulling objects is false?

(a) Push, rather than pull, whenever possible.
(b) Keep your back locked in and keep the line of pull through the center of the body by bending the knees.

(c) Keep the weight close to your body and push from the area between the waist and shoulder.
(d) If the weight is below your waist level, bend over at the waist to access it.
(e) Avoid pushing or pulling from an overhead position if possible.

272. An **emergency move** is when a patient is moved before thorough examination and without full spinal precautions. This type of move is indicated when there is an immediate danger to the patient or others if the patient is not **immediately** moved. All of the following are situations that would require an emergency move, except

(a) a fire or the danger of fire.
(b) the presence of explosives or other hazardous materials.
(c) the inability to gain access to another patient who needs lifesaving care.
(d) the patient is a "public spectacle" and should be moved before news cameras arrive (to avoid breaching patient confidentiality).
(e) the patient is in cardiac arrest and is sitting in a chair or lying on a bed.

273. An **urgent move** is when a patient is moved after only brief examination but with full spinal precautions. This type of move is indicated when there are signs of serious life-threat and the patient must be moved **quickly**. Which of the following is an example of such a situation?

(a) Altered level of consciousness.
(b) Inadequate breathing or ventilation.
(c) Shock (hypoperfusion).
(d) Answers (a) and (b) only.
(e) Answers (a), (b), and (c).

274. Which of the following statements regarding emergency moves is false?

(a) The greatest danger in moving a patient quickly is the possibility of aggravating a spine injury.
(b) In an emergency, every effort should be made to push (rather than pull) the patient in the direction of the long axis of the body to provide as much protection to the spine as possible.
(c) If the patient is on the floor or ground, she/he should be pulled to safety using the clothing of her/his neck and shoulder area.
(d) All of the above are false.
(e) None of the above are false.

275. Which of the following statements regarding patient positioning is false?

(a) An unresponsive patient without spine injury should be moved into the "recovery position" by rolling the patient onto her/his side (preferably the left).
(b) A patient with chest pain or discomfort or difficulty breathing should sit in a position of comfort as long as hypotension is not present.
(c) A patient with suspected spine injury should be immobilized on a long backboard.
(d) A patient in shock (hypoperfusion) should have her/his legs elevated 8 to 12 inches.
(e) None of the above are false.

The answer key for Test Section One is on pages 347 through 352.

Test Section Two

This test section covers the following subjects:

* Respiration Anatomy Review
* Opening the Airway
* Techniques of Artificial Ventilation
* Airway Adjuncts
* Suctioning and Suction Devices
* Oxygen Therapy
* Special Airway Considerations

1994 Revised EMT-Basic National Standards Review Self-Test

1. The respiratory system is responsible for the

    (a) introduction of carbon dioxide to the bloodstream and excretion of oxygen.
    (b) introduction of oxygen to the bloodstream and excretion of carbon dioxide.
    (c) the muscular function of inhalation and exhalation only.
    (d) Answers (a) and (c) only.
    (e) Answers (b) and (c) only.

2. When breathing through the mouth, air first enters the

    (a) pharynx.
    (b) nasopharynx.
    (c) larynx.
    (d) endopharynx.
    (e) oropharynx.

3. When breathing through the nose, air first enters the

    (a) pharynx.
    (b) nasopharynx.
    (c) larynx.
    (d) endopharynx.
    (e) oropharynx.

4. A leaf-shaped valve that prevents food and liquid from entering the windpipe is called the

    (a) cricoid cartilage.
    (b) larynx.
    (c) valecula.
    (d) epiglottis.
    (e) trachea.

5. The medical term for the windpipe is the

    (a) cricoid cartilage.
    (b) larynx.
    (c) valecula.
    (d) epiglottis.
    (e) trachea.

6. The firm ring that forms the lower portion of the voice box is the

    (a) cricoid cartilage.
    (b) larynx.

(c) valecula.
(d) epiglottis.
(e) trachea.

7. The medical term for the voice box is the

(a) cricoid cartilage.
(b) larynx.
(c) valecula.
(d) epiglottis.
(e) trachea.

8. The windpipe divides into two large air tubes at a junction called the **carina**. The medical term for these air tubes is the

(a) right or left rhonchi.
(b) right or left bronchi.
(c) right or left alveoli.
(d) anterior or posterior rhonchi.
(e) anterior or posterior bronchi.

9. At the end of the respiratory "tree" are groups of tiny sacs. These sacs are called the

(a) rhonchi.
(b) bronchi.
(c) alveoli.
(d) petechia.
(e) cilia.

10. When the diaphragm and rib (intercostal) muscles are activated,

(a) the larynx opens and air flows in.
(b) the chest cavity becomes smaller and air flows out.
(c) the larynx opens and air flows out.
(d) the chest cavity enlarges and the lungs fill with air.
(e) None of the above.

11. When the diaphragm and rib (intercostal) muscles relax,

(a) the larynx opens and air flows in.
(b) the chest cavity becomes smaller and air flows out.
(c) the larynx opens and air flows out.
(d) the chest cavity enlarges and the lungs fill with air.
(e) None of the above.

12. The inhalation phase of respiration is considered _____ phase of respiration because it requires energy to accomplish.

    (a) an active
    (b) a passive
    (c) the second
    (d) the formal
    (e) None of the above.

13. The exhalation phase of respiration is considered _____ phase of respiration because it requires energy to accomplish.

    (a) an active
    (b) a passive
    (c) the first
    (d) an informal
    (e) None of the above.

14. The respiratory gas exchange of oxygen and carbon dioxide occurs in the

    (a) alveoli only.
    (b) rhonchi and bronchi only.
    (c) cells of the body (via capillaries) only.
    (d) alveoli and the cells of the body (via capillaries) only.
    (e) rhonchi, bronchi, alveoli, and the cells of the body.

15. For an adult, an adequate rate of respiration at rest is considered to be _____ breaths per minute.

    (a) 10 to 12
    (b) 12 to 20
    (c) 15 to 30
    (d) 25 to 35
    (e) 25 to 50

16. For an infant, an adequate rate of respiration at rest is considered to be _____ breaths per minute.

    (a) 10 to 12
    (b) 12 to 20
    (c) 15 to 30
    (d) 25 to 35
    (e) 25 to 50

17. For a child, an adequate rate of respiration at rest is considered to be _____ breaths per minute.

    (a) 10 to 12
    (b) 12 to 20

(c) 15 to 30
(d) 25 to 35
(e) 25 to 50

18. The complete assessment of respiration includes assessing the rate of breathing, the rhythm of breathing (is it regular or irregular?), and the

    (a) clarity and equality of breath sounds.
    (b) equality and fullness of chest expansion.
    (c) use of accessory muscles.
    (d) Answers (a) and (b) only.
    (e) Answers (a), (b), and (c).

19. Which of the following statements regarding pediatric airway anatomy considerations is false?

    (a) In general, all pediatric airway structures are smaller and more easily obstructed than adult airway structures.
    (b) The trachea is harder and less flexible in children, providing greater protection from direct injury.
    (c) Children's tongues take up proportionally more space in the mouth than adults'.
    (d) All of the above are false.
    (e) None of the above are false.

20. Which of the following statements regarding pediatric airway anatomy considerations is true?

    (a) Children have narrower tracheas that can be obstructed more easily by swelling.
    (b) Like other cartilage in the child, the cricoid cartilage is less developed and less rigid than in the adult.
    (c) The chest wall is softer, and children tend to depend more heavily on the diaphragm for breathing.
    (d) All of the above are true.
    (e) None of the above are true.

21. Which of the following statements regarding measuring the respiratory rate of a patient is false?

    (a) The patient should be told that her/his respiratory rate is being counted so that the patient will cease talking or crying and perform "normal" respiration.
    (b) Respiratory rates are assessed by observing the patient's chest rise and fall.
    (c) The quality of respirations should be determined simultaneously with the rate of respiration.
    (d) All of the above are false.
    (e) None of the above are false.

22. The medical term for a fast respiratory rate is

(a) normopnea.
(b) apnea.
(c) tachypnea.
(d) bradypnea.
(e) dyspnea.

23. The medical term for a slow respiratory rate is

(a) normopnea.
(b) apnea.
(c) tachypnea.
(d) bradypnea.
(e) dyspnea.

24. The medical term for difficulty breathing is

(a) normopnea.
(b) apnea.
(c) tachypnea.
(d) bradypnea.
(e) dyspnea.

25. The medical term for absence of breathing is

(a) normopnea.
(b) apnea.
(c) tachypnea.
(d) bradypnea.
(e) dyspnea.

26. To obtain an accurate respiratory rate per minute, you should count the number of breaths (each inhalation and exhalation cycle) the patient makes in

(a) 10 seconds, then multiply that number by 6.
(b) 15 seconds, then multiply that number by 4.
(c) 30 seconds, then multiply that number by 2.
(d) a full 60 seconds.
(e) Any of the above.

27. Determining the *quality* of respiratory effort includes assessing all of the following, except

(a) rate of chest movement.
(b) equality of chest wall movement.

(c) depth of chest excursion.
(d) effort of chest excursion (use of accessory muscles).
(e) noisy respirations (snoring, wheezing, gurgling, crowing, or the like).

28. In the adult patient, the assessment of accessory muscle use includes observing any or all of the following, except

   (a) pulling in of the shoulder or neck muscles when inhaling (suprasternal retractions).
   (b) excessive abdominal movement when inhaling.
   (c) pulling in of the skin between the ribs when inhaling (intercostal retractions).
   (d) grasping of the neck with both hands while inhaling.
   (e) widening of the nostrils (nasal flaring) while inhaling.

29. Noisy breathing can indicate some sort of respiratory obstruction. Snoring respirations generally indicate

   (a) the presence of fluid in the upper airway, indicating a need for suction.
   (b) obstruction of inhalation in the upper airway, usually relieved with airway-opening maneuvers.
   (c) difficulty exhaling past clogged lower airways, a condition that may respond to inhaled medications.
   (d) obstruction of inhalation in the upper airway that often will not respond to airway-opening maneuvers or treatments rendered by EMTs.
   (e) a normal respiratory manifestation that is not a concern for prehospital care providers.

30. Wheezing respirations generally indicate

   (a) the presence of fluid in the upper airway, indicating a need for suction.
   (b) obstruction of inhalation in the upper airway, usually relieved with airway-opening maneuvers.
   (c) difficulty exhaling past clogged lower airways, a condition that may respond to inhaled medications.
   (d) obstruction of inhalation in the upper airway that often will not respond to airway-opening maneuvers or treatments rendered by EMTs.
   (e) a normal respiratory manifestation that is not a concern for prehospital care providers.

31. Gurgling respirations generally indicate
    (a) the presence of fluid in the upper airway, indicating a need for suction.
    (b) obstruction of inhalation in the upper airway, usually relieved with airway-opening maneuvers.
    (c) difficulty exhaling past clogged lower airways, a condition that may respond to inhaled medications.
    (d) obstruction of inhalation in the upper airway that often will not respond to airway-opening maneuvers or treatments rendered by EMTs.
    (e) a normal respiratory manifestation that is not a concern for prehospital care providers.

32. Crowing respirations generally indicate
    (a) the presence of fluid in the upper airway, indicating a need for suction.
    (b) obstruction of inhalation in the upper airway, usually relieved with airway-opening maneuvers.
    (c) difficulty exhaling past clogged lower airways, a condition that may respond to inhaled medications.
    (d) obstruction of inhalation in the upper airway that often will not respond to airway-opening maneuvers or treatments rendered by EMTs.
    (e) a normal respiratory manifestation that is not a concern for prehospital care providers.

33. Which of the following statements regarding respiratory rhythm is true?
    (a) Even and regular respirations are the only respirations considered "normal."
    (b) In an unconscious patient, irregular respirations are a cause for concern.
    (c) In the conscious patient, irregular respirations are common (and not a cause for concern) because things such as speech, mood, and physical activity normally cause irregular respiratory patterns.
    (d) Both answers (a) and (b) are true.
    (e) Both answers (b) and (c) are true.

34. The definition of **cyanosis** is
    (a) the absence of respiratory effort.
    (b) the absence of oxygen in the blood.
    (c) pale nail beds, palms, and skin.
    (d) a grayish-blue discoloration of the skin.
    (e) a lack of oxygen in the lungs.

35. Cyanosis usually indicates inadequate perfusion (lack of oxygen in the tissues) because of
- (a) poor ventilation.
- (b) poor circulation.
- (c) poor cardiac function.
- (d) Answers (a) and/or (b) only.
- (e) Answers (a), (b), and/or (c).

36. To open the airway when no spine injury is suspected, the EMT should use the
- (a) head-tilt, neck-lift technique.
- (b) head-tilt, chin-lift technique.
- (c) jaw-thrust maneuver.
- (d) Any of the above.
- (e) None of the above.

37. To open the airway when a spine injury is suspected, the EMT should use the
- (a) head-tilt, neck-lift technique.
- (b) head-tilt, chin-lift technique.
- (c) jaw-thrust maneuver.
- (d) Any of the above.
- (e) None of the above.

38. When administering mouth-to-mask ventilations, if the pocket face mask has an oxygen inlet, oxygen tubing should be attached and oxygen should be run at _____ liters per minute (lpm).
- (a) 2 to 6
- (b) 6 to 8
- (c) 8 to 10
- (d) 10 to 12
- (e) 12 to 15

39. The pocket face mask should be positioned on an adult patient with the apex of the mask
- (a) over the bridge of the nose.
- (b) under the chin.
- (c) between the lower lip and the chin.
- (d) Any of the above.
- (e) None of the above.

40. When exhaling into the pocket face mask to ventilate an adult patient, each exhalation (ventilation) should last

    (a) ½ to 1 second.
    (b) 1 to 1½ seconds.
    (c) 1½ to 2 seconds.
    (d) 2 to 2½ seconds.
    (e) 2½ to 3 seconds.

41. When exhaling into the pocket face mask to ventilate a pediatric patient, each exhalation (ventilation) should last

    (a) ½ to 1 second.
    (b) 1 to 1½ seconds.
    (c) 1½ to 2 seconds.
    (d) 2 to 2½ seconds.
    (e) 2½ to 3 seconds.

42. The bag-valve-mask (BVM) device should be equipped with all of the following, except

    (a) a non-jam valve that allows a maximum of oxygen inlet flow of 15 lpm.
    (b) a pop-off valve.
    (c) standardized 15/22 mm fittings (to fit face masks or endotracheal tubes).
    (d) a "true" valve for nonrebreathing.
    (e) a self-refilling bag.

43. The BVM device should be

    (a) equipped with an oxygen inlet and a reservoir (bag or tube) to allow for a high concentration of oxygen.
    (b) easy to clean and sterilize, or disposable after a single-patient use.
    (c) available in adult, pediatric, and infant sizes.
    (d) Answers (a) and (c) only.
    (e) Answers (a), (b), and (c).

44. Which of the following statements regarding the BVM device is false?

    (a) The BVM provides less volume than mouth-to-mask ventilation.
    (b) The volume of the BVM bag is approximately 1600 ml of air.
    (c) At least 800 ml of air should be delivered to the patient.
    (d) Use of adjunct airways (oropharyngeal or nasopharyngeal) is unnecessary when using the BVM correctly.
    (e) Obtaining an effective seal with the patient's face, while still maintaining an open airway, is the most difficult aspect of delivering effective BVM ventilations.

45. When delivering BVM ventilations to an adult, ventilate the patient every ___ seconds.

   (a) 10
   (b) 8
   (c) 5
   (d) 3
   (e) 2

46. When delivering BVM ventilations to children and infants, ventilate the patient every ___ seconds.

   (a) 10
   (b) 8
   (c) 5
   (d) 3
   (e) 2

47. Without an oxygen reservoir, when supplemented with 15 lpm of oxygen, the BVM device will deliver approximately ____ percent oxygen.

   (a) 100
   (b) 90
   (c) 70
   (d) 50
   (e) 25

48. With an oxygen reservoir, when supplemented with 15 lpm of oxygen, the BVM device will deliver approximately ____ percent oxygen.

   (a) 100
   (b) 90
   (c) 70
   (d) 50
   (e) 25

49. Some ventilation techniques and devices provide better oxygenation and ventilation than others. Place the following in the order of their effectiveness, from the most effective to the least effective.

   1. Single-person-operated BVM with supplemental oxygen
   2. Two-person-operated BVM with supplemental oxygen
   3. A flow-restricted, oxygen-powered ventilation device
   4. Mouth-to-mask ventilation with supplemental oxygen

   (a) 1, 3, 2, 4
   (b) 4, 2, 3, 1
   (c) 2, 1, 3, 4
   (d) 2, 1, 4, 3
   (e) 1, 2, 3, 4

50. When using a BVM, in the absence of spinal injury suspicion, if the chest does not rise and fall with each ventilation,

(a) reposition the patient's head and ensure an open airway.
(b) reposition fingers and mask, evaluating for air escaping from under the mask.
(c) evaluate for airway obstruction or obstruction of the BVM.
(d) Answers (a) and (b) only.
(e) Answers (a), (b), and (c).

51. When using a BVM, in the presence of spinal injury suspicion, if the chest does not rise and fall with each ventilation,

(a) reposition the patient's jaw and ensure an open airway.
(b) reposition fingers and mask, evaluating for air escaping from under the mask.
(c) evaluate for airway obstruction or obstruction of the BVM.
(d) Answers (a) and (b) only.
(e) Answers (a), (b), and (c).

52. If the chest still does not rise with each BVM ventilation,

(a) continue repositioning the head and/or jaw.
(b) continue repositioning fingers and mask to obtain a better seal.
(c) use an alternative method of ventilation, such as mouth-to-mask or a manually triggered device.
(d) Answers (a) and (b) only.
(e) None of the above.

53. When using a flow-restricted, oxygen-powered ventilation device to deliver ventilations to an adult, ventilate the patient every ___ seconds.

(a) 10
(b) 8
(c) 5
(d) Either answer (a) or (b).
(e) None of the above.

54. When using a flow-restricted, oxygen-powered ventilation device to deliver ventilations to a pediatric patient, ventilate the patient every ___ seconds.

(a) 8
(b) 5
(c) 3
(d) Either answer (a) or (b).
(e) None of the above; these devices are not to be used on children.

55. Oropharyngeal (oral) airways may be used to assist an open airway
    (a) for deeply unresponsive patients without a gag reflex.
    (b) for patients who are responsive and have a gag reflex, but need assistance keeping their tongue from obstructing the airway.
    (c) in either adult or pediatric patients, as long as the appropriate size is selected.
    (d) Answers (a) and (c) only.
    (e) Answers (a), (b), and (c).

56. Nasopharyngeal (nasal) airways may be used to assist an open airway
    (a) for deeply unresponsive patients without a gag reflex.
    (b) for patients who are responsive and have a gag reflex, but need assistance keeping their tongue from obstructing the airway.
    (c) in any adult, as long as the appropriate size is selected.
    (d) Answers (a) and (c) only.
    (e) Answers (a), (b), and (c).

57. To select the appropriate size of an oral airway, measure from the
    (a) corner of the patient's lips to the bottom of the earlobe.
    (b) tip of the patient's nose to the bottom of the earlobe.
    (c) corner of the patient's lips to the angle of the jaw.
    (d) Either answer (a) or (c).
    (e) None of the above.

58. To select the appropriate size of a nasal airway, measure from the
    (a) corner of the patient's lips to the bottom of the earlobe.
    (b) tip of the patient's nose to the bottom of the earlobe.
    (c) corner of the patient's lips to the angle of the jaw.
    (d) Either answer (a) or (c).
    (e) None of the above.

59. Which of the following statements regarding insertion of an oral airway is false?
    (a) Insert the airway upside down, with the tip facing toward the roof of the patient's mouth.
    (b) Insert the airway in the position of its function, with the tip facing the posterior oropharnyx, and advance it gently into the airway.
    (c) Advance the airway gently, rotating the airway 180 degrees, so that it comes to rest with the flange on the patient's teeth.
    (d) Both answers (a) and (c) are false.
    (e) None of the above are false.

60. The preferred method for oral airway insertion in an infant or child is

  (a) the same as that for adult insertion.
  (b) using a tongue depressor to lift the tongue up and forward, while inserting the airway with the tip facing the posterior oropharnyx, and advancing it gently into the airway.
  (c) the same as that for adult insertion, but rotating the airway only 90 degrees.
  (d) Either answer (a) or (c).
  (e) None of the above.

61. Which of the following statements regarding the insertion of a nasal airway is false?

  (a) Lubricate the airway with an oil-based lubricant.
  (b) Insert the airway with the bevel away from the base of the nare (away from the nasal septum).
  (c) If the airway cannot be gently inserted in one nostril, try the other nostril.
  (d) Both answers (a) and (b) are false.
  (e) None of the above are false.

62. When a gurgling sound is heard with the first ventilation of a patient, it indicates that the

  (a) patient requires immediate hyperventilation.
  (b) patient needs immediate suction.
  (c) ventilation device is not adequately sealing to the patient's face. Reseal the device and continue ventilations
  (d) airway adjunct is an incorrect size and should be immediately removed.
  (e) patient is being successfully ventilated.

63. Other names for hard or rigid "Yankauer" suction-tipped catheters include

  (a) "tonsil sucker" or "tonsil tip."
  (b) "rigid sucker" or "rigid tip."
  (c) "French" catheter.
  (d) Either answer (a) or (c).
  (e) Either answer (b) or (c).

64. Other names for soft suction catheters include

  (a) "tonsil sucker" or "tonsil tip."
  (b) "rigid sucker" or "rigid tip."
  (c) "French" catheter.
  (d) Either answer (a) or (c).
  (e) Either answer (b) or (c).

65. Which of the following statements regarding a rigid "Yankauer" suction-tipped catheter is false?
   (a) It is useful for suctioning the nasopharynx.
   (b) It is used to suction the mouth and oropharynx of an unresponsive patient.
   (c) It should be inserted only as far as you can see.
   (d) It may be used for pediatric patients, but caution should be exercised to avoid touching the back of the airway.
   (e) None of the above are false.

66. Which of the following statements regarding a soft suction catheter is true?
   (a) It is useful for suctioning the nasopharynx.
   (b) When suctioning the oropharnyx, it should be measured so that it is inserted only as far as the base of the tongue.
   (c) It may be used to suction through an endotracheal tube.
   (d) Both answers (b) and (c) are true.
   (e) Answers (a), (b), and (c) are true.

67. Which of the following statements regarding suctioning with either a rigid or soft suction catheter is false?
   (a) Apply suction only during insertion of the catheter.
   (b) Suction an adult for no more than 15 seconds at a time.
   (c) Rinse the catheter with water as needed, to prevent tubing obstruction.
   (d) If secretions or emesis cannot be removed quickly and easily by suctioning, logroll the patient to her/his side for manual clearance of the oropharynx.
   (e) When applying suction, move the catheter tip from side to side.

68. At sea level, the atmosphere provides an adequately breathing person with _____ percent oxygen.
   (a) 100
   (b) 75
   (c) 33
   (d) 21
   (e) 10

69. The medical term for an inadequate supply of oxygen to the tissues of the body is
   (a) anoxia.
   (b) hyperpnea.
   (c) apnea.
   (d) hypoxemia.
   (e) hypoxia.

70. Even appropriately performed CPR is only _____ percent as effective as a patient's normal circulation.

    (a) 75 to 85
    (b) 55 to 75
    (c) 25 to 33
    (d) 10 to 15
    (e) 5 to 10

71. Which of the following statements regarding the hazards of oxygen therapy is false?

    (a) A punctured oxygen tank may become a destructive missile because of the compressed gas within.
    (b) An increased risk of fire accompanies oxygen use, because oxygen supports combustion, causing fire to burn more rapidly.
    (c) Oxygenation equipment must be oiled regularly to prevent dried connections from encouraging explosion.
    (d) Patients with chronic obstructive pulmonary disease (COPD) may lose their stimulus to breathe if supplemental oxygen is delivered over a long period of time. Yet supplemental oxygen should **not** be withheld from a COPD patient experiencing an emergency.
    (e) None of the above are false.

72. A full tank of oxygen contains approximately _____ pounds per square inch (psi).

    (a) 3,000
    (b) 2,000
    (c) 1,000
    (d) 500
    (e) 100

73. Oxygen cylinders come in many different sizes. The "D" cylinder contains _____ liters of oxygen.

    (a) 350
    (b) 625
    (c) 3,000
    (d) 5,300
    (e) 6,900

74. The "E" cylinder contains _____ liters of oxygen.

    (a) 350
    (b) 625
    (c) 3,000
    (d) 5,300
    (e) 6,900

75. The "M" cylinder contains _____ liters of oxygen.

(a) 350
(b) 625
(c) 3,000
(d) 5,300
(e) 6,900

76. The "G" cylinder contains _____ liters of oxygen.

(a) 350
(b) 625
(c) 3,000
(d) 5,300
(e) 6,900

77. The "H" cylinder contains _____ liters of oxygen.

(a) 350
(b) 625
(c) 3,000
(d) 5,300
(e) 6,900

78. Which of the following statements regarding the nonrebreather mask is false?

(a) The nonrebreather bag must be full before the mask is placed on the patient.
(b) The nonrebreather mask should never be used on COPD or pediatric patients.
(c) The flow rate should ensure that the nonrebreather bag does not collapse when the patient inhales.
(d) All of the above are false.
(e) None of the above are false.

79. The optimal oxygen flow rate for a nonrebreather mask is _____ lpm.

(a) 25 to 50
(b) 12 to 15
(c) 6 to 10
(d) 5 to 8
(e) 1 to 6

80. With the optimal flow rate of oxygen, a nonrebreather mask will deliver _____ percent of oxygen.

(a) 100
(b) 80 to 90
(c) 50 to 75
(d) 24 to 44
(e) 10 to 15

The following six (6) questions pertain to a single important subject regarding the physiology of breathing and the administration of oxygen to the prehospital emergency patient.

81. Normally, the body's stimulus to breathe is based on the level of _____ in the blood.

    (a) carbon monoxide
    (b) carbon dioxide
    (c) oxygen
    (d) Both answers (a) and (b).
    (e) Both answers (a) and (c).

82. Patients with COPD chronically have increased levels of _____ in their blood.

    (a) carbon monoxide
    (b) carbon dioxide
    (c) oxygen
    (d) Both answers (a) and (b).
    (e) Both answers (a) and (c).

83. Because of this chronic abnormality, the bodies of patients with COPD develop a stimulus to breathe based on the level of _____ in the blood.

    (a) carbon monoxide
    (b) carbon dioxide
    (c) oxygen
    (d) Both answers (a) and (b).
    (e) Both answers (a) and (c).

84. The development of this abnormal stimulus to breathe creates the abnormal condition known as

    (a) hypoxic drive.
    (b) carbon dioxide drive.
    (c) oxygen drive.
    (d) anoxia drive.
    (e) carbon monoxide drive.

85. This abnormal condition once was considered to be _____ the administration of high concentrations of oxygen (oxygen by nonrebreather mask).

    (a) a contraindication to
    (b) an indication for
    (c) a side effect of
    (d) Any of the above.
    (e) None of the above.

86. Now, however, it is widely believed that this condition is

   (a) not a valid contraindication to the administration of high concentrations of oxygen in the prehospital setting.
   (b) an even greater contraindication to the administration of high concentrations of oxygen in the prehospital setting than previously suspected, due to its encouragement of respiratory depression or arrest.
   (c) an even greater indication for the administration of high concentrations of oxygen in the prehospital setting than previously suspected.
   (d) a more prevalent side effect of the administration of high concentrations of oxygen in the prehospital setting.
   (e) None of the above.

87. According to DOT guidelines, the nasal cannula oxygen delivery device

   (a) is rarely the best method of delivering adequate oxygen to the prehospital emergency patient.
   (b) should be used only when the patient will not tolerate a nonrebreather mask.
   (c) is the only oxygen delivery device that should be used for COPD patients.
   (d) Both answers (a) and (b).
   (e) Both answers (b) and (c).

88. The maximum flow rate of oxygen when using a nasal cannula is _____ lpm.

   (a) 15
   (b) 10
   (c) 8
   (d) 6
   (e) 2

89. When using a nasal cannula, the oxygen concentration delivered to the patient varies from _____ percent oxygen.

   (a) 80 to 90
   (b) 50 to 75
   (c) 24 to 44
   (d) 13 to 22
   (e) 5 to 10

90. Special considerations regarding the airway management of patients with facial injuries include all except which of the following?

 (a) Because blood supply to the face is so rich, blunt injuries frequently result in severe swelling.
 (b) If facial injuries are present, no attempt should be made to insert an airway adjunct.
 (c) Bleeding into the airway from facial injuries can be a challenge to manage.
 (d) Frequent suctioning may be required in the presence of facial injuries.
 (e) Advanced airway management may be required if severe facial injuries are present.

91. Special considerations regarding the airway management of patients with obstructions include all except which of the following?

 (a) Many suction units or catheters are inadequate for removing large solid objects, such as teeth or food, from the airway.
 (b) Manual techniques for clearing the obstructed airway are important and include abdominal thrusts, chest thrusts, and/or finger sweeps.
 (c) Logrolling the patient to a laterally recumbent position may be necessary to clear the airway.
 (d) Dentures always pose an obstruction to ventilation of the unconscious patient. Thus, dentures always should be removed from the patient.
 (e) If a foreign-body airway obstruction persists, the EMT should continue to perform manual techniques for clearing the obstructed airway and transport the patient.

92. Special considerations regarding the airway management of pediatric patients include all except which of the following?

 (a) The smaller mouth and nose of pediatric patients are more easily obstructed.
 (b) A pediatric tongue takes up more space in the oropharynx than an adult tongue.
 (c) Excessive hyperextension of the head in pediatric patients should be avoided.
 (d) Because pediatric patients are "belly breathers" (depending more on the diaphragm for breathing), gastric distention indicates adequate ventilation and should be ignored.
 (e) Children should be ventilated only forcefully enough to produce a chest rise. More than this will result in gastric distention that will interfere with adequate ventilation.

93. Which of the following statements is not a special consideration for patients with laryngectomies?

(a) A breathing tube may be present. Do not suction it, as suctioning may increase the patient's lack of oxygenation.
(b) If the patient has a stoma, the head and neck may be left in a neutral position, as traditional airway positioning is not necessary.
(c) Some patients have only partial laryngectomies, causing ventilations delivered to the stoma to escape from the mouth and/or nose. In these cases, close the mouth and pinch the nostrils closed when ventilating.
(d) A pediatric-sized mask may be used to establish a seal around the stoma for ventilation.
(e) In a partial laryngectomy patient, if stoma ventilation is not effective, consider sealing the stoma, positioning the head in a traditional airway-opening manner, and ventilate the patient in a normal manner.

The answer key for Test Section Two is on pages 353 through 355.

Test Section Three

This test section covers the following subjects:

* Scene Size-up
* The Initial Assessment
* The Focused History and Physical Exam of Trauma Patients
* The Focused History and Physical Exam of Medical Patients
* The Detailed Physical Exam
* Ongoing Assessment
* Communications
* Documentation
* Elective Group of Medical Terminology and Abbreviations Questions

1994 Revised EMT-Basic National Standards Review Self-Test

1. Which of the following subjects are part of the EMT's **scene size-up** (assessment of the scene and surroundings)?

    (a) Scene safety considerations.
    (b) Consideration of the mechanism of injury or nature of illness.
    (c) Body-substance isolation precautions required.
    (d) Answers (a) and (b) only.
    (e) Answers (a), (b), and (c).

2. Which of the following statements regarding scene safety is false?

    (a) Scene safety considerations are focused only on ensuring the safety of the patient.
    (b) Personal protection of the care providers is the first scene safety consideration. (Is it safe to approach the patient?)
    (c) Protection of bystanders is an important aspect of scene safety considerations.
    (d) Scene safety considerations are not limited to the initial scene size-up, but continue throughout the call.
    (e) If a scene is unsafe, it should not be entered, for any reason, until it is made safe by appropriately trained and equipped personnel.

3. Diseases are caused by _____, such as viruses and bacteria.

    (a) halogens
    (b) carcinogens
    (c) pathogens
    (d) biogens
    (e) germogens

4. Infectious diseases may be spread by

    (a) direct contact with infected blood or other body fluids.
    (b) droplet infection from airborne organisms (coughing, sneezing, or breathing).
    (c) indirect contact via handling objects or materials contaminated with infectious secretions.
    (d) Answers (a) and (c) only.
    (e) Answers (a), (b), and (c).

5. Which of the following statements regarding personal protective equipment is false?
    (a) Hand washing before and after every patient contact is required only if protective gloves are not worn throughout the entire patient contact.
    (b) Protective gloves should be worn for every patient contact, and a separate pair should be used for each separate patient.
    (c) Eye protection should be worn whenever airborne droplet (or fluid splashing) contact is anticipated.
    (d) Masks should be worn whenever airborne droplet (or fluid splashing) contact is anticipated.
    (e) A gown should be worn whenever spilling or splashing of infectious fluid is anticipated.

6. Determining the mechanism of injury helps the EMT anticipate what injuries a patient may have. Which of the following statements regarding knowledge of the mechanism of injury is true?
    (a) Some injuries can be considered "common" to specific types of trauma.
    (b) Even though the patient's complaint is isolated to a single body part, the mechanism of injury may require suspicion of (and treatment for) "hidden" injuries in other body parts or areas.
    (c) If the mechanism of injury appears superficial, the EMT may officially "rule out" injuries to the patient, thus avoiding the necessity of expensive treatment and transportation (especially when the patient seems to be complaining of pain only in order to file a lawsuit against another party).
    (d) Both answers (a) and (b) are true.
    (e) None of the above are true.

7. Which of the following sources provide useful information regarding the patient's nature of illness?
    (a) The patient.
    (b) Family members or bystanders.
    (c) The patient's medication bottles.
    (d) Answers (a) and (b) only.
    (e) Answers (a), (b), and (c).

8. Part of every scene size-up is determining whether there are adequate resources present to deal with the emergency. Often, even with only one patient, the need for lift-assistance or extrication equipment will require a call for additional help. In multiple-patient situations, after recognizing that there are more patients than the responding unit can handle effectively, the EMT should

   (a) immediately begin treatment and call for additional resources only after life-threatening conditions have been stabilized.
   (b) immediately begin triage and call for additional resources only after patients with life-threatening conditions have been identified.
   (c) always call for additional resources before initiating treatment.
   (d) initiate treatment for one minute, and then call for additional resources.
   (e) do an initial walk-through, getting a specific and accurate count of the patients present, and then call for additional resources.

9. The *initial assessment* of a patient consists of six specific steps. Of the following possible steps, select the six initial assessment steps and place them in correct order (from first-performed to last-performed).

   1. Using the mnemonic SAMPLE, assess the patient's medical history.
   2. Using the mnemonic AVPU, assess the patient's level of consciousness.
   3. Determine a *general impression* of the patient.
   4. Inspect and palpate the abdomen for injuries or signs of injuries.
   5. Assess the patient's circulation.
   6. Identify *priority patients*.
   7. Assess the patient's breathing.
   8. Assess the patient's airway.

   (a) 8, 7, 5, 2, 3, 6
   (b) 3, 2, 8, 7, 5, 6
   (c) 8, 7, 5, 2, 1, 3
   (d) 6, 8, 7, 5, 2, 1
   (e) 2, 1, 8, 7, 5, 6

10. When assessing a patient's medical history, the "A" of the mnemonic (a memory aid) SAMPLE stands for

    (a) Aftereffects—complaints following the incident.
    (b) Allergies—to medications, foods, or environmental substances.
    (c) Altered level of consciousness.
    (d) Affect—What does the patient look like?
    (e) Anxiety—Is the patient upset?

11. When assessing a patient's level of consciousness, the "A" of the mnemonic AVPU stands for

    (a) Alert.
    (b) Altered level of consciousness.
    (c) Anxiety—Is the patient upset?
    (d) the fact that the patient is Awake but possibly confused.
    (e) the fact that Alcohol abuse is suspected.

12. When assessing a patient's level of consciousness, the "V" of the mnemonic AVPU stands for the fact that the patient is

    (a) Very unconscious.
    (b) Very alert.
    (c) responsive to Verbal stimuli.
    (d) Verbally unresponsive.
    (e) Verbally responsive (talkative) without stimuli.

13. When assessing a patient's medical history, the "P" of the mnemonic SAMPLE stands for

    (a) Plan—your planned course of treatment.
    (b) Potential—the suspected diagnosis.
    (c) Previous—the treatment already rendered.
    (d) pertinent Past medical history—medical, surgical, or trauma.
    (e) Pulse—Does the patient have a pulse?

14. When assessing a patient's level of consciousness, the "P" of the mnemonic AVPU stands for the fact that

    (a) the patient responds to Painful stimuli.
    (b) the patient is Partially unconscious.
    (c) the patient is Partially conscious.
    (d) the patient complains of Pain.
    (e) a Painful stimuli provokes no patient response.

15. When assessing a patient's level of consciousness, the "U" of the mnemonic AVPU stands for the fact that

    (a) Unusual circumstances are involved in this patient's situation.
    (b) the patient provides an Unreliable history.
    (c) the patient is Unresponsive but has an intact gag reflex or coughs when stimulated.
    (d) the patient is Unresponsive with no gag or cough reflex.
    (e) Any of the above, depending on the circumstances of the particular call.

16. A *general impression* of the patient must be developed. This general impression serves to

    (a) determine the exact nature of the patient's illness and/or injury (such as whether a spinal injury or a medical problem exists).
    (b) determine the patient's exact age, sex, and race.
    (c) develop a "gut" sense (or "sixth" sense) for whether the patient's condition is critical or not.
    (d) Answers (a) and (b) only.
    (e) Answers (a), (b), and (c).

17. Which of the following statements regarding the initial assessment of a patient's circulation is false?

    (a) For patients of all ages, assess the radial pulse first.
    (b) If no radial pulse is felt (on either side), palpate for a carotid pulse.
    (c) If no carotid pulse is felt, start CPR.
    (d) Assess for major bleeding and, if present, control the bleeding *now*.
    (e) None of the above are false.

18. The patient's skin color is assessed by looking at the patient's

    (a) nail beds.
    (b) lips or mucosal membranes.
    (c) conjunctiva of the eyes.
    (d) Answers (a) and (b) only.
    (e) Answers (a), (b), and/or (c).

19. Abnormal skin temperature or condition includes all of the following, except

    (a) warm and dry.
    (b) hot and dry.

(c) warm and wet.
(d) cold and dry.
(e) "clammy" (cool and moist).

20. Which of the following statements regarding capillary refill assessment is false?
    (a) Capillary refill should be assessed in patients of all ages.
    (b) Normal capillary refill is less than two seconds.
    (c) Abnormal capillary refill is greater than two seconds.
    (d) Capillary refill assessment should be performed only on pediatric patients.
    (e) Capillary refill assessment can be performed on any extremity.

21. Which of the following statements regarding assessment of the conscious and responsive patient's airway status is true?
    (a) It is important to note if the patient is talking or crying.
    (b) If the patient is able to talk or cry (even only weakly), adequate breathing is present and no further "airway" consideration is necessary.
    (c) Even when the patient is talking or crying, breathing may still be inadequate and require airway assistance.
    (d) Answers (a) and (c) are true.
    (e) None of the above are true.

22. Which of the following statements regarding assessment of breathing (and subsequent treatment) is false?
    (a) If breathing rate and depth are adequate and the patient is responsive, oxygen administration is never indicated.
    (b) All adult patients breathing greater than 24 times per minute should receive high-flow oxygen (15 liters per minute by a nonrebreather mask).
    (c) If the patient is unresponsive but with adequate breathing, the airway should be opened and maintained and high-concentration oxygen should be administered.
    (d) If the patient is unresponsive with inadequate breathing, the airway should be opened and maintained, ventilatory adjuncts should be used, the patient's breathing should be assisted, and high-concentration oxygen should be administered.
    (e) If the patient is complaining of shortness of breath, oxygen should be administered.

23. When a life-threatening problem is encountered during the initial assessment of a patient,

(a) make a special mental note of the problem and quickly proceed to the next initial assessment step (it is important that all steps are accomplished prior to beginning any treatment). Begin treatment of the noted problem only upon completion of the full initial assessment phase.
(b) attempt treatment of the problem for one minute only. It is important that the full initial assessment be performed prior to spending large amounts of time on any single problem.
(c) stop the assessment procedure and treat each life-threatening problem as it is discovered. Additional assessment is performed only after each step is successfully managed by the patient or EMT.
(d) begin transport immediately (this is a critical patient), continuing the assessment until all steps are performed. Treatment may be initiated en route to the hospital, but only after all assessment steps have been performed.
(e) call for ALS assistance but continue the assessment steps without treatment until all steps have been assessed.

24. Identifying the *priority* of patients means determining which patients require rapid transportation to the emergency department and/or a request for ALS backup. All of the following patients require rapid transport or ALS backup, except

(a) patients who generate a poor general impression (for whatever reason) on an EMT.
(b) patients with bleeding controlled by direct pressure.
(c) responsive patients who are unable to follow commands.
(d) patients with severe pain (anywhere).
(e) patients with chest pain and a systolic blood pressure less than 100 mmHg (millimeters of mercury).

After the initial assessment has been accomplished, a more in-depth assessment occurs. This assessment is called the Focused History and Physical Examination. This secondary assessment is divided into "trauma" and "medical" formats.

25. For the trauma patient, the first step of the Focused History and Physical Examination is

(a) treatment of any airway problems found during the initial assessment.
(b) reconsideration of the mechanism of injury.
(c) treatment of any breathing problems during the initial assessment.
(d) reconsideration of the patient's sex or race.
(e) None of the above.

26. Determining the mechanism of injury is an important aspect of assessment for hidden injuries. Of the following situations, which one describes the least serious mechanism of injury (poses the least risk of severe and/or hidden injury)?

    (a) Ejection from a vehicle during an accident.
    (b) An accident resulting in the death of another patient within the same compartment.
    (c) A 9-foot fall to the ground.
    (d) A rollover vehicular accident.
    (e) A high-speed vehicular collision.

27. Of the following patients, which one has the least serious mechanism of injury?

    (a) The pedestrian of an auto-pedestrian accident.
    (b) A helmeted motorcycle operator who "laid his/her bike down" to avoid subsequent impacts.
    (c) Any unresponsive patient, or one with an altered level of consciousness.
    (d) A patient who fell at least (if not more than) 20 feet.
    (e) A patient with penetrating injuries (gunshot wounds or stabbings) to a single extremity.

28. For pediatric patients, significant mechanisms of injury include all of the following, except

    (a) low-speed, bicycle-versus-bicycle collisions.
    (b) an accident resulting in the death of another patient within the same compartment.
    (c) falls from as low as 10 feet.
    (d) penetrating injuries (gunshot wounds or stabbings) of an isolated extremity.
    (e) any medium-speed vehicular collision.

29. Which of the following statements regarding the use of seat belts during a motor vehicle accident is true?

    (a) When worn appropriately, seat belts save lives.
    (b) Even when worn appropriately, seat belts may cause serious injuries to the bowel or other abdominal injuries.
    (c) If a patient was wearing an appropriately positioned seat belt, the patient will not have serious injuries.
    (d) Both answers (a) and (b) are true.
    (e) All of the above are true.

30. Which of the following statements regarding the use of airbags during a motor vehicle accident are true?

    (a) Airbags save more lives than seat belts.
    (b) Airbags are just as effective, with or without using a seat belt (thus they are much more convenient and effective).
    (c) Patients may impact the steering wheel after the airbag has deflated.
    (d) None of the above are true.
    (e) Answers (a), (b), and (c) are true.

31. When assessing a motor vehicle accident where the patient's airbag has been deployed, the EMT should

    (a) recognize that serious trauma to the patient's head, chest, or abdomen is highly unlikely, due to the efficiency of airbags.
    (b) "lift and look" under the airbag to determine if potentially serious patient injury may have occurred, as evidenced by a dented or deformed steering wheel.
    (c) "lift and look" under the airbag, but remember that steering wheel deformity often accompanies the normal deployment of airbags and is not a sign of patient injury.
    (d) treat the patient only for the minor abrasions that often accompany patient impact less with airbags.
    (e) None of the above.

32. The second step in the Focused History and Physical Examination for trauma patients with a significant mechanism of injury is to perform a Rapid Trauma Assessment. For the responsive patient, this assessment includes

    (a) continuing the spinal immobilization initiated in the initial assessment or after the mechanism-of-injury re-evaluation.
    (b) determining the patient's **chief complaint** (what the patient most complains of or what prompted the emergency call).
    (c) considering the request of ALS support.
    (d) reconsidering the transport priority decision.
    (e) All of the above.

A head-to-toe Rapid Trauma Assessment consists of inspection and palpation for injuries or signs of injury. To accomplish a thorough physical examination of each body part or area, the mnemonic DCAP-BTLS (pronounced "dee cap, BTLS") is helpful. It reminds the EMT of what to assess in each area.

33. The "D" of the Rapid Trauma Assessment mnemonic DCAP-BTLS represents examination for

    (a) a Disturbed area of skin.
    (b) a patient with Developmental disabilities.

(c) Degeneration of an area.
(d) Disabled parts.
(e) Deformities.

34. The "C" of the Rapid Trauma Assessment mnemonic DCAP-BTLS represents examination for

(a) Contusions.
(b) Contraindications to treatment.
(c) Chief Complaint factors.
(d) Cold skin temperature.
(e) Complications of examination findings.

35. The "A" of the Rapid Trauma Assessment mnemonic DCAP-BTLS represents examination for

(a) an Altered level of consciousness.
(b) any Alcohol involvement.
(c) Abrasions.
(d) Alignment alterations of the injured area or limb.
(e) any Aggravating circumstances.

36. The "P" of the Rapid Trauma Assessment mnemonic DCAP-BTLS represents examination for

(a) Partial avulsions or amputations.
(b) Punctures or Penetrations.
(c) Parietal skull injuries.
(d) Probable injury signs and symptoms.
(e) the Presence of any injury findings.

37. The "B" of the Rapid Trauma Assessment mnemonic DCAP-BTLS represents examination for

(a) a mechanism of injury involving Blunt injury.
(b) Borderline findings for injury.
(c) the Ballistic information required for reporting gunshot wounds.
(d) Burns.
(e) Bulging anatomical parts.

38. The "T" of the Rapid Trauma Assessment mnemonic DCAP-BTLS represents examination for

(a) Tenderness.
(b) Tremulousness (patient shaking or shivering).
(c) Total amputation of a part or area.
(d) Tearing of a body part.
(e) Tremendous (or devastating) evidence of injury.

39. The "L" of the Rapid Trauma Assessment mnemonic DCAP-BTLS represents examination for

    (a) Level of consciousness.
    (b) Location of injury.
    (c) Long bone injury findings (a potentially dire emergency).
    (d) Lacerations.
    (e) Loss of sensation or motor function.

40. The "S" of the Rapid Trauma Assessment mnemonic DCAP-BTLS represents examination for

    (a) loss of body part Stability.
    (b) Swelling.
    (c) Significant injury.
    (d) Stable injury.
    (e) Soreness.

41. In addition to the DCAP-BTLS steps of Rapid Trauma Assessment, the presence of crepitation (or "crepitus") should be noted as present or absent in all of the following areas, except the

    (a) head.
    (b) neck.
    (c) chest.
    (d) abdomen.
    (e) All of the above are areas where crepitation (or "crepitus") may be noted.

42. The presence of jugular vein distention should be evaluated in which of the following areas?

    (a) The head.
    (b) The neck.
    (c) The chest.
    (d) The abdomen.
    (e) All of the above are areas where jugular vein distention may be noted.

43. The presence of paradoxical motion should be evaluated in which of the following areas?

    (a) The head.
    (b) The neck.
    (c) The chest.
    (d) The extremities.
    (e) All of the above are areas where paradoxical motion may be noted.

44. The presence, absence, and/or equality of breath sounds should be evaluated at all of the following locations, except

   (a) the mid-axillary line of each lung's apex.
   (b) the mid-clavicular line of each lung's apex.
   (c) the mid-axillary line of each lung's base.
   (d) the midline of the abdomen.
   (e) All of the above are legitimate auscultation locations for breath sound evaluation.

45. In addition to the DCAP-BTLS steps of Rapid Trauma Assessment, the presence or absence of softness, firmness, or distention should be noted in which of the following areas?

   (a) The head.
   (b) The neck.
   (c) The chest.
   (d) The abdomen.
   (e) All of the above are areas regularly requiring assessment of softness, firmness, or distention.

46. In addition to the DCAP-BTLS steps of Rapid Trauma Assessment, the presence or absence of distal pulse, sensation, and motor function should be noted in which of the following areas?

   (a) The extremities.
   (b) The head and neck.
   (c) The chest.
   (d) The abdomen.
   (e) All of the above are areas regularly requiring assessment of distal pulse, sensation, and motor function.

47. After a Rapid Trauma Assessment, the EMT should next obtain a baseline set of vital signs. Which of the following statements regarding measuring the respiratory rate of a patient is false?

   (a) The patient should be told that her/his respiratory rate is being counted so that the patient will cease talking or crying and perform "normal" respiration.
   (b) Respiratory rates are assessed by observing the patient's chest rise and fall.
   (c) The quality of respiration should be determined simultaneously with the rate of respiration.
   (d) All of the above are false.
   (e) None of the above are false.

48. To obtain an accurate respiratory rate per minute, count the number of breaths (each inhalation and exhalation cycle) the patient makes in

    (a) 10 seconds, then multiply that number by 6.
    (b) 15 seconds, then multiply that number by 4.
    (c) 30 seconds, then multiply that number by 2.
    (d) a full 60 seconds.
    (e) Any of the above.

49. Determining the *quality* of respiratory effort includes assessing all of the following, except

    (a) rate of chest movement.
    (b) equality of chest wall movement.
    (c) depth of chest excursion.
    (d) effort of chest excursion (use of accessory muscles).
    (e) noisy respiration (snoring, wheezing, gurgling, crowing, or the like).

50. In the adult patient, the assessment of accessory muscle use includes observing any or all of the following, except

    (a) pulling in of the shoulder or neck muscles when inhaling (suprasternal retractions).
    (b) excessive abdominal movement when inhaling.
    (c) pulling in of the skin between the ribs when inhaling (intercostal retractions).
    (d) grasping of the neck with both hands while inhaling.
    (e) widening of the nostrils (nasal flaring) while inhaling.

51. In all patients over the age of 1 year, the radial pulse should be assessed first. Per the DOT EMT guidelines, the initial method of determining a patient's vital sign pulse rate per minute consists of counting the number of pulse beats that can be felt in

    (a) 10 seconds, then multiplying that number by 6.
    (b) 15 seconds, then multiplying that number by 4.
    (c) 30 seconds, then multiplying that number by 2.
    (d) a full 60 seconds.
    (e) Any of the above.

52. While counting the vital sign pulse rate, the *quality* of the pulse also should be assessed. Pulse quality is characterized by whether the pulse is

    (a) strong (normal or "full"), or weak and thin (abnormal or "thready").
    (b) regular in beat rhythm (normal) or irregular in beat rhythm (abnormal).

(c) fast or slow.
(d) Answers (a) and (b) only.
(e) Answers (a) and (c) only.

53. If the patient's pulse rate is noted to be irregular in rhythm, the pulse rate per minute should be obtained by counting the number of pulse beats that can be felt in

(a) 10 seconds, then multiplying that number by 6.
(b) 15 seconds, then multiplying that number by 4.
(c) 30 seconds, then multiplying that number by 2.
(d) a full 60 seconds.
(e) Any of the above.

54. In an average adult, the "normal" resting pulse rate is between

(a) 20 and 40 beats per minute.
(b) 40 and 60 beats per minute.
(c) 60 and 100 beats per minute.
(d) 80 and 120 beats per minute.
(e) 100 and 150 beats per minute.

55. Adult athletes usually have more developed, stronger heart muscle. Thus, for the adult athlete, the "normal" resting pulse rate may be between

(a) 20 and 40 beats per minute.
(b) 40 and 60 beats per minute.
(c) 60 and 100 beats per minute.
(d) 80 and 120 beats per minute.
(e) 100 and 150 beats per minute.

56. Emergency situations often cause the "normal" adult patient's pulse to be ***temporarily*** between _____. Thus, this finding should not be considered unusual, or a sign of serious injury, unless it is maintained throughout several pulse checks.

(a) 20 and 40 beats per minute
(b) 60 and 80 beats per minute
(c) 80 and 100 beats per minute
(d) 100 and 150 beats per minute
(e) 150 and 200 beats per minute

57. A sign of serious injury or illness is a ***maintained*** pulse rate that is slower than ___ ***or*** faster than ___ beats per minute.

(a) 20/80
(b) 50/120
(c) 40/150
(d) 150/200
(e) 80/250

58. Infants and children normally have different pulse rate ranges than adult patients. Which of the following general statements regarding infant and child pulse rates is false?

  (a) A maintained pulse rate of greater than 100 in an infant or child is a cause for serious illness or injury concern.
  (b) A maintained pulse rate of lower than 60 in an infant or child is not a cause for serious illness or injury concern.
  (c) In infants and children, maintenance of a faster pulse rate (100 to 120) is a much greater concern than maintenance of a slower pulse rate (40 to 60).
  (d) Only answers (a) and (b) are false.
  (e) All of the above are false.

59. An adult patient should be considered to have seriously low blood pressure when her/his systolic reading is less than _____ mmHg (millimeters of mercury).

  (a) 150
  (b) 120
  (c) 110
  (d) 90
  (e) Either answer (b) or (c).

60. An adult patient should be considered to have seriously high blood pressure when her/his systolic reading is greater than _____ mmHg (millimeters of mercury).

  (a) 150
  (b) 140
  (c) 120
  (d) 110
  (e) Either answer (b) or (c).

61. After the Rapid Trauma Assessment and obtaining baseline vital signs, the EMT should obtain a complete patient history, using the mnemonic SAMPLE to remember what questions to ask. The "S" of a SAMPLE history represents questions about

  (a) Signs and Symptoms—What is wrong with the patient?
  (b) Size—What is the weight and height of the patient?
  (c) Speech—How well does the patient speak?
  (d) Snoring—Does the patient have an airway?
  (e) Sleeping—Does the patient "pass out" often?

62. The "M" of a SAMPLE history stands for

  (a) Major—What are the patient's major complaints?
  (b) Minor—What are the patient's minor complaints?

(c) Multiple—What is the number of patient complaints?
(d) Married—Is the patient married, single, divorced, or widowed?
(e) Medications—current and/or recent prescription or non-prescription drugs.

63. The "L" of a SAMPLE history represents questions about the patient's

(a) Likes and dislikes.
(b) Last menstrual period.
(c) Last meal or oral intake—time, quantity, and substance(s).
(d) Looks—What is the patient's appearance? Does the patient appear sick or injured?
(e) Late-developing signs and symptoms, if any.

64. The "E" of a SAMPLE history stands for

(a) Equal—equality of grips, pupils, and movement.
(b) Energy—Is the patient fatigued?
(c) Events leading to the injury or illness.
(d) Extra—What extra things can you think to ask?
(e) Evaluation—the suspected diagnosis.

65. The term _____ is defined as a permanent or temporary opening of some portion of the intestine, connected to the abdominal wall, where an external bag is attached to collect feces.

(a) abdominal stoma
(b) colitis
(c) colostomy
(d) episiotomy
(e) thoracotomy

66. The term _____ is defined as the grating sound or feeling made by the movement of broken bone ends.

(a) aggravation
(b) crepitation (or "crepitus")
(c) phonation
(d) distention
(e) osteoporosis

67. The term _____ is defined as a condition of being larger than normal, stretched, or inflated.

(a) aggravation
(b) crepitation (or "crepitus")
(c) hypoextension
(d) distention
(e) hydration

68. The phrase _____ motion (or movement) is used to describe when one part of the chest moves opposite to the rest of the chest during respiration.

   (a) paradoxical
   (b) hypothetical
   (c) paranormal
   (d) hyperextension
   (e) inflation

69. A spinal cord injury may produce a persistent erection of the penis. This condition is called _____.

   (a) hypererection
   (b) priapism
   (c) penile hyperextension
   (d) Cushing's syndrome
   (e) primary erection

The first step of a medical patient's Focused History and Physical Examination is to obtain an in-depth history of the present illness (patient's chief complaint). The mnemonic O-P-Q-R-S-T is helpful for this history assessment.

70. The "O" of the present illness history mnemonic O-P-Q-R-S-T stands for the word(s)

   (a) Oxygen ("Do you use oxygen at home?").
   (b) Onset ("Describe the onset of this problem [time; activity during onset].").
   (c) Only ("Is this the only problem you have right now?").
   (d) Other or Old problems ("Do you have other problems than this one?" "Is this an old problem or a new one?").
   (e) Orientation (Does the patient know who she/he is, where she/he is, and the day and date?).

71. The "P" of the present illness history mnemonic O-P-Q-R-S-T stands for the word

   (a) Plan (What do *you* plan to do about the patient's problem?).
   (b) Previous ("Have you had this problem before? What was it?").
   (c) Part (What part of the patient does the problem involve?).
   (d) Provocation ("What brought the problem on? What makes it worse?").
   (e) Payment (What kind of medical insurance does the patient have?).

72. The "Q" of the present illness history mnemonic O-P-Q-R-S-T stands for the word

   (a) Qualify (Does the patient qualify for Medicare or Medicaid insurance?).
   (b) Quit ("When did the problem stop bothering you?").
   (c) Questions ("Do you have any questions for us or the doctor?").
   (d) Quick (Does the patient have a rapid heart rate or respiratory rate?).
   (e) Quality ("Describe the quality of your pain, discomfort, or difficulty. What does it feel like?").

73. The "R" of the present illness history mnemonic O-P-Q-R-S-T stands for the word

   (a) Radiation (Does the chief complaint "radiate," or spread, to other areas, or does the patient have complaints elsewhere that may be related to the chief complaint?).
   (b) Relatives ("Have any of your relatives had this problem?").
   (c) Respiration (Does the patient have any respiratory problems?).
   (d) Religion (What is the patient's religious preference?).
   (e) Reason (Why did the patient call?).

74. The "S" of the present illness history mnemonic O-P-Q-R-S-T stands for the word

   (a) Severity (How does the patient rate this problem's severity in relation to the most severe problem she/he has ever had?).
   (b) Solution ("What would you like us to do for you today?").
   (c) Single (Is this a single problem, or does the patient have other complaints?).
   (d) Separate ("Is this a separate incident of this problem, or have you had other incidents?").
   (e) Selection ("What hospital would you like to go to?").

75. The "T" of the present illness history mnemonic O-P-Q-R-S-T stands for the word(s)

   (a) Temperature (What is the patient's oral or rectal temperature?).
   (b) Treatment Tried (Did the patient do or take anything to alleviate the problem, and did it work?).
   (c) Time (What time did the problem start or how long has it lasted?)
   (d) Telephone (Has the patient called her/his private physician?).
   (e) Talk ("Tell me all about this problem. Describe it.").

76. The O-P-Q-R-S-T history is immediately followed by additionally obtaining

  (a) billing information to complete your medical documentation form.
  (b) a SAMPLE history.
  (c) an AVPU history.
  (d) Answers (a) and (c) only.
  (e) Answers (a), (b), and (c).

77. Which of the following statements regarding the performance of a focused Rapid Physical Exam on the responsive (conscious) medical patient is true?

  (a) It is necessary to perform an in-depth examination only of body areas that directly relate to the patient's medical complaint (if the patient's complaint is abdominal pain, a pupil exam is not necessary).
  (b) Every area of the responsive medical patient's body must be examined thoroughly.
  (c) Areas where the patient complains of pain should be palpated repeatedly to determine the patient's consistency of complaint.
  (d) All of the above are true.
  (e) None of the above are true.

78. Which of the following statements regarding the performance of a focused Rapid Physical Exam on the unresponsive (unconscious) medical patient is true?

  (a) It is necessary to perform an in-depth examination only of body areas that directly relate to what bystanders or family members describe as the patient's medical complaint prior to loss of consciousness (respect the patient's privacy).
  (b) Every area of the unresponsive medical patient's body must be examined thoroughly.
  (c) Areas where the patient seems to have a pain response should be palpated repeatedly to determine the patient's consistency of response.
  (d) All of the above are true.
  (e) None of the above are true.

79. The Focused History and Physical Exam for all patients includes searching for medical ID devices that identify the patient's medical problems and/or allergies. These devices can be found

  (a) on the patient's wrist or ankle (a bracelet ID).
  (b) around the patient's neck (a necklace ID).
  (c) in the patient's wallet (a medical ID card).
  (d) Answers (a) and (b) only.
  (e) Answers (a), (b), and (c).

80. Another form of medical information that may be present in a patient's home is called a "Vial of Life." This device is usually a small canister containing patient medical information and/or a list of the patient's medicines. The presence of this device usually is identified by a sticker mounted on the

    (a) patient's refrigerator door.
    (b) main door of the patient's residence.
    (c) window closest to the main door.
    (d) Answers (b) and (c) only.
    (e) Answers (a), (b), and (c).

81. Which of the following statements regarding the Detailed Physical Exam is true?

    (a) The Detailed Physical Exam is performed only if time permits, usually while en route to the emergency department.
    (b) For simple, isolated injuries, a Detailed Physical Exam of uninjured body areas is not required.
    (c) Treatment for critical or serious problems **always** precedes a Detailed Physical Exam.
    (d) Only answers (a) and (c) are true.
    (e) Answers (a), (b), and (c) are true.

*The only difference between the physical assessment portions of a **Focused History and Physical Exam** and a **Detailed Physical Exam** is a more in-depth examination of the patient's head.*

82. In the Detailed Physical Exam, assessment of the scalp and cranium includes a DCAP-BTLS inspection, in addition to an assessment for

    (a) paradoxical movement on respiration.
    (b) crepitation (or "crepitus").
    (c) hair color alterations.
    (d) Answers (a) and (c) only.
    (e) Answers (a), (b), and (c).

83. In the Detailed Physical Exam, assessment of the ears includes a DCAP-BTLS inspection, in addition to an assessment for

    (a) missing earrings.
    (b) paradoxical movement on respiration.
    (c) fluid drainage.
    (d) Answers (a) and (b) only.
    (e) Answers (a), (b), and (c).

84. In the Detailed Physical Exam, assessment of the eyes includes a DCAP-BTLS inspection, in addition to an assessment for

    (a) discoloration.
    (b) unequal pupils.
    (c) foreign bodies or blood in the anterior chamber.
    (d) Answers (b) and (c) only.
    (e) Answers (a), (b), and (c).

85. In the Detailed Physical Exam, assessment of the nose includes a DCAP-BTLS inspection, in addition to an assessment for

    (a) fluid drainage or bleeding.
    (b) paradoxical movement on respiration.
    (c) the presence of mucus.
    (d) Answers (b) and (c) only.
    (e) Answers (a), (b), and (c).

86. In the Detailed Physical Exam, assessment of the mouth includes a DCAP-BTLS inspection, in addition to an assessment for

    (a) loose or broken teeth or other objects that may obstruct the airway.
    (b) wounds, discoloration, or edema of the tongue.
    (c) breath odor.
    (d) Answers (a) and (b) only.
    (e) Answers (a), (b), and (c).

87. The Ongoing Assessment phase of prehospital care can be best defined as a procedure for

    (a) filling time until arrival at the patient's destination.
    (b) detecting changes in the patient's clinical presentation, vital signs, and/or response to treatment that may indicate underlying disease or injury processes.
    (c) documenting several sets of vital signs to fulfill basic vital sign documentation requirements.
    (d) Answers (a) and (c) only.
    (e) Answers (a), (b), and (c).

88. The term *trending* is best defined as the process of

    (a) assessing and documenting changes in the patient's clinical presentation, vital signs, and response to treatment that may indicate underlying disease or injury processes.
    (b) identifying the patient's involvement in a specific "subculture," by observing clothing and language trends (subculture trends may identify a patient at risk for specific illnesses or injuries).

(c) following current protocols and trends of patient care, even when radically different from long-standing, accepted protocols.
(d) Answers (b) and (c) only.
(e) Answers (a), (b), and (c).

89. Which of the following steps is not part of the Ongoing Assessment?

(a) Recheck the potential for life-threatening injury or illness by repeating the initial assessment.
(b) Reassess and record the patient's vital signs.
(c) Repeat the Focused Assessment regarding the patient's complaint or injuries.
(d) Assess and document the effectiveness of EMS interventions (adequacy of oxygen delivery or artificial ventilation, bleeding management, and other medical interventions) and the patient's response to those interventions.
(e) Reassess all vital signs and document them every 5 minutes for each patient transported.

90. All of the following are part of the initial and repeated initial patient assessment, except

(a) assessment/monitoring of mental status.
(b) assessment/monitoring of airway and breathing status.
(c) assessment/monitoring of pulse presence, rate, and quality.
(d) assessment/monitoring of skin color and temperature.
(e) documentation of verbal comments that a patient makes regarding criminal activities.

91. The best definition of the term (or phrase) _____ is a radio that is located at a stationary site, such as a hospital or public safety agency.

(a) portable radio
(b) base station
(c) repeater
(d) mobile two-way radio
(e) cellular telephone

92. The best definition of the term (or phrase) _____ is a transmitter/receiver that usually is mounted in a vehicle and typically transmits at 20 to 50 watts, with a general transmission range of 10 to 15 miles.

(a) portable radio
(b) base station
(c) repeater
(d) mobile two-way radio
(e) cellular telephone

93. The best definition of the term (or phrase) _____ is a radio that is handheld and typically transmits at a power of 1 to 5 watts, with a limited general range of transmission.

    (a) portable radio
    (b) base station
    (c) repeater
    (d) mobile two-way radio
    (e) cellular telephone

94. The best definition of the term (or phrase) _____ is a device that receives a transmission on one frequency and retransmits at a higher power on another frequency.

    (a) portable radio
    (b) base station
    (c) repeater
    (d) mobile two-way radio
    (e) cellular telephone

95. The best definition of the term (or phrase) _____ is a device that transmits through the air instead of over wires so that its range is expanded; it has the advantage of simultaneous, two-way conversation (allowing for interruptions, questions, and answers during communication).

    (a) portable radio
    (b) base station
    (c) repeater
    (d) mobile two-way radio
    (e) cellular telephone

96. Radio frequencies are assigned, licensed, and monitored by

    (a) the Federal Communications Commission (FCC).
    (b) the County Communications Commission (CCC).
    (c) the Federal Aviation Association (FAA).
    (d) the County Aviation Association (CAA).
    (e) the provider's local Communications Association ([city's initials]CA).

97. Communication with medical direction occurs when

    (a) the receiving facility is contacted regarding the patient.
    (b) a separate (primary) facility is contacted regarding the patient and then relays that information to the actual receiving facility.
    (c) the EMT contacts the medical director for consultation and/or receipt of patient care instructions or orders.
    (d) Answers (b) and (c) only.
    (e) Answers (a), (b), and/or (c).

98. The content of radio transmissions needs to be

(a) sketchy and nonspecific (to save on "air time") and can be made in any order, as long as information about the patient's complaints is relayed.
(b) organized and concise, relaying any information pertinent to the patient's immediate medical needs and any questions or concerns the EMT may have about the patient's care.
(c) as brief as possible, with only patient medical history and chief complaint information relayed (consultations and questions about care should **not** be necessary if the EMT is well trained).
(d) Answers (a) and (c) only.
(e) Answers (a), (b), and (c).

99. Which of the following statements regarding EMT/physician radio communication is false?

(a) The medical director's orders and recommendations will be based solely upon the EMT's transmitted patient information; therefore, this information must be accurate.
(b) After receiving a medication or procedure order, the EMT should repeat that order back to the medical director.
(c) After receiving a denial of orders for medication or procedure performance, the EMT should repeat the denial of orders back to the medical director.
(d) Even if the medical director's orders are unclear or appear to be inappropriate, the EMT should never question such orders. The sole responsibility for patient care lies with the medical director.
(e) EMTs' radio reports provide information that allows hospitals to prepare for a patient's arrival by having the right room, equipment, and personnel prepared.

100. Which of the following statements regarding radio communication principles is false?

(a) Ensure that the radio is on and the volume is properly adjusted.
(b) Listen to the frequency before transmitting to be sure that it is clear of other radio traffic.
(c) Begin speaking immediately upon pressing the "press to talk" (PTT) button to avoid excessive obstruction of air time.
(d) Speak with your lips approximately two to three inches from the microphone (too close, and your transmission becomes garbled; too far away, and your transmission is too faint).
(e) Address the unit being called; then give the name (and/or number) of the calling unit.

101. Which of the following statements regarding radio communication principles is false?

 (a) Speak clearly and slowly, using clear text, avoiding meaningless phrases such as "Be advised."
 (b) Transmit as long as necessary before pausing to allow for other radio traffic (the interruption of other radio transmissions may confuse the receiving party).
 (c) Avoid codes; use plain English (codes may confuse the receiving party).
 (d) Courtesy is assumed when speaking on a radio, so there is no need to say "please," "thank you," and/or "you're welcome."
 (e) None of the above are false.

102. Which of the following statements regarding radio communication principles is false?

 (a) When transmitting a number that might be confused (for example, a number in the "teens," such as 15 being confused for 50), give the number first; then give the individual digits ("one-five").
 (b) To ensure appropriate reception of the patient, always transmit the patient's full name and the name of the patient's physician.
 (c) An EMT may be sued for slander for airing biased, derogatory, or injurious patient information over radio waves.
 (d) An EMT may be fined for using profanity over the air.
 (e) Avoid words that may be difficult to hear, such as "yes" or "no." Instead, use "affirmative" or "negative."

103. Which of the following statements regarding radio communication principles is false?

 (a) Standard formats of order for radio transmission of patient information are unnecessary as long as all important patient information is transmitted.
 (b) Indicate the end of radio transmission by saying "over," and then get confirmation that the message was received.
 (c) Avoid offering a diagnosis of the patient's problem.
 (d) Use EMS frequencies only for EMS communication.
 (e) Reduce background noise as much as possible by closing windows during transmission.

104. Place the following essential elements of a radioed patient medical report in the order they should be given.

 1. Mental status
 2. Chief complaint

3. Emergency medical care given
4. Estimated time of arrival at the emergency department (ETA)
5. Patient's age and sex
6. Brief, pertinent history of the patient's present illness or injury
7. Major past illnesses or injuries
8. Baseline vital signs
9. Pertinent physical exam findings
10. Response to emergency medical care given
11. Identification of calling unit and level of care provider

   (a) 11, 4, 5, 2, 6, 7, 1, 8, 9, 3, 10
   (b) 1, 2, 3, 4, 5, 6, 7, 8, 9, 10, 11
   (c) 11, 10, 9, 8, 7, 6, 5, 4, 3, 2, 1
   (d) 10, 3, 11, 4, 5, 2, 6, 7, 1, 8, 9
   (e) 5, 4, 3, 2, 1, 11, 10, 9, 8, 7, 6

105. Which of the following statements regarding EMT activity after the patient care radio report is false?

   (a) The EMT should continue to assess the patient and relay any additional pertinent information via additional radio contact.
   (b) A deterioration in the patient's condition should be relayed to the receiving facility.
   (c) The receiving hospital will be busy preparing for the patient's arrival (especially a critical patient). The EMT should not distract them with any additional radio contact.
   (d) Additional patient vital signs should be obtained and the patient's condition reassessed en route to the emergency department.
   (e) In some systems, particularly during long transport times, updated patient vital signs or any new information obtained that is pertinent to the patient's condition should be relayed to the receiving facility via additional radio contact.

106. Ambulance dispatch should be notified of all of the following, except

   (a) the receipt of the call information, that the unit is en route, and the unit's arrival on the scene.
   (b) any need for notification and/or dispatch of other agencies.
   (c) the patient's medical condition upon arrival at the scene.
   (d) when the unit leaves the incident scene and/or returns to available service.
   (e) when the unit arrives at the receiving facility.

107. Which of the following statements regarding the verbal report to the emergency department staff upon arrival is true?

(a) The patient should be introduced by name (if known).
(b) A summary of the same information relayed by radio should be given.
(c) Additional vital signs (taken after the radio report) and any additional history or treatment/responses to treatment should be reported.
(d) All of the above are true.
(e) None of the above are true.

108. Which of the following statements regarding interpersonal communication with the patient is true?

(a) Avoid causing patients emotional discomfort by avoiding direct eye contact.
(b) As often as possible, position yourself above the patient. This identifies you as an authority figure and provides the emotional relief that someone *else* is now in charge.
(c) When you anticipate the truth being negative, frightening, or uncomfortable for the patient to hear, assure the patient of a pleasant and positive outcome.
(d) All of the above are true.
(e) None of the above are true.

109. Which of the following statements regarding interpersonal communication with the patient is true?

(a) Use medical terminology as often as possible to demonstrate that you are an expert at emergency care. This will reassure frightened patients.
(b) Use the patient's first name only after obtaining the patient's permission to do so.
(c) It is often quite helpful to use pleasant nicknames for pediatric patients, such as "Sonny" (for boys), "Missy" (for girls), or the like. This reassures the child that you are older, wiser, and able to take good care of her/him.
(d) Both answers (a) and (c) are true.
(e) All of the above are true.

110. Which of the following statements regarding the prehospital patient care written report is false?

(a) The prehospital written report provides for continuity of care. Although it may not be read immediately, it may be referred to later for important patient information.
(b) A good written report documents what emergency medical care was provided and any changes in the patient's status.

TEST SECTION THREE

(c) Because the patient care report is a legal document, if the person who completed it did so thoroughly, a court appearance usually is avoided by simply submitting the report to the lawyers (much like a "deposition").
(d) Prehospital documentation aids in EMT evaluation and quality improvement efforts.
(e) Prehospital documentation aids in billing the patient, is a source for service statistics, and is helpful for prehospital research.

111. Written documentation of each patient contact should include all of the following information, except every patient's
   (a) chief complaint.
   (b) level of consciousness (AVPU) and mental status.
   (c) capillary refill status.
   (d) skin color, condition, and temperature.
   (e) respiratory rate and effort, and pulse rate and quality.

112. Documentation of things the EMT observes about a patient during the physical examination is called _____ information.
   (a) approximated
   (b) objective
   (c) subjective
   (d) pertinent negative
   (e) unreliable

113. Documentation of symptoms or sensations a patient complains of is called _____ information.
   (a) approximated
   (b) objective
   (c) subjective
   (d) pertinent negative
   (e) unreliable

114. Documentation of patient information reported by bystanders or family members is called _____ information.
   (a) approximated
   (b) objective
   (c) subjective
   (d) pertinent negative
   (e) unreliable

115. Documentation of symptoms or sensations the patient denies having is called _____ information.

   (a) approximated
   (b) objective
   (c) subjective
   (d) pertinent negative
   (e) unreliable

116. Documentation of a patient's vital signs or physical assessment findings is called _____ information.

   (a) approximated
   (b) objective
   (c) subjective
   (d) pertinent negative
   (e) unreliable

117. The narrative section of a prehospital patient care document is the section that

   (a) provides space to write patient information that supplements check box or fill-in-the-blank information sections.
   (b) consists of check boxes regarding patient condition.
   (c) is available only to providers who dictate their reports over a telephone dictation service.
   (d) consists of check boxes and fill-in-the-blank boxes for patient vital signs.
   (e) consists of check boxes and fill-in-the-blank boxes regarding patient condition and/or patient vital signs.

118. Which of the following statements regarding written documentation of patient condition, assessment, or treatment information is false?

   (a) Like the use of medical abbreviations, radio codes should be used on the written report as often as possible. This saves space and allows room for more complete documentation of important patient information.
   (b) Describe your findings in detail, but avoid drawing conclusions or documenting personal opinions.
   (c) Include all pertinent negatives regarding the patient's complaints and condition.
   (d) Record important scene observations, such as mechanism of injury descriptions, suicide notes, weapons, the presence of empty medication or alcohol containers, and the like.
   (e) None of the above are false.

119. Which of the following statements regarding the use of medical abbreviations is true?

(a) Because the documenter must always appear in court along with the prehospital patient care record, EMTs are free to compose their own, personal system of medical abbreviations.
(b) Even standard medical abbreviations may be confused with other meanings. Consequently, **any** use of medical abbreviations is discouraged. Always write it out!
(c) Although medical abbreviations greatly improve the ability to document large amounts of patient information in small spaces, only standard medical abbreviations should be used (some services provide lists of acceptable abbreviations).
(d) Radio codes are a widely accepted form of standard medical abbreviations.
(e) Both answers (a) and (d) are true.

120. Which of the following statements regarding written documentation of patient condition, assessment, or treatment information is true?

(a) When information of a sensitive nature (such as communicable diseases) is documented, note the source of that information.
(b) If you do not know how to spell a word, look up the correct spelling or use another word.
(c) Spelling is not important to patient care; therefore, it also is not important to patient care documentation. As long as any reader can determine your intended message, spelling is not an issue.
(d) Both answers (a) and (b) are true.
(e) Both answers (a) and (c) are true.

121. Which of the following statements regarding written documentation of patient condition, assessment, or treatment information is true?

(a) "If you didn't write it down, it wasn't done."
(b) All of the information on the prehospital patient documentation form is considered to be confidential.
(c) Only the patient's name, address, and billing information is considered to be confidential.
(d) Both answers (a) and (b) are true.
(e) Both answers (a) and (c) are true.

122. An *error of omission* is defined as
    (a) not doing something that should have been done.
    (b) not noticing something that should have been noticed.
    (c) performing a procedure that should not have been performed.
    (d) Answers (a) and/or (b) only.
    (e) Answers (a), (b), and/or (c).

123. An *error of commission* is defined as
    (a) not doing something that should have been done.
    (b) not noticing something that should have been noticed.
    (c) performing a procedure that should not have been performed.
    (d) Answers (a) and/or (b) only.
    (e) Answers (a), (b), and/or (c).

124. When an error of omission or commission occurs, the EMT should
    (a) remember that the written patient care document is the only legal record of the patient's care and should take advantage of the opportunity to avoid punishment or prosecution by documenting things as they **should** have been done.
    (b) carefully document all appropriate assessments and/or treatments, leaving the inappropriate or injurious portions out of the written document.
    (c) document what did or did not happen, exactly as it occurred, and what steps were taken (if any) to correct the situation.
    (d) Answers (a) or (b) only.
    (e) Answers (a), (b), or (c).

125. Which of the following statements regarding falsification of information on the prehospital care report is false?
    (a) Suspension or revocation of the EMT's certification/license may occur.
    (b) Poor patient care may occur because other health care providers have a false impression of which assessment findings were discovered or what treatment was performed.
    (c) False vital sign documentation may detrimentally affect continuing patient care.
    (d) If a treatment was overlooked (such as application of oxygen) and then falsely documented as having occurred, such documentation may detrimentally affect continuing patient care.
    (e) Falsified information on the prehospital care report is rarely discovered because these reports are rarely actually read.

126. If a patient refuses treatment, the EMT should

(a) try again to persuade the patient to allow treatment and transportation.
(b) ensure that the patient is able to make a rational, informed decision (Does the patient have an altered level of consciousness because of drugs or the effects of illness/injury?).
(c) inform the patient specifically why she/he should allow treatment and transportation and what may happen to her/him if she/he does not.
(d) seek medical direction as required by local protocol, perhaps allowing the medical director to speak directly with the refusing patient (via radio or phone contact).
(e) do all of the above.

127. If the patient continues to refuse treatment, the EMT should

(a) document any assessment findings and emergency medical care given.
(b) have the patient sign a refusal form.
(c) have a family member, bystander, or police officer sign the form as a witness to the patient's refusal.
(d) document the complete patient assessment, the care the EMT wished to provide, a statement that the EMT explained to the patient possible consequences of care refusal and then encourage alternative methods of gaining care (also encouraging the patient or family members to call the EMT back to the scene as needed).
(e) do all of the above.

128. When an error is made while writing the prehospital patient report form, the EMT should

(a) draw a single horizontal line through the error, initial above the line, and write the correct information beside it.
(b) carefully obliterate (darkly scribble over) the written error, so that its presence will not confuse future readers of the report.
(c) carefully obliterate the error, write the word "error" over the obliteration, and then continue with the correct information.
(d) leave the error as is, making a note at the end of the document regarding the error, and then supply the correct information.
(e) Any of the above.

129. If a written error is discovered at **any** time after the report form is submitted, the EMT should

(a) remember that there is no way to legally alter a previously submitted document.
(b) notify a supervisor to substitute a correct report form.
(c) write an entirely new patient report form, find and destroy the form with the error, and substitute the correct form in its place.
(d) draw a single line though the error, initial and date the line, write a note with the correct information at the end of the report (initialing and dating the note), and distribute corrected copies to all appropriate personnel.
(e) find all submitted forms and destroy them.

130. Which of the following statements regarding multiple casualty incidents (MCIs) and report writing is false?

(a) All prehospital patient care documentation is exactly the same for MCIs as for any other patient contact.
(b) There probably will not be enough time for the EMT to complete the patient care report during MCIs. Thus, it often must be completed at a later time.
(c) The local MCI plan should have some means of temporarily recording important medical information (such as a triage tag), which can be used later to complete each patient's care form.
(d) The standard for completing the patient care form in an MCI is not the same as that of a typical call.
(e) Local MCI preparedness plans should have altered guidelines established for what information is required on the final patient prehospital care documentation for MCI patients.

The following 59 questions are an elective group of Medical Abbreviations and Symbols questions. These symbols and abbreviations do not represent DOT-required knowledge for the EMT-Basic.[*] Page numbers keyed to Brady's Emergency Care, 7th ed., are not provided for these questions. Instead, reference the Common Medical Abbreviations and Symbols available in the appendix to this text (page 383).

131. The medical abbreviation/symbol $\bar{a}$ means

(a) before.
(b) after.
(c) every.
(d) with.
(e) without.

---

* All DOT-required medical **terminology** will be presented in appropriate test sections of this text. The DOT does not list specific, "standard" medical abbreviations or symbols.

132. The medical abbreviation/symbol $\bar{s}$ means

    (a) before.
    (b) after.
    (c) every.
    (d) with.
    (e) without.

133. The medical abbreviation/symbol $\bar{c}$ means

    (a) before.
    (b) after.
    (c) every.
    (d) with.
    (e) without.

134. The medical abbreviation/symbol $\bar{p}$ means

    (a) before.
    (b) after.
    (c) every.
    (d) with.
    (e) without.

135. The medical abbreviation/symbol $\bar{q}$ means

    (a) before.
    (b) after.
    (c) every.
    (d) with.
    (e) without.

136. The medical abbreviation **abd** means

    (a) airway, breathing, disability.
    (b) always buy disposable items.
    (c) abdomen or abdominal.
    (d) abnormal (appearance), bleeding, deformity.
    (e) alcohol, barbiturates, or other drugs.

137. The medical abbreviation for a sudden heart attack is

    (a) AMA (acute myocardial attack).
    (b) AHA (acute heart attack).
    (c) SHA (sudden heart attack).
    (d) AMI (acute myocardial infraction).
    (e) AMI (acute myocardial infarction).

138. The medical abbreviation for "two times a day" is

    (a) qd or q.d. (initials for the Latin *quaque die*).
    (b) bid or b.i.d. (initials for the Latin *bis in die*).
    (c) hs or h.s. (initials for the Latin *hora somni*).
    (d) qid or q.i.d. (initials for the Latin *quarter in die*).
    (e) tid or t.i.d. (initials for the Latin *ter in die*)

139. The medical abbreviation for "every day" is

    (a) qd or q.d. (initials for the Latin *quaque die*).
    (b) bid or b.i.d. (initials for the Latin *bis in die*).
    (c) hs or h.s. (initials for the Latin *hora somni*).
    (d) qid or q.i.d. (initials for the Latin *quarter in die*).
    (e) tid or t.i.d. (initials for the Latin *ter in die*)

140. The medical abbreviation for "four times a day" is

    (a) qd or q.d. (initials for the Latin *quaque die*).
    (b) bid or b.i.d. (initials for the Latin *bis in die*).
    (c) hs or h.s. (initials for the Latin *hora somni*).
    (d) qid or q.i.d. (initials for the Latin *quarter in die*).
    (e) tid or t.i.d. (initials for the Latin *ter in die*)

141. The medical abbreviation for "at bedtime" is

    (a) qd or q.d. (initials for the Latin *quaque die*).
    (b) bid or b.i.d. (initials for the Latin *bis in die*).
    (c) hs or h.s. (initials for the Latin *hora somni*).
    (d) qid or q.i.d. (initials for the Latin *quarter in die*).
    (e) tid or t.i.d. (initials for the Latin *ter in die*)

142. The medical abbreviation for "three times a day" is

    (a) qd or q.d. (initials for the Latin *quaque die*).
    (b) bid or b.i.d. (initials for the Latin *bis in die*).
    (c) hs or h.s. (initials for the Latin *hora somni*).
    (d) qid or q.i.d. (initials for the Latin *quarter in die*).
    (e) tid or t.i.d. (initials for the Latin *ter in die*)

143. The medical abbreviation **BS** means

    (a) bovine scat.
    (b) breath sounds.
    (c) blood sugar.
    (d) Answers (b) or (c).
    (e) None of the above.

144. The medical abbreviation **BM** means

    (a) bowel movement.
    (b) basic mobility (of extremities).

(c) basic movement (of extremities).
(d) borderline mechanism.
(e) blood measurement.

145. The medical abbreviation **BVM** means

(a) basic voluntary movement (of extremities).
(b) bag-valve-mask.
(c) borderline vector of mobility (of extremities).
(d) believable version of mechanism.
(e) None of the above.

146. The medical abbreviation **CA** means

(a) coronary attack.
(b) cumulative assessment.
(c) coronary artery.
(d) cancer.
(e) caught in the act.

147. The medical abbreviation **CHF** means

(a) chronic heart failure.
(b) coronary heart failure.
(c) chronic heart fatigue.
(d) cardiac/hepatic (kidney) failure.
(e) congestive heart failure.

148. The medical abbreviation **CHI** means

(a) congestive heart injury.
(b) coronary heart injury.
(c) chronic heart injury.
(d) chronic head injury.
(e) closed head injury.

149. The medical abbreviation **CNS** means

(a) chronic nervous syndrome.
(b) congested nervous syndrome.
(c) central nervous system.
(d) coronary node, sinus.
(e) coughing, nausea, sputum.

150. The medical abbreviation **COPD** means

(a) cold or pneumonia disease.
(b) coronary obstruction with pulmonary disease.
(c) chronic obstructive pulmonary disease.
(d) crazy old person's disease.
(e) careful observation, palpation, and detection.

151. The medical abbreviation **CVA** means

    (a) chronic ventricular activity.
    (b) cerebrovascular accident.
    (c) cardiovascular accident.
    (d) cerebrovascular activity.
    (e) chronic vascular accidents.

152. The medical abbreviation **GI** means

    (a) grossly intact.
    (b) gastrointestinal.
    (c) gradually increasing (pain).
    (d) growth injury.
    (e) great injury.

153. The medical abbreviation **GSW** means

    (a) growth spurt wound.
    (b) gradual signs of wounds (developing).
    (c) good sensation within (extremities).
    (d) gunshot wound.
    (e) gross signs of wounds.

154. The medical abbreviation **GU** means

    (a) genitourinary.
    (b) grossly unwell.
    (c) growing upward.
    (d) gastrourinary.
    (e) growing underneath.

155. The medical abbreviation **HA** means

    (a) helpful activity.
    (b) hardly any.
    (c) help arrives.
    (d) headache.
    (e) head accident.

156. The medical abbreviation **Hx** means

    (a) hare traction.
    (b) head exam.
    (c) history.
    (d) Any of the above.
    (e) None of the above.

157. The medical abbreviation **JVD** means

    (a) junior vascular disease.
    (b) jugular vein distention.

(c) journeying vascular disease.
(d) James Victor disease.
(e) John Vincent disease.

158. The medical abbreviation **LBB** means

 (a) long backboard.
 (b) little bundle branch.
 (c) long bone broken.
 (d) little baby buggy.
 (e) None of the above.

159. The medical abbreviation **LLQ** means

 (a) light or little quality (of pain).
 (b) long or lasting quality (of pain).
 (c) less lethal quality (of pain).
 (d) left lung quadrant.
 (e) left lower quadrant (of the abdomen).

160. The medical abbreviation **LMP** means

 (a) last menstrual period.
 (b) less movement or pain.
 (c) light movement pain.
 (d) lower margin of parietal skull.
 (e) lower margin of peritoneum.

161. The medical abbreviation **lpm** means

 (a) little pain with movement.
 (b) liters per minute.
 (c) lower part of mediastinum.
 (d) lightly palpated motion.
 (e) little palpated motion.

162. The medical abbreviation **LUQ** means

 (a) less than usual quality (of pain).
 (b) lung's upper quadrant.
 (c) lasting unusual quality (of pain).
 (d) left upper quadrant (of the abdomen).
 (e) lessening unusual quality (of pain).

163. The medical abbreviation **LOC** means

 (a) level of consciousness.
 (b) little of consequence.
 (c) lasting obstructive coronary (disease).
 (d) Any of the above.
 (e) None of the above.

164. The medical abbreviation **nc** means

   (a) non-chronic.
   (b) not counted (pulse or respiratory rate).
   (c) nasal cannula.
   (d) north corner.
   (e) no crepitus.

165. The medical abbreviation **NRB** means

   (a) no rotation or bulges (of the hip or leg).
   (b) normal return of breathing.
   (c) normal return of beats (pulse).
   (d) never returned to breathing.
   (e) nonrebreather mask.

166. The medical abbreviation **NTG** means

   (a) numbness and tingling.
   (b) nitroglycerine.
   (c) non-toxic gas.
   (d) normal teenage growth.
   (e) non-tenting (skin condition).

167. The medical abbreviation **n/v** means

   (a) no volition.
   (b) non-vomiting.
   (c) nausea and vomiting.
   (d) non-violent.
   (e) normal ventilations.

168. The medical abbreviation **n/v/d** means

   (a) normal ventilation and delivery (of oxygen).
   (b) nocturnal vascular disease.
   (c) normal ventricular delivery (of pulse).
   (d) nausea, vomiting, and dehydration.
   (e) nausea, vomiting, and diarrhea.

169. The medical abbreviation **PE** means

   (a) pulmonary embolism.
   (b) pulmonary edema.
   (c) partially eaten.
   (d) potential emergency.
   (e) pediatric emergency.

170. The medical abbreviation **PID** means

   (a) pulmonary interruption disease.
   (b) pediatric intelligence disease.

(c) partial intelligence disruption.
(d) pelvic inflammatory disease.
(e) pulmonary injury or disease.

171. The medical abbreviation **PNS** means

(a) pulmonary nocturnal symptoms.
(b) partially normal signs.
(c) peripheral nervous system.
(d) pain and numbness signs.
(e) pain symptoms.

172. The medical abbreviation **PTOA** means

(a) pulmonary tingling or obstruction assessment.
(b) previous times of assessments.
(c) partial obstruction accident.
(d) painful tingling or aches.
(e) prior to our arrival.

173. The medical abbreviation **R/O** means

(a) rule out.
(b) rollover (accident).
(c) renal obstruction (kidney stone).
(d) relatives or others.
(e) rings (and other jewelry) off.

174. The medical abbreviation **RLQ** means

(a) relatively less in quality (of pain).
(b) right lower quadrant (of the abdomen).
(c) radiating and lasting quality (of pain).
(d) right lung quadrant.
(e) ridiculously low quality (of pain).

175. The medical abbreviation **RUQ** means

(a) relatively unusual quality (of pain).
(b) relatively usual quality (of pain).
(c) right upper quadrant (of lungs).
(d) radiating, unusual quality (of pain).
(e) None of the above.

176. The medical abbreviation **SOB** means

(a) shortness of breath.
(b) signs of breathing.
(c) symptoms of breathing.
(d) Either answer (b) or (c).
(e) None of the above.

177. The medical abbreviation **TIA** means

    (a) tingling in abdomen.
    (b) times in accidents (previous MVA history).
    (c) transient ischemic attack.
    (d) telephoned in assessment.
    (e) trauma injury assessment.

178. The medical abbreviation **URI** means

    (a) unknown reasons for injury.
    (b) upper respiratory infection.
    (c) unknown respiratory infection.
    (d) unreasonable reasons for injury.
    (e) urinary injury.

179. The medical abbreviation **UTI** means

    (a) unknown time of injury.
    (b) upper thoracic injury.
    (c) urinary tract infection.
    (d) unusual treatment of injury.
    (e) uterus intact.

180. The medical abbreviation **WNL** means

    (a) weeping, necrotic lesions.
    (b) with no loss (of).
    (c) wandering neural loss.
    (d) with normal length.
    (e) within normal limits.

181. The medical abbreviation **y/o** means

    (a) yellow.
    (b) yards of (travel).
    (c) yours/ours.
    (d) years old.
    (e) young or old.

182. The medical symbol ∿∿ stands for

    (a) change.
    (b) less than or equal to.
    (c) approximately.
    (d) more than or equal to.
    (e) unequal to.

183. The medical symbol △ stands for

    (a) change.
    (b) sorority or fraternity member.

(c) approximately
(d) angulated.
(e) triangulated.

184. The medical symbol $>$ stands for

(a) less than.
(b) greater than.
(c) smaller than.
(d) taller than.
(e) above.

185. The medical symbol $<$ stands for

(a) less than.
(b) greater than.
(c) smaller than.
(d) taller than.
(e) above.

186. The medical symbol ♀ stands for a _____ patient.

(a) pediatric
(b) male
(c) female
(d) adult
(e) psychiatric

187. The medical symbol ♂ stands for a _____ patient.

(a) pediatric
(b) male
(c) female
(d) adult
(e) psychiatric

188. The medical symbol ↑ stands for

(a) above or taller than.
(b) below or shorter than.
(c) above or increased.
(d) below or decreased.
(e) up and away from.

189. The medical symbol ↓ stands for

(a) above or taller than.
(b) below or shorter than.
(c) above or increased.
(d) below or decreased.
(e) down and away from.

The answer key for Test Section Three is on pages 356 through 360.

Test Section Four

This test section covers the following subjects:

* General Pharmacology
* Respiratory Emergencies
* Cardiac Emergencies
* Diabetes and Altered Mental Status
* Allergies
* Poisonings and Overdoses
* Environmental Emergencies
* Behavioral Emergencies
* Obstetrics and Gynecology

1994 Revised EMT-Basic National Standards Review Self-Test

1. The study of sources, characteristics, effects, and administration of medications (drugs) is called
   (a) medicology.
   (b) anatomy.
   (c) pharmacology.
   (d) physiology.
   (e) pharmacy.

2. Which of the following statements regarding EMT-Basic drug administration is false?
   (a) Activated charcoal is carried on the basic EMS unit for administration to patients.
   (b) With the medical director's approval, EMT-Basics may assist patients in using their own (prescribed) respiratory medication inhalers.
   (c) Oral glucose is carried on the basic EMS unit for administration to patients.
   (d) Nitroglycerin is carried on the basic EMS unit for administration to patients with chest pain who have run out of their own nitroglycerin.
   (e) Oxygen is a drug and is carried on the basic EMS unit for administration to patients.

3. With the medical director's approval, EMT-Basics may assist patients in using **their own** (prescribed)
   (a) nitroglycerin.
   (b) epinephrine auto-injectors.
   (c) insulin.
   (d) Answers (a) and (b) only.
   (e) Answers (a), (b), and (c).

4. When a drug is developed, its name is listed in the **U.S. Pharmacopedia**, a governmental publication listing all drugs in the United States, with the initials "U.S.P." following it. This drug name (without the U.S.P. initials) is called the drug's
   (a) generic name (such as "epinephrine hydrochloride").
   (b) chemical name (such as "beta-[3,4-dihydroxyphenl]-a-methylaminoethanol").
   (c) trade, proprietary, or brand name (such as "Adrenalin" or "Epi-Pen").
   (d) slang or abbreviated name (such as "epi").
   (e) official name (such as "epinephrine").

5. When a manufacturer markets the drug, another name is created. This name is called the drug's
    (a) generic name (such as "epinephrine hydrochloride").
    (b) chemical name (such as "beta-[3,4-dihydroxyphenl]-a-methylaminoethanol").
    (c) trade, proprietary, or brand name (such as "Adrenalin" or "Epi-Pen").
    (d) slang or abbreviated name (such as "epi").
    (e) official name (such as "epinephrine").

6. The reasons for administering a medication (its most common uses) are called the drug's
    (a) contraindications.
    (b) effects.
    (c) side effects.
    (d) indications.
    (e) toxic effects.

7. Situations in which a medication should not be given (because it may cause harm to the patient or offer no improving effect) are called the drug's
    (a) contraindications.
    (b) effects.
    (c) side effects.
    (d) indications.
    (e) toxic effects.

8. Actions of a drug other than those desired are called _____. Some of these actions may be predictable.
    (a) contraindications
    (b) desired effects
    (c) side effects
    (d) indications
    (e) cosmic effects

9. Medications come in different forms. Activated charcoal is an example of a medication that comes in _____ form.
    (a) sublingual spray
    (b) compressed powder or tablet
    (c) suspension
    (d) Either answer (a) or (b), depending on the form carried.
    (e) None of the above.

10. Nitroglycerin is an example of a medication that comes in _____ form.

    (a) sublingual spray
    (b) compressed powder or tablet
    (c) suspension
    (d) Either answer (a) or (b), depending on the form carried.
    (e) None of the above.

11. Epinephrine is an example of a medication that comes in _____ form.

    (a) gel
    (b) injectable liquid
    (c) gas
    (d) a fixed dose of liquid for vaporization
    (e) a metered dose of fine powder for inhalation

12. Glucose is an example of a medication that comes in _____ form.

    (a) gel
    (b) injectable liquid
    (c) gas
    (d) a fixed dose of liquid for vaporization
    (e) a metered dose of fine powder for inhalation

13. Oxygen is an example of a medication that comes in _____ form.

    (a) gel
    (b) injectable liquid
    (c) gas
    (d) a fixed dose of liquid for vaporization
    (e) a metered dose of fine powder for inhalation

14. An EMT-B may assist with the administration of a particular respiratory medication (one that the patient has by prescription, usually for the treatment of asthma). This medication comes in _____ form.

    (a) gel
    (b) injectable liquid
    (c) gas
    (d) sublingual spray
    (e) a metered dose of fine powder for inhalation

15. A sublingual medication is a drug that is administered by

    (a) an auto-injector device.
    (b) intravenous injection.

(c) inhalation.
(d) oral ingestion.
(e) placing it under the tongue.

16. All of the following signs indicate that an EMT is providing adequate artificial ventilation, except
    (a) when the chest rises and falls with each artificial ventilation.
    (b) when the abdomen rises with each artificial ventilation.
    (c) when the ventilation rate is between 12 and 20 per minute for adults, or greater than 20 per minute for children and infants.
    (d) when the patient's heart rate returns to normal.
    (e) when the patient's skin becomes warm and dry, with pink mucous membranes.

17. Of the following signs, which does not indicate difficulty breathing?
    (a) Restlessness.
    (b) Increased pulse rate.
    (c) Increased respiratory rate (from normal).
    (d) Decreased respiratory rate (from normal).
    (e) Any of the above may be signs of difficulty breathing.

18. Of the following signs, which does not indicate difficulty breathing?
    (a) Frantically complaining of difficulty breathing in such long, wordy, and anxious phrases that it is difficult to get the patient's attention.
    (b) Retractions—the use of accessory muscles.
    (c) Altered level of consciousness, usually with signs of fatigue.
    (d) Abdominal breathing.
    (e) Any of the above may be signs of difficulty breathing.

19. The **tripod position** may be observed in children or adults and often indicates that they are having serious difficulty breathing. This position is best described as when the patient
    (a) lays on her/his side, bent at the waist, with legs straight out (also called the lateral "V" position).
    (b) leans forward while sitting upright, with arms straight, hands resting on knees (or another surface), and neck extended.
    (c) is slumped over in a large easy chair with her/his feet elevated.
    (d) assumes a semi-fowler's position with legs straight out and elevated (also called the "V" position).
    (e) stands upright with legs spread apart, but bent over at the waist and dangling her/his head, while leaning one hand on a supportive surface (creating a "tripod" appearance).

20. Observing that the patient has a **barrel chest** often indicates that the patient has a history of chronic lung disease. A barrel chest is best described as

    (a) an obesity problem (where the chest and abdomen are large and rounded, creating the impression that the patient's torso looks like a barrel).
    (b) an enlarged chest diameter with a shallow and fixed amount of expansion (creating the impression that the patient's chest looks like a barrel).
    (c) excessive chest expansion with inspiration and excessive chest deflation with expiration (creating the impression that the patient "blows up like a barrel" when she/he inhales).
    (d) Either answer (a) or (b).
    (e) Either answer (b) or (c).

21. The term (or phrase) _____ is best described as a harsh sound heard during both inspiration and expiration, usually indicating that an upper airway obstruction is present.

    (a) crowing
    (b) audible wheezing
    (c) gurgling
    (d) snoring
    (e) stridor

22. The term (or phrase) _____ is best described as a harsh, musical sound, heard without the use of a stethoscope, which usually is most profound (loudest, harshest) when the patient is exhaling. This sound is associated with lower airway obstruction.

    (a) crowing
    (b) audible wheezing
    (c) gurgling
    (d) snoring
    (e) stridor

23. Your patient complains of trouble breathing, has signs and symptoms of trouble breathing, but does not have a prescribed medication inhaler. Which of the following treatment measures should be taken, and in what order?

1. Assess baseline vital signs.
2. Apply oxygen by nonrebreather mask at 15 lpm (using a nasal cannula at 4 to 6 lpm only if the patient does not tolerate a nonrebreather mask).
3. Apply oxygen by nonrebreather mask at 15 lpm (unless the patient has a history of COPD; then use a nasal cannula at only 4 lpm).

4. Apply oxygen by nasal cannula at 4 lpm.
5. Consult the medical director regarding assisted administration of a prescribed medication inhaler (one prescribed to another family member or close friend).
6. Repeat the inhaler administration as indicated.
7. Continue focused assessment.
8. Prepare to assist the patient with ventilatory support.

   (a) 1, 3, 7, 8.
   (b) 1, 2, 5, 6, 7, 8.
   (c) 2, 1, 7, 8.
   (d) 8, 1, 4, 7.
   (e) 3, 1, 7, 8.

24. Your patient complains of trouble breathing, has signs and symptoms of trouble breathing, and has a prescribed medication inhaler. Which of the following treatment measures should be taken, and in what order?

    1. Assess baseline vital signs.
    2. Apply oxygen by nonrebreather mask at 15 lpm (using a nasal cannula at 4 to 6 lpm only if the patient does not tolerate a nonrebreather mask).
    3. Apply oxygen by nonrebreather mask at 15 lpm (unless the patient has a history of COPD; then use a nasal cannula at only 4 lpm).
    4. Apply oxygen by nasal cannula at 4 lpm.
    5. Consult the medical director regarding assisted administration of the patient's prescribed medication inhaler.
    6. Repeat the inhaler administration as indicated.
    7. Continue focused assessment.
    8. Prepare to assist the patient with ventilatory support.

       (a) 1, 3, 5, 6, 7, 8
       (b) 1, 2, 5, 6, 2, 8
       (c) 2, 1, 5, 6, 7, 8
       (d) 8, 7, 1, 4
       (e) 4, 1, 7, 5, 8

25. Generic names for a patient's prescribed inhaler include all of the following, except

    (a) albuterol.
    (b) Alupent.
    (c) isoetharine.
    (d) metaproteranol.
    (e) All of the above are generic names for prescribed inhalers.

26. Trade (or proprietary) names for a patient's prescribed inhaler include all of the following, except

    (a) Proventil.
    (b) Ventolin.
    (c) Bronkosol.
    (d) Metaprel.
    (e) All of the above are trade names for prescribed inhalers.

27. In order for an EMT-B to assist with the administration of a patient's prescribed inhaler, which of the following criteria must be met?

    (a) The patient must exhibit signs and symptoms of a respiratory emergency.
    (b) The patient must have her/his own prescribed inhaler present.
    (c) The EMT-B must have specific authorization by the medical director to administer a respiratory inhaler.
    (d) Answers (a) and (c) only.
    (e) Answers (a), (b), and (c).

28. Contraindications for EMT-B assistance with the administration of a patient's prescribed inhaler include all except which of the following?

    (a) The medical director denies the inhaler administration assistance request.
    (b) The patient already has used the inhaler the maximum times allowed.
    (c) The patient is unable to use the device, even with assistance (can't follow directions).
    (d) The patient has wheezes that can be heard only with a stethoscope.
    (e) The inhaler is prescribed for a person other than the patient.

29. Which of the following statements regarding inhaler dosage (the number of times the EMT-B may assist the patient with inhalation) is true?

    (a) The number of EMT-assisted inhalations is based on the medical director's orders.
    (b) The number of EMT-assisted inhalations is based on the number of doses the patient already has inhaled.
    (c) Only one EMT-assisted inhalation may be administered to any prehospital patient.
    (d) Both answers (a) and (b) are true.
    (e) Answers (a), (b), and (c) are true.

30. After an order has been received from the medical director, the EMT should do all of the following, except

(a) assure that the patient is alert enough to use the inhaler.
(b) check the expiration date of the inhaler.
(c) avoid shaking or disturbing the inhaler's contents prior to inhalation.
(d) assure that the inhaler is at room temperature or warmer.
(e) shake the inhaler vigorously, several times.

31. Patients with difficulty breathing are often anxious and may neglect to perform one or more steps of using the inhaler. This minimizes the inhaler's effectiveness. Thus, the EMT-B may need to coach the patient through the correct steps. Choose the correct directions from the following selection, and place your selected directions in their correct order.

1. Have the patient exhale deeply.
2. Instruct the patient to hold her/his breath for as long as she/he comfortably can (so the medication can be absorbed as much as possible).
3. Assist the patient by pinching her/his nose closed (this prevents escape of medication through the nasal pharynx).
4. Have the patient depress the handheld inhaler as she/he begins to inhale deeply.
5. Have the patient put her/his lips around the opening of the inhaler.
6. If a second dose is to be administered, have the patient breathe normally a few times, and then repeat the administration steps.
7. Immediately after depressing the handheld inhaler, instruct the patient to exhale deeply (the patient should not be allowed to hold her/his breath, as too much medication will be retained).
8. Ensure that the patient holds the inhaler with the opening **directed at** her/his open mouth (not **in** her/his mouth) before depressing the inhaler. The medication should "shoot" into the patient's open mouth. Do not allow the nervous patient to actually place her/his lips on the inhaler and "suck" in the medication, as this may result in an overdose.

(a) 1, 5, 4, 2, 6
(b) 8, 1, 3, 4, 7
(c) 1, 8, 4, 2
(d) 5, 3, 4, 7, 6
(e) 3, 8, 4, 7

32. A _____ is an attachment placed between the inhaler and the patient that allows for more effective use of the medication. If the patient has one (not all patients do), it should be used.

(a) spirometer
(b) bronchometer
(c) spacer device
(d) buff-cap
(e) medimeter

33. Narrowing or blockage of the tubes that lead from the trachea to the farthest portions of each lung's respiratory "tree" is called

(a) bronchodilation.
(b) bronchoalleviation.
(c) bronchoexcursion.
(d) bronchoconstriction.
(e) bronchoscopy.

34. Widening or opening of the tubes that lead from the trachea to the farthest portions of each lung's respiratory "tree" is called

(a) bronchodilation.
(b) bronchoalleviation.
(c) bronchoexcursion.
(d) bronchoconstriction.
(e) bronchoscopy.

35. Prescription respiratory inhalers contain _____ medication. This means that the inhaled medication will expand the patient's bronchioles, reducing airway resistance and increasing the patient's ability to exchange oxygen and carbon dioxide.

(a) alpha agonist bronchoconstriction
(b) beta agonist bronchodilator
(c) alpha antagonist bronchodilator
(d) beta antagonist bronchoconstriction
(e) alpha agonist bronchodilator

36. Anticipated side effects of prescribed respiratory inhaler medication administration include

(a) increased pulse rate.
(b) tremors.
(c) nervousness.
(d) Answers (a) and (c) only.
(e) Answers (a), (b), and (c).

37. After assisting the patient with self-administration of a prescribed respiratory inhaler medication, the EMT should

  (a) gather additional sets of vital signs and repeat a focused assessment.
  (b) anticipate the potential for deterioration of the patient's condition in spite of the medication administration, and be prepared to perform positive pressure artificial ventilation.
  (c) continue high-flow oxygenation of the patient.
  (d) Answers (a) and (c) only.
  (e) Answers (a), (b), and (c).

38. Which of the following illnesses are classified as chronic obstructive pulmonary disease (COPD)?

  (a) Emphysema.
  (b) Chronic bronchitis.
  (c) Asthma.
  (d) Answers (a) and (b) only.
  (e) Answers (a), (b), and (c).

39. Which of the following illnesses affect the patient episodically (at irregular intervals) only?

  (a) Emphysema.
  (b) Chronic bronchitis.
  (c) Asthma.
  (d) All of the above.
  (e) None of the above.

The following six (6) questions pertain to a single important subject regarding the physiology of breathing and the administration of oxygen to the prehospital emergency patient.

40. Normally, the body's stimulus to breathe is based on the level of _____ in the blood.

  (a) carbon monoxide
  (b) carbon dioxide
  (c) oxygen
  (d) Both answers (a) and (b).
  (e) Both answers (a) and (c).

41. Patients with chronic obstructive pulmonary diseases chronically have increased levels of _____ in their blood.

  (a) carbon monoxide
  (b) carbon dioxide
  (c) oxygen
  (d) Both answers (a) and (b).
  (e) Both answers (a) and (c).

42. Because of this chronic abnormality, the bodies of patients with chronic obstructive pulmonary disease develop a stimulus to breathe based on the level of _____ in the blood.

    (a) carbon monoxide
    (b) carbon dioxide
    (c) oxygen
    (d) Both answers (a) and (b).
    (e) Both answers (a) and (c).

43. The development of this abnormal stimulus to breathe creates the abnormal condition known as

    (a) hypoxic drive.
    (b) carbon dioxide drive.
    (c) oxygen drive.
    (d) anoxia drive.
    (e) carbon monoxide drive.

44. This abnormal condition once was considered to be _____ the administration of high concentrations of oxygen (oxygen by nonrebreather mask).

    (a) a contraindication to
    (b) an indication for
    (c) a side effect of
    (d) Any of the above.
    (e) None of the above.

45. Now, however, it is widely believed that this condition is

    (a) not a valid contraindication to the administration of high concentrations of oxygen in the prehospital setting.
    (b) an even greater contraindication to the administration of high concentrations of oxygen in the prehospital setting than previously suspected, due to its encouragement of respiratory depression or arrest.
    (c) an even greater indication for the administration of high concentrations of oxygen in the prehospital setting than previously suspected.
    (d) a more prevalent side effect of the administration of high concentrations of oxygen in the prehospital setting.
    (e) None of the above.

46. A respiratory disease that primarily restricts bronchial airflow on exhalation is

    (a) emphysema.
    (b) chronic bronchitis.

(c) asthma.
(d) Both answers (a) and (b).
(e) Answers (a), (b), and (c).

47. _____ is a disease that mainly affects middle-aged and older patients, rarely affecting children and teenagers.

(a) Emphysema
(b) Chronic bronchitis
(c) Asthma
(d) Both answers (a) and (b).
(e) Answers (a), (b), and (c).

48. Inflammation of the bronchioles with development of excess mucus is a primary aspect of the respiratory disease _____. Normally, the cilia (fine hairs) along the interior lining of the bronchioles are able to "sweep" away this excess mucus. However, when the patient develops this disease, the cilia are damaged or destroyed and become unable to perform their sweeping, airway-clearing job.

(a) emphysema
(b) chronic bronchitis
(c) asthma
(d) Either answer (a) or (b).
(e) Either answer (b) or (c).

49. Breakdown of the alveolar wall surface is a primary aspect of the respiratory disease _____. When this occurs, the functional surface area of the alveoli (where gas exchange occurs) is greatly diminished. Also, the lungs begin to lose their elasticity and excessive mucus is secreted in both the alveoli and bronchioles (further reducing the ability to exchange air). The combination of these factors contributes to "trapped" air within the lungs, with progressive reduction in normal breathing effectiveness.

(a) emphysema
(b) chronic bronchitis
(c) asthma
(d) Either answer (a) or (b).
(e) Either answer (b) or (c).

50. COPD patients are rarely "purists." Often, a COPD patient will exhibit signs and symptoms of

(a) emphysema.
(b) chronic bronchitis.
(c) asthma.
(d) Both answers (a) and (b).
(e) Both answers (b) and (c).

51. The respiratory disease _____ often is triggered by inhalation, ingestion, or injection of a substance the patient is allergic to (such as air pollutants, foods, or insect stings).

   (a) emphysema
   (b) chronic bronchitis
   (c) asthma
   (d) Both answers (a) and (b).
   (e) Both answers (b) and (c).

52. An accurate identification of the *specific* respiratory disease the patient is suffering from is

   (a) essential to all prehospital care procedures.
   (b) essential to all prehospital care oxygen administration decisions.
   (c) essential to all prehospital medication administration decisions.
   (d) essential to all prehospital transportation and hospital destination decisions.
   (e) relatively unessential. Prehospital care and transportation decisions are based on the immediate needs of each particular patient, during each individual emergency, and not upon the specific identification of the patient's current disease or diagnosis.

53. The right atrium receives blood from the _____ and directs (pumps) blood flow to the _____.

   (a) body and heart / left ventricle
   (b) lower extremities / upper extremities
   (c) pulmonary veins (the lungs) / left ventricle
   (d) body and heart / right ventricle
   (e) upper extremities / lower extremities

54. The left atrium receives blood from the _____ and directs (pumps) blood flow to the _____.

   (a) body and heart / left ventricle
   (b) lower extremities / upper extremities
   (c) pulmonary veins (the lungs) / left ventricle
   (d) body and heart / right ventricle
   (e) upper extremities / lower extremities

55. The left ventricle directs (pumps) blood flow to the

   (a) body, via the aorta.
   (b) lungs, via the pulmonary arteries.
   (c) lungs, via the pulmonary veins.
   (d) right ventricle.
   (e) right atrium.

56. The right ventricle directs (pumps) blood flow to the

    (a) body, via the aorta.
    (b) lungs, via the pulmonary arteries.
    (c) lungs, via the pulmonary veins.
    (d) left ventricle.
    (e) left atrium.

57. The valves within the circulatory system (including the cardiac valves) serve to

    (a) pump blood forward.
    (b) pump blood upward.
    (c) propel blood backward.
    (d) stop blood from flowing forward.
    (e) prevent the backflow of blood.

58. Which of the following statements regarding the cardiac conductive system is true?

    (a) The heart is composed of specialized contractile tissue.
    (b) The heart contains specialized electrical impulse conduction tissue.
    (c) Specialized areas of the heart are able to generate their own electrical impulses.
    (d) Only answers (a) and (b) are true.
    (e) Answers (a), (b), and (c) are true.

59. The medical abbreviation (initials) **ACLS** stands for

    (a) Always C-spine and Lay (the patient) Supine.
    (b) Advanced Controlled Lung Support (tracheal intubation with positive pressure ventilation).
    (c) Advanced Cardiac Life Support.
    (d) Alpha, Charly, Lima, Sierra.
    (e) Anxiousness, Clammy skin, Low (blood pressure), Sweating (the cardinal signs of shock).

60. The medical abbreviation (initials) **CHF** stands for

    (a) Cardiac Heart Function.
    (b) Compromised Heart Function.
    (c) Coronary Heart Failure.
    (d) Complex Heart Fluctuation (another term for irregular heartbeat).
    (e) Congestive Heart Failure.

61. The medical abbreviation (initials) **CAD** stands for

   (a) Carotid Artery Dysfunction.
   (b) Coronary Artery Disease.
   (c) Chronic Atherosclerosis Disease.
   (d) Congestive Artery Disease.
   (e) Complex Arterial Dysfunction.

62. The condition _____ results from the buildup of fatty deposits on the inner walls of blood vessels.

   (a) angioplasty
   (b) ascites
   (c) asystole
   (d) atherosclerosis
   (e) arterial stenography

63. The condition _____ results from the buildup of fat and calcium deposits on the inner walls of ateries, causing them to become hard and unable to dilate or constrict well.

   (a) arteriosclerosis
   (b) angiography
   (c) asystole
   (d) atherosclerosis
   (e) arterial petrification

64. When a section of the wall of an artery becomes weakened, the layers of the wall may split, becoming ballooned with blood. This condition is called

   (a) an aortic bypass.
   (b) an embolism.
   (c) an aneurysm.
   (d) a cardiac bypass.
   (e) grafting.

65. A blood clot (sometimes including plaque) that becomes attached to the inner wall of an artery, obstructing some or all of the blood flow, is called a

   (a) coronary impasse.
   (b) hemobolus.
   (c) hemocoagulant.
   (d) hemo-obstruction.
   (e) thrombus.

66. An object composed of clotted blood, fat, and/or plaque that breaks loose from the wall of an artery and travels the circulatory system is called

   (a) a thrombophlebitis.
   (b) an aneurysm.
   (c) an embolism.
   (d) a coronary.
   (e) an arterial shunt.

67. The term _____ is often used when referring to obstruction of blood flow through an artery or a blockage of a blood vessel.

   (a) occlusion
   (b) aneurysm
   (c) coronary
   (d) asystole
   (e) arrhythmia

68. The phrase **cardiac compromise** may be used to describe

   (a) only those patients who are in congestive heart failure.
   (b) only those patients who have low blood pressure.
   (c) only those patients who have irregular heartbeats.
   (d) only those patients who complain of chest pain and shortness of breath.
   (e) any patient with signs and symptoms of any heart problem.

69. The condition called **cardiac compromise** may be indicated by the patient's complaint or physical signs of

   (a) dull and/or squeezing pressure in the chest.
   (b) chest pain radiating down the arms or into the jaw.
   (c) a sudden onset of sweating.
   (d) Answers (a) and/or (b) only.
   (e) Answers (a), (b), and/or (c).

70. The condition called **cardiac compromise** may be indicated by the patient's complaint or physical signs of

   (a) difficulty breathing (dyspnea).
   (b) anxiety, irritability, and an altered level of consciousness.
   (c) a feeling of impending doom.
   (d) Answers (a) and/or (b) only.
   (e) Answers (a), (b), and/or (c).

71. The condition called **cardiac compromise** may be indicated by the patient's complaint or physical signs of any of the following, except

    (a) an abnormal pulse rate (which may or may not be irregular).
    (b) an abnormal blood pressure.
    (c) epigastric pain.
    (d) an abnormal feeling of peacefulness or euphoria.
    (e) nausea, with or without vomiting.

72. The literal translation of the medical phrase **angina pectoris** is

    (a) heart palpitations.
    (b) heart pain.
    (c) pain in the chest.
    (d) a heart attack.
    (e) agony of the heart.

73. When heart tissue is deprived of oxygen, the most frequent result is an episode of angina pectoris (angina). Angina is caused by the

    (a) narrowing and/or obstruction of coronary arteries.
    (b) increased cardiac workload that accompanies stress, when the patient has coronary artery disease.
    (c) increased cardiac workload that accompanies physical exertion, when the patient has coronary artery disease.
    (d) Answers (a) and/or (c) only.
    (e) Answers (a), (b), and/or (c).

74. Which of the following statements regarding angina is true?

    (a) Since a cause of angina is physical exertion, rest often relieves the pain.
    (b) Normal attacks of angina usually last two to four hours.
    (c) Patients with a previous history of angina often are prescribed nitroglycerin to take when an attack occurs.
    (d) Only answers (a) and (c) are true.
    (e) Answers (a), (b), and (c) are true.

75. Nitroglycerin dilates coronary arteries, increasing oxygenated blood flow to injured or obstructed areas of the heart. This often relieves or decreases angina. Nitroglycerin further reduces or relieves angina by dilating the body's blood vessels, which

    (a) decreases the amount of blood the heart must pump.
    (b) increases the amount of blood the heart must pump.
    (c) decreases the amount of oxygen required by the heart muscle.
    (d) Both answers (a) and (c).
    (e) Both answers (b) and (c).

TEST SECTION FOUR

76. Which of the following statements regarding nitroglycerin is true?
    (a) Nitroglycerin comes in tablet or spray form and is placed under the patient's tongue, where it is absorbed.
    (b) Nitroglycerin comes in patches that stick to the patient's skin, slowly releasing nitroglycerin throughout the day.
    (c) Nitroglycerin is available in capsule form that the patient breaks open with his teeth before swallowing it to achieve the maximum benefit.
    (d) Both answers (a) and (b) are true.
    (e) Answers (a), (b), and (c) are true.

77. Acute myocardial infarction (AMI) may occur when
    (a) a portion of the heart dies from lack of oxygen.
    (b) the narrowing or obstruction of a coronary artery prevents enough oxygenated blood from reaching an area of heart tissue.
    (c) a coronary artery ruptures.
    (d) Answers (a) and/or (b) only.
    (e) Answers (a), (b), and/or (c).

78. The majority of sudden death incidents occur outside of the hospital. Which of the following situations may be considered a definition of **sudden death**?
    (a) A cardiac arrest without any preceding signs and symptoms.
    (b) A person with no history of heart problems who goes into cardiac arrest within one hour of developing AMI signs and symptoms.
    (c) A person with no history of heart problems who goes into cardiac arrest within two hours of developing AMI signs and symptoms.
    (d) Answers (a) and/or (b) only.
    (e) Answers (a), (b), and/or (c).

79. Cardiac arrest may result from CAD or an acute respiratory problem. Additional causes of cardiac arrest include
    (a) high levels of emotional stress.
    (b) COPD.
    (c) unusual exertion.
    (d) Answers (b) and/or (c) only.
    (e) Answers (a), (b), and/or (c).

80. Since clot obstruction of a coronary artery is a frequent cause of AMI, _____ medications have been developed. The nickname for these medications is "clot busters," because they dissolve clots.
    (a) hemodialysis
    (b) prohemorrhage
    (c) thrombolytic
    (d) blood-thinning
    (e) anticlot

81. The medical term **edema** is best defined as
    (a) the accumulation of fluid in the legs or lungs.
    (b) the "goose-egg" swelling caused by blunt injury.
    (c) a localized or general accumulation of excessive fluid within body tissues.
    (d) a localized or general accumulation of excessive blood within body tissues.
    (e) None of the above define the term **edema.**

82. Edema that occurs in the feet and/or ankles is called
    (a) orthopedic edema.
    (b) pedal edema.
    (c) pediatric edema.
    (d) gout.
    (e) pregnancy edema.

83. Edema that occurs in the abdomen is called
    (a) obesity.
    (b) abdominal rigidity (or a "hot abdomen").
    (c) ascites.
    (d) peritonitis.
    (e) None of the above; edema does not occur in the abdomen.

84. Edema that occurs in the lungs is called
    (a) pulmonary edema.
    (b) pleurisy.
    (c) COPD.
    (d) peripheral edema.
    (e) pneumonia.

85. CHF is a condition that can result in edema of
    (a) the feet and/or ankles.
    (b) the lungs.
    (c) a variety of body organs or parts.
    (d) Answers (a) and/or (b) only.
    (e) Answers (a), (b), and/or (c).

86. Which of the following statements regarding CHF is false?

 (a) One of the primary signs and symptoms is nasal congestion (hence, the term "congestive").
 (b) CHF may result from lung function failure.
 (c) Lung function failure may be caused by CHF.
 (d) CHF may result from heart function failure.
 (e) Heart function failure may be caused by CHF.

87. The medical term **diuretic** is best defined as an agent that

 (a) decreases the secretion of urine, retaining the body's fluid volume.
 (b) normalizes the body's fluid volume. (If the patient is hypovolemic, the agent acts to retain fluid, decreasing urine output. If the patient has too much body fluid, the agent encourages the secretion of urine.)
 (c) increases the secretion of urine, decreasing the body's fluid volume.
 (d) Either answer (a) or (b), depending on the type of diuretic.
 (e) None of the above define the term **diuretic**.

88. After an initial assessment and the focused history and physical exam are performed, the patient with cardiac compromise should be placed in a position of comfort. Which of the following statements regarding the cardiac compromise position of comfort is false?

 (a) Especially for patients with shortness of breath or dyspnea, the cardiac compromise position of comfort most often will be sitting up.
 (b) The vast majority of cardiac compromise patients prefer to lay flat (supine) with their feet elevated eight to ten inches. This "shock" positioning reduces the workload of the heart (immediately relieving or diminishing chest pain) and especially relieves or diminishes shortness of breath.
 (c) Hypotensive cardiac compromise patients (those with a systolic blood pressure less than 90 mmHg) may feel dizzy or become confused when sitting up. These patients may feel better lying down (supine).
 (d) If the cardiac compromise patient is hypotensive and complains of shortness of breath, a position of comfort may be difficult to find.
 (e) None of the above are false.

89. For a patient with signs and symptoms of cardiac compromise, oxygen should be administered by a

(a) nasal cannula, at 2 liters per minute.
(b) nasal cannula, at 8 liters per minute.
(c) nonrebreather mask, at 12 to 15 liters per minute.
(d) nonrebreather mask, at 12 to 15 liters per minute (unless the patient has a history of COPD; then oxygen should be administered by a nasal cannula at only 2 or 3 liters per minute to avoid respiratory arrest).
(e) a nonrebreather mask, at 6 to 10 liters per minute.

90. Patients with cardiac compromise may benefit from the administration of nitroglycerin (NTG). Which of the following conditions **must** be met before an EMT-B may assist the patient with taking NTG?

1. Chest pain must be one of the patient's complaints.
2. Either the patient's own nitroglycerin **or** a friend or family member's nitroglycerin must be present.
3. Shortness of breath must be one of the patient's chief complaints.
4. The EMT must have on-line or off-line authorization from the medical director to assist the patient with nitroglycerin administration.
5. The nitroglycerin must already be prescribed by the patient's private physician.
6. The patient must be alert.
7. The patient must have her/his own nitroglycerin with her/him.
8. The patient's diastolic blood pressure must be greater than 100 mmHg.
9. The patient's systolic blood pressure must be greater than 90 mmHg.
10. The patient's systolic blood pressure must be less than 100 mmHg.

(a) Conditions 1, 2, 3, 4, 5, and 6 must be met.
(b) Conditions 1, 4, 5, 6, and 7 must be met.
(c) Conditions 2, 3, 4, and 8 must be met.
(d) Conditions 1, 3, 4, 5, 6, 7, and 9 must be met.
(e) Conditions 1, 3, 4, 5, 6, 7, and 10 must be met.

91. Contraindications to nitroglycerin administration include

(a) hypotension or systolic blood pressure less than 100 mmHg.
(b) signs and symptoms of head injury.

(c) when the patient already has taken the maximum number of prescribed doses.
(d) Answers (a) and (c) only.
(e) Answers (a), (b), and (c).

92. More than one dose of nitroglycerin may be required to alleviate chest pain. Which of the following conditions **must** be met before an EMT-B may assist the patient with taking **another** dose of NTG?

   1. A period of 3 to 5 minutes must have passed without the patient receiving relief.
   2. Authorization for additional assisted NTG administrations must be obtained.
   3. Some relief must have been obtained from the first assisted dose (proving that the medication is having an effect on the patient).
   4. The maximum number of NTG doses must not have been administered.
   5. The patient must be alert.
   6. The patient must continue to complain of shortness of breath (alleviation of dyspnea indicates that the nitroglycerin has reached its maximum effectiveness, and no further doses are indicated).
   7. The patient must specifically request an additional dose of NTG (the EMT-B **may not** suggest it).
   8. The patient's systolic blood pressure must be above 100 mmHg.

   (a) Conditions 2, 3, 4, 6, and 7 must be met.
   (b) Conditions 1, 3, 5, 6, and 8 must be met.
   (c) Conditions 1, 2, 3, 4, 5, 6, 7, and 8 must be met.
   (d) Conditions 1, 2, 4, 5, and 8 must be met.
   (e) Conditions 1, 2, 3, and 8 must be met.

93. Side effects of nitroglycerin administration may include all of the following, except

   (a) hypotension (nitroglycerin lowers blood pressure).
   (b) headache.
   (c) increased pulse rate.
   (d) hypertension (decreased workload often seriously increases cardiac output).
   (e) decreased pulse rate.

94. Which of the following statements regarding reassessment of the patient's blood pressure after nitroglycerin administration is true?

    (a) Recheck the patient's blood pressure within 2 minutes of NTG administration.
    (b) Because NTG is a strong and fast-acting medication, the patient's blood pressure should be rechecked every 30 seconds for the first 5 minutes following administration (leave the blood pressure cuff on the patient's arm).
    (c) The patient's system must become adjusted to the effects of NTG. Wait at least 5 minutes following administration before rechecking the patient's blood pressure (readings taken earlier will be falsely low).
    (d) Every system rechecks blood pressures at different times. There is no set standard for the timing of blood pressure rechecks when administering NTG.
    (e) None of the above are true.

95. Which of the following statements regarding cardiac arrest is false?

    (a) The vast majority of chest-pain patients will deteriorate into cardiac arrest. Be prepared to start CPR.
    (b) The earlier the EMS system is activated, the more likely it is that the patient will survive cardiac arrest.
    (c) The earlier CPR is started, the more likely it is that the patient will survive cardiac arrest.
    (d) The most important factor in improving chances of survival from cardiac arrest is early defibrillation (within 8 minutes following cardiac arrest).
    (e) Early ALS performance improves the likelihood of cardiac arrest survival.

96. There are two types of automated external defibrillators (AEDs). _____ operate(s) without action by the EMT (except to turn on the power and place the monitor-defibrillation pads on the patient).

    (a) The fully automated defibrillator
    (b) The incompletely automated defibrillator
    (c) The semiautomated defibrillator
    (d) Both the fully automated defibrillator and the semiautomated defibrillator
    (e) Both the fully automated defibrillator and the incompletely automated defibrillator

97. _____ use(s) three monitor-defibrillation pads to sense the electrical activity of the patient's heart and/or to deliver an electrical shock.

   (a) The fully automated defibrillator
   (b) The incompletely automated defibrillator
   (c) The semiautomated defibrillator
   (d) Neither the fully automated defibrillator nor the semiautomated defibrillator
   (e) Both the fully automated defibrillator and the incompletely automated defibrillator

98. _____ use(s) two monitor-defibrillation pads to sense the electrical activity of the patient's heart and/or to deliver an electrical shock.

   (a) The fully automated defibrillator
   (b) The incompletely automated defibrillator
   (c) The semiautomated defibrillator
   (d) Both the fully automated defibrillator and the semiautomated defibrillator
   (e) Both the fully automated defibrillator and the incompletely automated defibrillator

99. _____ has (have) a computer microprocessor that evaluates the patient's electrical rhythm and determines what action should be taken (to shock or not to shock).

   (a) The fully automated defibrillator
   (b) The incompletely automated defibrillator
   (c) The semiautomated defibrillator
   (d) Both the fully automated defibrillator and the semiautomated defibrillator
   (e) Both the fully automated defibrillator and the incompletely automated defibrillator

100. _____ use(s) a computer voice synthesizer to advise the EMT whether or not to press the button for a shock delivery, based on its (their) analysis of the patient's cardiac rhythm.

   (a) The fully automated defibrillator
   (b) The incompletely automated defibrillator
   (c) The semiautomated defibrillator
   (d) Both the fully automated defibrillator and the semiautomated defibrillator
   (e) Both the fully automated defibrillator and the incompletely automated defibrillator

101. Based on its analysis of the patient's cardiac rhythm, _____ deliver(s) an electrical shock without any assistance from the EMT.

(a) the fully automated defibrillator
(b) the incompletely automated defibrillator
(c) the semiautomated defibrillator
(d) neither the fully automated defibrillator nor the semiautomated defibrillator
(e) both the fully automated defibrillator and the incompletely automated defibrillator

102. AEDs have been researched extensively and found to have a

(a) high degree of accuracy in the ability to detect rhythms requiring electrical shock.
(b) low degree of accuracy in the ability to detect rhythms that should not be shocked.
(c) high degree of accuracy in the ability to detect rhythms that should not be shocked.
(d) Both answers (a) and (b).
(e) Both answers (a) and (c).

103. Although mechanical error is always possible, research has found that the most frequent cause of an inappropriate shock delivered by the AED is human error. AED-related human errors that may contribute to the delivery of an inappropriate shock include all of the following, except

(a) application of the AED when the patient has a radial pulse but does not have any respiratory effort.
(b) inaccurate placement of the third monitor-defibrillation pad.
(c) application of the AED when the patient has respiratory effort but does not have a radial pulse.
(d) improper AED operation.
(e) improper AED maintenance.

104. Completely disorganized and chaotic electrical activity best describes the cardiac rhythm called

(a) ventricular tachycardia.
(b) ventricular fibrillation.
(c) asystole.
(d) Both answers (a) and (b).
(e) Both answers (a) and (c).

105. The absence of electrical activity (sometimes called "flatline") best describes the cardiac rhythm called

   (a) ventricular tachycardia.
   (b) ventricular fibrillation.
   (c) asystole.
   (d) Either answer (a) or (b).
   (e) Either answer (a) or (c).

106. The cardiac rhythm _____ can be described as the presence of organized electrical activity that shows unusually wide and very rapid complexes.

   (a) ventricular tachycardia
   (b) ventricular fibrillation
   (c) asystole
   (d) Either answer (a) or (b).
   (e) Either answer (a) or (c).

107. The cardiac rhythm _____ is always an indication for delivery of an electrical shock.

   (a) ventricular tachycardia
   (b) ventricular fibrillation
   (c) asystole
   (d) Both answers (a) and (b).
   (e) Both answers (a) and (c).

108. The cardiac rhythm _____ is a rhythm that never should be shocked.

   (a) ventricular tachycardia
   (b) ventricular fibrillation
   (c) asystole
   (d) Both answers (a) and (b).
   (e) Both answers (a) and (c).

109. The cardiac rhythm _____ should be shocked only when the patient is not breathing and has no carotid pulse.

   (a) ventricular tachycardia
   (b) ventricular fibrillation
   (c) asystole
   (d) Either answer (a) or (b).
   (e) Either answer (a) or (c).

110. The cardiac rhythm called ***pulseless electrical activity*** (PEA) is best described as

    (a) any cardiac rhythm with or without a pulse.
    (b) ventricular tachycardia, with a pulse.
    (c) any organized, coordinated (usually slow) cardiac rhythm that generates no pulse.
    (d) any cardiac electrical activity without a pulse.
    (e) ventricular fibrillation, with a pulse.

111. If EMS responders arrive within 8 minutes of the patient's cardiac arrest, 50 to 60 percent of the time the patient will be in

    (a) ventricular tachycardia.
    (b) ventricular fibrillation.
    (c) asystole.
    (d) Either answer (a) or (b).
    (e) Either answer (a) or (c).

112. A patient in the cardiac rhythm _____ may have a pulse.

    (a) ventricular tachycardia
    (b) ventricular fibrillation
    (c) asystole
    (d) Any of the above.
    (e) None of the above (patients in these rhythms never have a pulse).

113. The most important rule to remember when considering the application of any AED model type is that

    (a) every medical patient should have an AED applied for cardiac rhythm diagnosis.
    (b) any unconscious patient should have an AED applied for cardiac rhythm diagnosis.
    (c) any nonbreathing patient should have an AED applied for cardiac rhythm diagnosis.
    (d) any patient with no palpable radial pulse should have an AED applied for cardiac rhythm diagnosis.
    (e) only unresponsive, nonbreathing, pulseless patients should have an AED applied for cardiac rhythm diagnosis.

114. Which of the following statements regarding AED use and interruption of CPR is false?

    (a) No CPR should be performed at the time a shock is delivered.
    (b) No person should be touching the patient at the time the patient's rhythm is being analyzed by the AED.

(c) No person should be touching the patient (or touching any devices that are in contact with the patient, such as a bag-valve-mask) at the time a shock is delivered by the AED.
(d) Chest compressions and artificial ventilations must be discontinued when the patient's rhythm is being analyzed by the AED.
(e) None of the above are false.

115. Which of the following statements regarding AED use and interruption of CPR is false?
    (a) Chest compressions and artificial ventilations must be discontinued when shocks are delivered by the AED.
    (b) Defibrillation is less effective than correctly performed CPR. Thus, application of the AED should be delayed until at least 5 minutes of CPR has been performed.
    (c) CPR may be stopped for up to 90 seconds if the delivery of 3 shocks is necessary.
    (d) Defibrillation is more effective than correctly performed CPR. Thus, stopping CPR during the process of AED analysis and shock delivery is not detrimental to the patient's outcome.
    (e) Resume CPR only after the first 3 shocks have been delivered (without success).

116. If no on-scene ALS is available, the patient should be transported when which of the following occurs?
    (a) The patient regains a pulse.
    (b) After 6 shocks have been administered.
    (c) After the AED has given 3 consecutive messages (separated by one minute of CPR) that no shock is advised.
    (d) Answers (a) and/or (b) only.
    (e) Answers (a), (b), and/or (c).

117. When the patient is apneic (not breathing) and pulseless, which of the following statements regarding defibrillation (administration of electrical shock) is true?
    (a) When only two EMTs are present, one operates the AED defibrillator and one does CPR.
    (b) Defibrillation comes first. The EMT should not administer oxygen or do anything else that may delay analysis of the patient's rhythm or administration of defibrillation.
    (c) All contact with the patient must be avoided during analysis of the cardiac rhythm, and the statement "Clear the patient" must be announced before delivering shocks.
    (d) Only answers (a) and (c) are true.
    (e) Answers (a), (b), and (c) are true.

118. Which of the following statements regarding age and weight considerations regarding the application of an AED is true?

  (a) There are no age and/or weight contraindications to the application of an AED when a patient is apneic and pulseless.
  (b) Patients less than 12 years old should not have an AED applied, even when they are apneic and pulseless.
  (c) Patients weighing less than 90 pounds should not have an AED applied, even when they are apneic and pulseless.
  (d) Both answers (b) and (c) are true.
  (e) None of the above are true.

119. Some AEDs have built-in voice recorders. These voice recorders are designed to

  (a) catch EMTs making mistakes so that they may be reprimanded.
  (b) assist in documentation of call activities.
  (c) represent the EMT's actions in a court of law, so that the EMT will not have to appear (a recorded "deposition").
  (d) Answers (a) and (c) only.
  (e) Answers (a), (b), and (c).

120. If your AED has a voice recorder, you should begin speaking to it

  (a) en route to the call; providing the call number, responding unit number, names of responding crew, and so on.
  (b) after the call is over (before you have forgotten the circumstances and activities).
  (c) after turning on the AED's power button.
  (d) after turning off the AED's power button (the voice recorder comes on automatically after AED use is terminated).
  (e) never. The voice recorder should never be specifically addressed, as this would distract the EMT from performing assessments and treatments.

121. After baring the patient's chest, the AED pad that attaches to the white cable should be placed

  (a) over the lower left area of the patient's chest (on the ribs).
  (b) just beneath the right clavicle, to the right of the patient's sternum.
  (c) over the lower right area of the patient's chest (on the ribs).
  (d) just beneath the left clavicle, to the left of the patient's sternum.
  (e) on the lower third of the patient's sternum (this pad also serves as a chest compression marker for CPR).

122. The AED pad that attaches to the red cable should be placed

    (a) over the lower left area of the patient's chest (on the ribs).
    (b) just beneath the right clavicle, to the right of the patient's sternum.
    (c) over the lower right area of the patient's chest (on the ribs).
    (d) just beneath the left clavicle, to the left of the patient's sternum.
    (e) on the lower third of the patient's sternum (this pad also serves as a chest compression marker for CPR).

123. The third AED pad should be placed

    (a) on the patient's back (this acts as a "grounding" pad).
    (b) just beneath the left clavicle, to the left of the patient's sternum.
    (c) over the lower right area of the patient's chest (on the ribs).
    (d) on the lower third of the patient's sternum (this pad also serves as a chest compression marker for CPR).
    (e) nowhere. AEDs do not have a third pad or cable.

124. A handy phrase to help the EMT remember the correct placement of the colored cables attached to AED pads is

    (a) "when red is right, what's left is white."
    (b) "when red is right, what's left is white, and third goes down to ground."
    (c) "white to right, red to ribs."
    (d) "white to right, red to ribs, and third goes down to ground."
    (e) not recommended. EMTs should be able to remember where to place the pads without any assistance, and if they cannot remember, they can read the directions that come with the AED.

AUTHORS' NOTE: Questions 125 and 127 will require an unusual amount of time to answer. If you are timing your test performance, stop timing now. These questions are much too long and involved to be used on an actual test. However, "normal-sized" questions regarding any of these questions' steps (and their correct order of performance) may appear on an actual test.

AUTHORS' TIP: Rather than trying to sort through all the steps provided (19 steps in question 125!), just read through them first. Then, on lined paper, write out the correct sequence of AED operation as you remember it (without using the provided steps). Write one performance activity on each line, leaving a margin on the left side of your paper. Now look at the steps provided in this text. Find the step that most closely corresponds to each of your performance activities, and put that step's number in the margin to the left of each line. When you are done, compare the numbered sequence of your performance activities to the available answers.

125. Place the following AED steps in their correct order of performance. *All steps should be used at least once. Some steps should be used more than once.*

1. "Clear" the patient.
2. Attach the AED pads and cables.
3. Begin or resume CPR.
4. Check for a carotid pulse.
5. If patient does not have a pulse, resume CPR for 1 minute.
6. If patient does not have a pulse, resume CPR and transport.
7. If the AED has a voice recorder, begin speaking to it now.
8. If the machine advises "Deliver shock," deliver the first shock.
9. If the machine advises "Deliver shock," deliver a second shock.
10. If the machine advises "Deliver shock," deliver a third shock.
11. If the machine advises "Deliver shock," deliver a fourth shock.
12. If the machine advises "Deliver shock," deliver a fifth shock.
13. If the machine advises "Deliver shock," deliver a sixth shock.
14. If the patient qualifies for AED application, turn on the defibrillator power.
15. Press the analysis button to re-analyze the rhythm.
16. Press the analysis button.
17. Stop CPR if in progress prior to your arrival.
18. Stop CPR.
19. Verify that the patient is not breathing and has no pulse.

(a) 17, 19, 3, 14, 7, 2, 18, 1, 16, 8, 15, 9, 15, 10, 15, 4, 5, 18, 1, 16, 11, 15, 12, 15, 13, 15, 4, 6
(b) 7, 17, 19, 3, 14, 2, 16, 8, 15, 9, 15, 10, 15, 4, 5, 16, 11, 15, 12, 15, 13, 15, 4, 6, 18, 1
(c) 17, 19, 3, 14, 2, 18, 1, 16, 8, 15, 9, 15, 10, 15, 11, 15, 12, 15, 13, 15, 4, 5, 4, 6, 7
(d) Both answers (a) and (b) show possibly correct sequences.
(e) Both answers (a) and (c) show possibly correct sequences.

126. ____ shocks may be delivered without pulse checks or CPR between them, followed by a pulse check and/or one minute of CPR performance before shocking again.

(a) Two
(b) Three
(c) Five
(d) Six
(e) None of the above. Only one shock should be delivered at a time, and a pulse check and/or one minute of CPR should be performed between each shock.

TEST SECTION FOUR

127. You (and the EMT driving) are transporting a conscious patient who has been having chest pain unrelieved by oxygen or the maximum dose of nitroglycerin. Suddenly your patient becomes unconscious. You evaluate the patient and discover that he has stopped breathing and has no pulse. Using **some or all** of the following steps, indicate the correct order of care performance. ***None of the following steps should be repeated.***

   1. Analyze the patient's rhythm.
   2. Continue transportation, providing AED application and/or CPR en route.
   3. Deliver up to 2 **stacked shocks** (shocks delivered without pulse checks or CPR between them), if indicated.
   4. Deliver up to 3 **stacked shocks** (shocks delivered without pulse checks or CPR between them), if indicated.
   5. Deliver up to 5 **stacked shocks** (shocks delivered without pulse checks or CPR between them), if indicated.
   6. Deliver up to 6 **stacked shocks** (shocks delivered without pulse checks or CPR between them), if indicated.
   7. If indicated, deliver only one shock, followed by a pulse check and/or 1 minute of CPR.
   8. Provide additional resuscitation efforts as per protocol.
   9. Start CPR if the AED is not immediately available.
   10. Stop CPR and "clear" the patient.
   11. Stop the vehicle.

   (a) 2, 9, 10, 1, 4, 8.
   (b) 2, 9, 1, 6, 8.
   (c) 9, 10, 1, 4, 8.
   (d) 11, 9, 1, 10, 4, 8.
   (e) 2, 9, 10, 1, 5, 8.

AUTHORS' NOTE: Now that you have finished question number 127, reward yourself with a break! Resume timing your performance when you continue with question number 128.

128. A fully automatic defibrillator will deliver different amounts of energy for different shocks. 360 joules of energy are delivered for the

   (a) first shock.
   (b) second shock (in a row).
   (c) third shock (in a row).
   (d) fourth shock (in a row).
   (e) fifth shock (in a row).

129. A fully automatic defibrillator will deliver 200 to 300 joules of energy for the

   (a) first shock.
   (b) second shock (in a row).
   (c) third shock (in a row).
   (d) fourth shock (in a row).
   (e) fifth shock (in a row).

130. A fully automatic defibrillator will deliver 200 joules of energy for the

   (a) first shock.
   (b) second shock (in a row).
   (c) third shock (in a row).
   (d) fourth shock (in a row).
   (e) fifth shock (in a row).

131. When the AED provides a "no shock" message after an analysis, the EMT should

   (a) call medical control to pronounce the patient "DOA" (dead on arrival).
   (b) immediately resume CPR.
   (c) check the patient's pulse and breathing.
   (d) immediately have CPR resumed by others while calling medical control to pronounce the patient "DOA" (dead on arrival).
   (e) do none of the above. The AED always will shock the patient.

132. Which of the following statements regarding coordination of ALS personnel (EMT-Intermediates or Paramedics) is false?

   (a) ALS should be summoned and notified of cardiac arrest events as soon as possible.
   (b) The use of an AED does not require the presence of ALS personnel on scene.
   (c) BLS personnel should never transport a cardiac arrest patient prior to the arrival of ALS personnel on the scene, for any reason.
   (d) All of the above are false.
   (e) None of the above are false.

133. Which of the following statements regarding the safe use of an AED and the administration of electric shock (defibrillation) to a patient is true?

    (a) It is not safe to defibrillate with an AED in a moving ambulance.

    (b) When the AED defibrillates a patient, it delivers an electrical shock that travels a straight line between the pads with red and white cables attached. As long as no responders are actually touching these pads (or the space between them), no harm will come to a person in contact with the patient during defibrillation.

    (c) Even if the patient receiving defibrillation is lying in a pool of water or on a metal surface, as long as no responders are actually touching the pads (or the space between them), no harm will come to a person in contact with the patient during defibrillation.

    (d) Both answers (b) and (c) are true.

    (e) None of the above are true.

134. Artificial cardiac pacemakers are implanted in patients whose natural pacemaker no longer functions appropriately. Which of the following statements regarding implanted artificial pacemakers is true?

    (a) If a patient in cardiac arrest has an implanted artificial pacemaker, the AED should **not** be used. The patient's implanted device will interfere with the AED's ability to correctly analyze the patient's cardiac rhythm and safely deliver appropriate shocks.

    (b) The battery that powers the patient's artificial pacemaker may be imbedded beneath the patient's skin, below the right or left clavicle.

    (c) If a lump that feels like an implanted artificial pacemaker's battery is found in the area where you normally would put an AED pad, place the pad several inches away from the battery lump. Then continue operation of the AED as usual.

    (d) Both answers (a) and (b) are true.

    (e) Both answers (b) and (c) are true.

135. Although not as commonly seen as patients with pacemakers, patients with surgically implanted automatic defibrillators[*] are encountered by EMTs. These patients have had a tiny defibrillator implanted in their bodies because they have a high risk for developing ventricular tachycardia or ventricular fibrillation. Which of the following statements regarding emergency care, CPR, and AED use for these patients is true?

(a) Since they already have a defibrillator implanted, the AED is not used on these patients, even when they are in cardiac arrest.
(b) It is extremely dangerous for anyone to be in contact with these patients when their defibrillator shocks them. Avoid all physical contact with these patients at all times.
(c) Because of the physical contact danger, a voice synthesizer also is implanted in the patient (usually in the abdomen, where there is more room). Just prior to administering a shock, the implanted defibrillator will activate the voice synthesizer and the message "Stand back!" will be broadcast 3 times before the shock is given.
(d) All of the above are true.
(e) None of the above are true.

136. The condition of **hypoglycemia** can be determined by a routine blood test and is defined as a

(a) high level of sugar in the blood.
(b) low level of sugar in the blood.
(c) low level of insulin in the blood.
(d) high level of insulin in the blood.
(e) low level of hormones in the blood.

137. The condition of **hyperglycemia** can be determined by a routine blood test and is defined as a

(a) high level of sugar in the blood.
(b) low level of sugar in the blood.
(c) low level of insulin in the blood.
(d) high level of insulin in the blood.
(e) low level of hormones in the blood.

138. The medical term **idiopathic** means

(a) a condition or disease that causes the patient to deteriorate in level of intelligence.
(b) a person with very low levels of intelligence, who abnormally excels in one or two areas of function (such as math or the arts).

---

* Automatic implantable cardioverter-defibrillator (AICD).

(c) a condition or disease without a clear cause.
(d) a condition or disease that causes severe mental deficiency.
(e) a person with mental retardation who fixates on ideas of perversion.

139. The rapid onset of an altered level of consciousness (or altered mental status) may be caused by all of the following, except

   (a) hypoglycemia.
   (b) hyperglycemia.
   (c) poisoning.
   (d) head trauma.
   (e) hypoxia.

140. The medical term **diabetes** is derived from the Greek language, meaning "passing through." Technically, this is a general term indicating any of several diseases characterized by excessive urination. However, the specific condition of **diabetes mellitus** is often referred to, simply, as **diabetes**. In this case, **diabetes** is defined as a disorder caused by the

   (a) inadequate production or utilization of the hormone insulin.
   (b) inadequate production of the polysaccharide glycogen.
   (c) inadequate production of the hormone glucose.
   (d) overproduction of the hormone insulin.
   (e) overproduction of the polysaccharide glycogen.

141. Because _____ cannot move from the blood into cells without assistance, _____ is required to allow transport into the cells.

   (a) insulin/oxygen
   (b) glucose/insulin
   (c) oxygen/insulin
   (d) oxygen/glucose
   (e) insulin/glucose

142. The most common diabetes-related medical emergency is

   (a) hypoinsulemia.
   (b) hyperinsulemia.
   (c) hyperglycemia.
   (d) hypoglycemia.
   (e) gluconeogenesis.

143. Diabetes-related altered mental status may occur without any identifiable factors preceding the event. However, which of the following situations normally would not be responsible for a sudden onset of diabetes-related altered mental status?

(a) The patient took her/his daily prescribed insulin and then missed a single meal.
(b) The patient took her/his daily prescribed insulin but then vomited and did not eat again.
(c) The patient engaged in an unusual amount of exercise or physical work.
(d) The patient ate normally and engaged in normal activities but forgot to take her/his daily prescribed insulin.
(e) The patient forgot to take her/his prescribed insulin the previous day, so she/he doubled the daily dose and then ate normally and engaged in normal activities.

144. All of the following signs and symptoms are associated with hypoglycemia ("insulin shock"), except

(a) slurred speech and staggering (as though intoxicated by alcohol or drugs).
(b) tachycardia with cool, pale, and/or clammy skin.
(c) abnormal thirst, with increased fluid intake and frequent urination.
(d) seizures.
(e) anxiousness, combativeness, or other uncharacteristic behaviors.

145. To administer oral glucose to a patient, the EMT-B first must determine that the patient has a probable history of diabetes. This is often a very tricky and difficult assessment. Of the following scenarios, which one demonstrates the least amount of likelihood that a patient is a diabetic (and should quickly be given oral glucose)?

(a) The patient is slightly confused, is wearing a medical alert diabetes bracelet, but strongly denies being a diabetic.
(b) The patient has slurred speech and is slightly confused, has no medical alert identification, but is found in a house where prescription diabetes medications are present.

(c) The patient is acting merely "drunk and silly," but her friends strongly insist that "She's a diabetic! She takes insulin shots!"
(d) The patient has slurred speech, has a strong odor of alcohol on her breath, has no medical alert identification, and is grossly well oriented (to person, place, and time), but insists that she has a diabetic problem after being arrested for "drunken driving."
(e) The patient has slurred speech, has a strong odor of alcohol on her breath, has no medical alert identification, is grossly well oriented (to person, place, and time), and denies having a diabetic problem after being arrested for "drunken driving."

146. A patient who has been previously diagnosed as having diabetes mellitus may be treated with any of the following medications, except

   (a) the oral medication insulin (Humulin®, Lente®).
   (b) the oral medication Orinase®.
   (c) the oral medication Micronase®.
   (d) the subcutaneously injected medication insulin (Humulin®, Lente®).
   (e) the oral medication Diabinese®.

147. The diabetes medication insulin (Humulin®, Lente®) most often is found in the patient's

   (a) refrigerator.
   (b) pants pocket.
   (c) bathroom medicine cabinet.
   (d) purse.
   (e) dresser drawer or on a bedside table.

148. Once it is determined that the patient has a history of diabetes, the EMT-B must have on-line or off-line ("standing orders") permission from the medical director for the administration of oral glucose. Even after those two factors have been met, however, oral glucose may be administered only if the patient also

   (a) is conscious.
   (b) is unconscious.
   (c) can swallow.
   (d) Either answer (a) or (b).
   (e) Both answers (a) and (c), only.

149. Which of the following methods of oral glucose administration is contraindicated?

    (a) Have the patient squeeze the tube between her/his own cheek and gum.
    (b) Place the gel on a tongue depressor and hold it between the conscious patient's cheek and gum.
    (c) Properly insert an oral airway in the unconscious patient's mouth; then squeeze the gel between the patient's cheek and gum.
    (d) Place the gel on a tongue depressor and have the conscious patient hold it between her/his own cheek and gum.
    (e) None of the above are contraindicated (all are acceptable methods of oral glucose administration).

150. Oral glucose administration acts to

    (a) increase the patient's blood sugar levels.
    (b) decrease the patient's blood sugar levels.
    (c) increase the patient's insulin levels.
    (d) Both answers (b) and (c).
    (e) Both answers (a) and (c).

151. Which of the following statements regarding hyperglycemia is false?

    (a) A fruity or nail-polish-remover-like breath odor ("acetone breath" or "ketone breath") may accompany hyperglycemia.
    (b) Deep inhalations with a rapid respiratory rate often accompany hyperglycemia.
    (c) Extreme thirst with excessive fluid intake and frequent urination often accompanies hyperglycemia.
    (d) Hyperglycemia has a very rapid onset of signs and symptoms.
    (e) Hyperglycemia may progress to unconsciousness and/or death.

152. Which of the following statements regarding seizures is false?

    (a) Seizures in children who have a chronic seizure disorder are rarely ever life-threatening. Reassure the parents and have them call the child's pediatrician during regular office hours. Ambulance treatment and transportation is not needed.
    (b) All seizures, including "febrile seizures" in infants and children, should be treated by the EMT as if they could be life-threatening.
    (c) Seizures may be brief or prolonged.
    (d) All of the above are false.
    (e) None of the above are false.

153. Seizures may be caused by any of the following, except

(a) fever.
(b) hypoglycemia.
(c) poisoning.
(d) excessive oxygen administration (such as nonrebreather mask use for hyperventilation or COPD patients).
(e) trauma.

154. Seizures may be caused by any of the following, except

(a) infection.
(b) electrolyte imbalances (such as excessive water ingestion).
(c) missing a single dose of diabetes medication.
(d) a brain tumor or congenital brain defect.
(e) hypoxia.

155. Idiopathic seizures are produced by

(a) unknown causes.
(b) severe mental retardation.
(c) missing a dose of diabetic medication.
(d) excessive oxygen administration (such as nonrebreather mask use for hyperventilation or COPD patients).
(e) prolonged lack of oxygen.

156. The most common cause of seizures in an adult is

(a) idiopathic.
(b) hypoglycemia.
(c) poisoning.
(d) failure to take prescribed seizure medications.
(e) excessive oxygen administration (such as nonrebreather mask use for hyperventilation or COPD patients).

157. The most common cause of seizures in infants and young children (ages 6 months to 3 years) is

(a) idiopathic.
(b) high fever.
(c) epilepsy.
(d) hypoglycemia.
(e) hypoxia.

158. The condition called **epilepsy** is used to describe

   (a) any patient who has any kind of seizure.
   (b) a patient who has had seizures since birth or since a traumatic head injury.
   (c) a patient who has seizures whenever excessive oxygen is administered.
   (d) any patient who has never had a seizure before (the term is used only as a temporary diagnosis).
   (e) None of the above.

159. If a seizure patient becomes cyanotic,

   (a) do not be concerned, this is a normal seizure phase. Simply roll the patient to her/his side and wait for her/his color to improve.
   (b) assure an airway and artificially ventilate the patient.
   (c) restrain the patient manually (hold all extremities still) and apply oxygen by a nonrebreather mask.
   (d) Both answers (a) and (c).
   (e) Both answers (b) and (c).

160. Which of the following statements regarding positioning of a patient immediately after a full-body seizure is true?

   (a) Roll the patient to her/his side to allow for fluid drainage and airway protection only if there is no mechanism of injury that suggests spine trauma.
   (b) If there is a mechanism of injury that suggests spine trauma, keep the patient supine and manually suction the airway.
   (c) The patient must not remain supine (even if the mechanism of injury suggests spine trauma) because the patient may swallow her/his tongue and choke. Roll the patient to her/his side as a unit and place a bite block between the teeth before suctioning.
   (d) Both answers (a) and (b).
   (e) Both answers (a) and (c).

161. Which of the following statements regarding the condition **status epilepticus** is false?

   (a) Status epilepticus is a high-priority, life-threatening condition. Immediate transportation with an ACLS intercept en route to the emergency department should be considered.
   (b) Any patient who has two or three seizures within a 24-hour period is considered to be in status epilepticus.

(c) Status epilepticus requires airway control, suctioning, and artificial ventilation.
(d) Some EMS systems consider any patient who is still seizing when the EMTs arrive to be in status epilepticus.
(e) Any patient who has two or more seizures in a row without regaining consciousness between them can be considered to be in status epilepticus.

162. Some patients describe experiencing an aura before having a seizure. Which of the following best describes the term *aura*?

(a) A strange taste sensation or unusual feeling (often in the patient's stomach) prior to the seizure.
(b) The hallucination of bright bursts of colors or lights prior to the seizure.
(c) An odd or out-of-place smell experienced just prior to the seizure.
(d) Only answers (a) and/or (b).
(e) Either answers (a), (b), and/or (c).

163. There are several different kinds of seizures that usually are grouped into two different classification types: partial seizures and generalized seizures. Which of the following would be classified as partial seizures?

(a) "Jacksonian" or "focal motor" seizures, which involve only one body part or one side of the body. They consist of a tingling sensation, stiffening, and/or uncontrollable jerking of that body portion. There is no loss of consciousness unless the seizure progresses to involve the entire body.
(b) "Psychomotor" or "temporal lobe" seizures, which involve various forms of uncontrollable abnormal behavior. The patient may act as though intoxicated or on drugs, may struggle or fight with responders, or may scream and cry out while running around disrobing or engaging in other bizarre behavior. There is no loss of consciousness unless the seizure develops into a generalized seizure, and the patient may have confusion and/or no memory of the incident when it is over.
(c) "Petit mal" seizures, which usually last only 1 to 10 seconds and often may not be noticed by those around or near the patient. Also called "absence seizures," they do not involve any kind of dramatic physical movement, slumping, or falling. There is simply a temporary loss of awareness that may be noticed only by the patient (after the seizure is over).
(d) Only answers (a) and (b).
(e) Only answers (b) and (c).

164. Which of the following would be classified as generalized seizures?

(a) "Jacksonian" or "focal motor" seizures, which involve only one body part or one side of the body. They consist of a tingling sensation, stiffening, and/or uncontrollable jerking of that body portion. There is no loss of consciousness unless the seizure progresses to involve the entire body.

(b) "Tonic-clonic" or "grand mal" seizures, which produce unconsciousness and involve uncontrollable motor activity of the entire body. In the brief tonic phase (usually about 30 seconds), the patient becomes rigid and may stop breathing. Tongue or cheek biting and/or incontinence of bladder or the bowels may occur. The clonic phase consists of violent flexion/contraction and extension of the body and may last for 1 to 5 minutes.

(c) "Petit mal" seizures, which usually last only 1 to 10 seconds and often may not be noticed by those around or near the patient. Also called "absence seizures," they do not involve any kind of dramatic physical movement, slumping, or falling. There is simply a temporary loss of awareness that may be noticed only by the patient (after the seizure is over).

(d) Only answers (a) and (b).

(e) Only answers (b) and (c).

165. An altered level of consciousness (mental status) also may be caused by a "stroke." The medical term for a stroke is abbreviated **CVA,** which stands for

(a) cardiovascular accident.
(b) cerebral-vascular accident.
(c) cardiovertebral accident (also known as "spinal shock").
(d) Either answer (a) or (b).
(e) None of the above.

166. A CVA may be caused by

(a) bleeding in the brain due to head trauma.
(b) a blocked artery in the brain (either from fat or tissue emboli or a blood clot).
(c) a ruptured artery in the brain.
(d) Only answers (b) and/or (c).
(e) Answers (a), (b), and/or (c).

167. Which of the following statements regarding patients having a CVA is true?

(a) Although most CVA patients do not experience (or are unable to complain of) a headache, the complaint of having a headache may be the only immediate symptom.
(b) Partial or complete inability to speak often accompanies CVA.

(c) Inability to hear or understand the speech of others may accompany a CVA, but the patient may be unable to communicate this symptom.
(d) Only answers (a) and (b) are true.
(e) Answers (a), (b), and (c) are true.

168. Classic signs and symptoms of a CVA include all of the following, except

(a) numbness, weakness, and/or paralysis (usually of only one side of the body).
(b) unequal pupils.
(c) a mental euphoria and comments of extreme happiness, without any physical signs and symptoms of abnormal function (often accompanied by nymph-like dancing about the room or scene).
(d) single-sided facial muscle droop.
(e) slurred and/or nonsensical speech patterns.

169. The medical term **allergen** is best defined as

(a) an exaggerated but localized immune response.
(b) a severe and life-threatening, exaggerated immune response, involving dilation of the body's blood vessels (causing low blood pressure) and edema of the respiratory tissues (which may threaten the patient's airway).
(c) something that causes an exaggerated immune response.
(d) a hormone produced by the body that constricts blood vessels and dilates respiratory passages.
(e) an electrolyte produced by the body that dilates blood vessels and constricts respiratory passages

170. The medical phrase **allergic reaction** is best defined as

(a) an exaggerated but localized immune response.
(b) a severe and life-threatening, exaggerated immune response, involving dilation of the body's blood vessels (causing low blood pressure) and edema of the respiratory tissues (which may threaten the patient's airway).
(c) something that causes an exaggerated immune response.
(d) a hormone produced by the body that constricts blood vessels and dilates respiratory passages.
(e) an electrolyte produced by the body that dilates blood vessels and constricts respiratory passages

171. The medical term ***anaphylaxis*** (or ***anaphylactic shock***) is best defined as

    (a) an exaggerated but localized immune response.
    (b) a severe and life-threatening, exaggerated immune response, involving dilation of the body's blood vessels (causing low blood pressure) and edema of the respiratory tissues (which may threaten the patient's airway).
    (c) something that causes an exaggerated immune response.
    (d) a hormone produced by the body that constricts blood vessels and dilates respiratory passages.
    (e) an electrolyte produced by the body that dilates blood vessels and constricts respiratory passages

172. The medical term ***epinephrine*** is best defined as

    (a) an exaggerated but localized immune response.
    (b) a severe and life-threatening, exaggerated immune response, involving dilation of the body's blood vessels (causing low blood pressure) and edema of the respiratory tissues (which may threaten the patient's airway).
    (c) something that causes an exaggerated immune response.
    (d) a hormone produced by the body that constricts blood vessels and dilates respiratory passages.
    (e) an electrolyte produced by the body that dilates blood vessels and constricts respiratory passages

173. People can develop allergic reactions or anaphylactic shock to almost any foreign substance. However, classic substances that often cause allergic reactions or anaphylactic shock include all of the following, except

    (a) oral contact (such as kissing) with a person infected with rabies or syphilis.
    (b) insect bites or stings (bees, wasps, and the like).
    (c) food ingestion such as nuts (especially peanuts), shellfish, milk, or the like.
    (d) exposure to various kinds of plants or animals.
    (e) exposure to particular medications.

174. The medical term ***erythema*** is also referred to as ***flushing*** and is best described as

    (a) a generalized redness of the skin.
    (b) a sensation of heat and/or tingling in the face, mouth, chest, feet, and hands.
    (c) a generalized itching sensation.
    (d) itchy, reddened bumps or bulges.
    (e) generalized tissue swelling of the face, neck, hands, feet, and/or tongue.

175. The medical term **urticaria** is also referred to as **hives** and is best described as

   (a) a generalized redness of the skin.
   (b) a sensation of heat and/or tingling in the face, mouth, chest, feet, and hands.
   (c) a generalized itching sensation.
   (d) itchy, reddened bumps or bulges.
   (e) generalized tissue swelling of the face, neck, hands, feet, and/or tongue.

176. Which of the following statements regarding allergic reactions (or anaphylactic shock) is true?

   (a) The first exposure to a foreign substance may result in the body's creation of antibodies (substances designed specifically to attack the foreign substance).
   (b) First exposure to an allergen will result in an immediate allergic reaction.
   (c) An allergic reaction does not occur until the second exposure to an allergen.
   (d) Both answers (a) and (b) are true.
   (e) Both answers (a) and (c) are true.

177. Which of the following statements regarding the primary differences between an allergic reaction and anaphylactic shock is false?

   (a) Localized allergic reactions do not present a life-threat to the patient and are not commonly treated by EMT-assisted epinephrine auto-injector use in the field.
   (b) Anaphylaxis may include any or all of the signs of a localized allergic reaction.
   (c) Localized allergic reactions often cause seriously low blood pressure. Because of this, low blood pressure is not an indication for EMT-assisted epinephrine auto-injector use in the field.
   (d) Wheezing (or any other signs of respiratory compromise) indicates an anaphylactic reaction and justifies seeking an order for EMT-assisted epinephrine auto-injector use in the field.
   (e) With an allergic reaction, if the patient also begins to develop an altered mental status and/or (simply) a profound sense of impending doom, this indicates the possibility of an anaphylactic reaction. These symptoms justify seeking an order for EMT-assisted epinephrine auto-injector use in the field.

178. Skin signs and symptoms of anaphylaxis may include

    (a) a warm, tingling sensation in the face, mouth, chest, feet, and hands.
    (b) itching.
    (c) hives and/or flushing.
    (d) edema of the face, neck, hands, feet, and/or tongue.
    (e) Any of the above.

179. Respiratory signs and symptoms of anaphylaxis may include all of the following, except

    (a) the patient's complaint of hoarseness or a "tightness" in her/his throat or chest.
    (b) coughing or labored breathing.
    (c) slow, relaxed, and even respiratory patterns.
    (d) stridor.
    (e) wheezing (audible with or without a stethoscope).

180. Cardiac signs and symptoms of anaphylaxis include

    (a) tachycardia.
    (b) bradycardia.
    (c) hypotension.
    (d) Both answers (a) and (c).
    (e) Both answers (b) and (c).

181. Generalized signs and symptoms of anaphylaxis include all of the following, except

    (a) euphoria and increased energy.
    (b) the patient's complaint of itchy, watery eyes and/or a runny nose.
    (c) the patient's complaint of headache.
    (d) the patient's sense of impending doom.
    (e) deteriorating mental status.

182. The focused history interview of an allergic reaction or anaphylaxis patient should include all except which of the following questions?

    (a) Does the patient have a history of allergies? To what?
    (b) When was the patient's last tetanus shot?
    (c) What was the patient exposed to, and how did exposure occur?
    (d) What are the patient's complaints, and how have they changed since exposure?
    (e) What has the patient already done to seek relief, and how successful was it?

183. Oxygen should be administered to an allergic reaction or anaphylaxis patient

   (a) only if respiratory complaints are present.
   (b) by nasal cannula at 4 liters per minute.
   (c) by nonrebreather mask at 4 liters per minute.
   (d) by nonrebreather mask at 12 to 15 liters per minute.
   (e) by nasal cannula at 12 to 15 liters per minute.

184. Prior to contacting the medical director to request an order for assisting the patient with use of an epinephrine auto-injector, the EMT must determine that the patient meets which of the following criteria for assisted injection?

   (a) The patient must have a history of previous allergic reactions to the same substance causing this exposure incident.
   (b) The patient must be complaining of respiratory distress or exhibit signs and symptoms of shock (hypoperfusion).
   (c) The patient must have a prescribed epinephrine auto-injector with him.
   (d) Only answers (a) and/or (b) are required for assisted injection orders.
   (e) Answers (a), (b), and (c) are required for assisted injection orders.

185. Your patient has a history of previous allergic reactions to the same substance causing this exposure incident and has signs and symptoms of shock, but he has left his prescribed epinephrine auto-injector at another location. A bystander offers the use of her prescribed epinephrine auto-injector, and the patient identifies the brand and dose as being the same as his own prescription. The EMT-B should

   (a) contact the medical director and request an order to assist the patient with administration of the bystander's prescribed epinephrine auto-injector.
   (b) transport the patient immediately, treating the patient for shock en route to the emergency department.
   (c) transport the patient to the location of his prescribed epinephrine auto-injector, only if that location is less than 10 minutes away, and proceed with protocol from there.
   (d) consider the fact that the patient is in a life-threatening situation. Since the patient has the same prescription as the bystander, do not tell the medical director that the prescribed epinephrine auto-injector present is not actually the patient's own.
   (e) immediately assist the patient with administration of the bystander's prescribed epinephrine auto-injector, and contact the medical director only after the fact.

186. Your patient has a history of previous allergic reactions to the same substance causing this exposure incident, has his prescribed epinephrine auto-injector present, but does not have signs and symptoms of respiratory distress or shock. The EMT-B should

(a) contact the medical director for a consultation. If the medical director orders it, assist the patient with administration of his prescribed epinephrine auto-injector.
(b) contact the medical director only to report the situation and provide your ETA. If the medical director orders it, remind her/him of protocol and refuse to assist with administration of the patient's prescribed epinephrine auto-injector until the patient develops respiratory distress or shock signs and symptoms.
(c) continue with the focused assessment and oxygen treatment.
(d) Both answers (a) and (c).
(e) Both answers (b) and (c).

187. If the adult patient continues to deteriorate after the first EMT-B-assisted epinephrine auto-injector use, the EMT-B should

(a) remember that only one EMT-B–assisted auto-injector use (0.3 mg of medication) is allowed.
(b) remember that two simultaneous auto-injector uses (0.6 mg of medication) may be given for the second injection.
(c) obtain a medical control order for another assisted auto-injector use (administration of an additional 0.3 mg of medication).
(d) automatically assist with two simultaneous auto-injector uses (0.6 mg of medication), for any repeat administration, until the patient's injectors are all used or you arrive at the emergency department (but only if the patient has **both** respiratory distress and signs and symptoms of shock).
(e) Any of the above, depending on patient complaints and local protocols.

188. The dosage protocol for EMT-B–assisted infant or child epinephrine auto-injector use is which of the following?

(a) Assist with only one infant/child auto-injector use (0.15 mg of medication).
(b) If the patient has **both** respiratory distress and signs and symptoms of shock, assist with two simultaneous infant/child auto-injector uses (0.3 mg of medication, total).

(c) Assist with one infant/child auto-injector use (0.15 mg of medication), followed by another assisted injection (if ordered) every 5 minutes until the patient's injectors are all used or you arrive at the emergency department.
(d) If the patient has **both** respiratory distress and signs and symptoms of shock, assist with two simultaneous infant/child auto-injector uses (0.6 mg of medication) every 5 minutes until the patient's injectors are all used or you arrive at the emergency department.
(e) None of the above. Infants and children are not prescribed epinephrine auto-injectors.

189. What is the location for epinephrine auto-injector administration?
    (a) On the patient's right or left hip, alternating sites with subsequent administrations (every 5 minutes).
    (b) On the patient's right or left shoulder, alternating sites with subsequent administrations (every 5 minutes).
    (c) On the lateral portion of the patient's right or left thigh, midway between the waist and the knee.
    (d) On the medial portion of the patient's right or left thigh, midway between the waist and the knee.
    (e) Either answer (c) or (d), alternating sites with subsequent administrations (every 5 minutes).

190. Common side effects of epinephrine auto-injector administration include any of the following, except
    (a) dizziness, excitement, and/or anxiousness.
    (b) hypotension (systolic blood pressure of less than 90 mmHg).
    (c) tachycardia and/or pale skin color.
    (d) chest pain and/or nausea and vomiting.
    (e) headache.

191. During transport, if the patient's condition continues to deteriorate after a single assisted auto-injection of epinephrine, the EMT-B should treat the patient for shock and
    (a) refrain from repeating the epinephrine injections.
    (b) consult the medical director for an order to assist with the administration of another epinephrine auto-injection.
    (c) anticipate the potential need for ventilatory assistance and/or CPR.
    (d) Both answers (a) and (c).
    (e) Both answers (b) and (c).

192. The focused history interview of a poisoning or overdose patient should include all except which of the following questions?

(a) What was the patient exposed to, and how did exposure occur?
(b) How much of the substance was consumed, and over what time period?
(c) When was the patient's last tetanus shot?
(d) How much does the patient weigh?
(e) What has the patient already done to seek relief, and how successful was it?

193. A medication that EMT-Bs may administer to an ingested poisoning or overdose patient is known by several trade names, such as SuperChar®, InstaChar®, Actidose®, and LiquiChar®. The generic name for this medication is

(a) activated carbon.
(b) liquid residue of charcoal.
(c) activated charcoal.
(d) crushed charcoal briquettes.
(e) liquid charcoal briquettes.

194. Contraindications to the administration of SuperChar® include

(a) altered mental status.
(b) ingestion of acids or alkali substances.
(c) inability to swallow.
(d) Only answers (a) and (c).
(e) Answers (a), (b), and (c).

195. SuperChar®, InstaChar®, Actidose® and the like are available

(a) premixed in an alcohol solution containing 12.5 or 25 grams of the medication.
(b) premixed in a water solution containing 12.5 or 25 grams of the medication.
(c) in a powder form that should be avoided for field use.
(d) Both answers (a) and (c).
(e) Both answers (b) and (c).

196. The universal administration dose of SuperChar®, InstaChar®, Actidose®, and the like is 1 gram of the medication per kilogram of body weight. However, the basically accepted dose range for adult administration is

(a) 50 to 100 grams of medication.
(b) 25 to 50 grams of medication.
(c) 12.5 to 25 grams of medication.
(d) Either answer (a) or (b).
(e) Either answer (a) or (c).

197. The universal administration dose of SuperChar®, InstaChar®, Actidose®, and the like is 1 gram of the medication per kilogram of body weight. However, the basically accepted dose range for pediatric administration is

  (a) 50 to 100 grams of medication.
  (b) 25 to 50 grams of medication.
  (c) 12.5 to 25 grams of medication.
  (d) Either answer (a) or (b).
  (e) Either answer (a) or (c).

198. Which of the following statements regarding administration of medication such as SuperChar®, InstaChar®, and Actidose® is false?

  (a) An on-line or off-line order for administration must be obtained from the medical director.
  (b) The medication container must be shaken thoroughly before administration.
  (c) If the patient takes too long to drink the medication, the medication may lose its potency. A new container should be opened and the patient should continue drinking until the appropriate dose is ingested.
  (d) A covered container with a straw may improve the patient's speed at drinking the medication, since she/he will not be able to see it.
  (e) The time of administration and the specific amount administered should be recorded.

199. Which of the following statements regarding the actions of medication such as Super-Char®, InstaChar®, and Actidose® is true?

  (a) This medication binds to certain poisons and prevents them from being excreted from the body.
  (b) This medication deactivates most poisons, turning them into nontoxic substances.
  (c) This medication coats the stomach to prevent the ingested substance from poisoning the patient.
  (d) None of the above are true.
  (e) All of the above are true.

200. Which of the following statements regarding the side effects of medication such as Super-Char®, InstaChar®, and Actidose® is true?

  (a) The medication may cause black stools.
  (b) Some patients, particularly those who have ingested poisons that cause nausea and vomiting, may vomit.
  (c) If the patient vomits, the dose should be repeated (but only one time).
  (d) Only answers (a) and (b) are true.
  (e) Answers (a), (b), and (c) are true.

201. Administration of medications such as Super-Char®, InstaChar®, and Actidose® to a patient with an altered level of consciousness

   (a) may be accomplished by squirting very small amounts at a time under the patient's tongue. Administration may take some time but should be continued until arrival at the emergency department.
   (b) is vitally important because of the seriousness of the patient's poisoning or overdose. Upon arrival at the emergency department, the amount of medication instilled in the field should be carefully documented.
   (c) is **always** contraindicated.
   (d) is contraindicated only if the patient appears to choke when small amounts of the medication are squirted under the patient's tongue.
   (e) Both answers (a) and (b).

202. The medical term **hypothermia** is best defined as having

   (a) a body temperature below normal.
   (b) the sensation of chills or shivering.
   (c) a body temperature above normal.
   (d) a headache.
   (e) the sensation of a fever.

203. The medical term **hyperthermia** is best defined as having

   (a) a body temperature below normal.
   (b) the sensation of chills or shivering.
   (c) a body temperature above normal.
   (d) a headache.
   (e) the sensation of a fever.

204. Heat loss that occurs by simply losing heat to the atmosphere (space) around you is called

   (a) radiation.
   (b) convection.
   (c) conduction.
   (d) evaporation.
   (e) breathing (respiration).

205. Heat loss that occurs because perspiration or a moist body surface acts to cool the body as it dries is called

   (a) radiation.
   (b) convection.
   (c) conduction.
   (d) evaporation.
   (e) breathing (respiration).

206. Warm air being expelled by the body (and not being returned) describes the process of heat loss from

    (a) radiation.
    (b) convection.
    (c) conduction.
    (d) evaporation.
    (e) breathing (respiration).

207. Heat loss that occurs because of direct contact with a cold object drawing heat out of the body is called

    (a) radiation.
    (b) convection.
    (c) conduction.
    (d) evaporation.
    (e) breathing (respiration).

208. Heat loss that occurs because of moving air or flowing liquids passing over the body, carrying away the body's heat, is called

    (a) radiation.
    (b) convection.
    (c) conduction.
    (d) evaporation.
    (e) breathing (respiration).

209. Body temperature is measured by degrees (°) and is based on one of two scales: the Fahrenheit (F) scale or the Celsius (C) scale. Normal body temperatures vary, depending on the site at which the temperature is measured. The normal, oral body temperature for an adult is considered to be

    (a) 99.2° F (37.3° C).
    (b) 98.8° F (37.1° C).
    (c) 98.6° F (37° C).
    (d) 96.8° F (36° C).
    (e) 90.6° F (32.5° C).

210. The normal, oral body temperature for a child is considered to be

    (a) 99.2° F (37.3° C).
    (b) 98.8° F (37.1° C).
    (c) 98.6° F (37° C).
    (d) 96.8° F (36° C).
    (e) 90.6° F (32.5° C).

211. The phrase *generalized hypothermia* is best defined as
   (a) the presence of a freezing injury to any single body part (if one part is frozen, the entire body **must** be hypothermic).
   (b) the cooling of the entire body (with or without localized freezing injuries).
   (c) any body temperature different from normal body temperature.
   (d) Either answer (a) or (b).
   (e) Either answer (a) or (c).

212. Which of the following statements regarding factors that increase a patient's susceptibility to generalized hypothermia is false?
   (a) Atmospheric temperatures at or below freezing are required before generalized hypothermia can occur in a dry adult.
   (b) Elderly patients often exist on low incomes and cannot afford to adequately heat their environment. Thus, they are more susceptible to generalized hypothermia.
   (c) Chronic illness will increase a patient's susceptibility to generalized hypothermia.
   (d) A poor diet may increase a patient's susceptibility to generalized hypothermia.
   (e) Certain medications may increase a patient's susceptibility to generalized hypothermia.

213. Which of the following statements regarding factors of an infant or pediatric patient's susceptibility to generalized hypothermia is false?
   (a) Infants and children are small in size, but their body surface area is larger when compared to their entire body mass. Thus, they are more susceptible to generalized hypothermia than adults.
   (b) Children actually have a larger muscle mass (compared to total body mass) than adults. Thus, they are better able to effectively generate heat by shivering. This is the one factor that makes them **less** susceptible to generalized hypothermia than adults.
   (c) Children have a smaller muscle mass than adults. Thus, they are less able to effectively generate heat by shivering and more susceptible to generalized hypothermia than adults.
   (d) Infants may be unable to shiver at all. Thus, they are even more susceptible to generalized hypothermia than children.
   (e) Infants and children have less body fat to insulate them from heat loss. Thus, they are more susceptible to generalized hypothermia than adults.

214. Which of the following conditions may increase any patient's susceptibility to generalized hypothermia?

    (a) Shock (hypoperfusion).
    (b) Head injury.
    (c) Burns.
    (d) Only answers (a) and (c).
    (e) Answers (a), (b), and (c).

215. Which of the following conditions may increase any patient's susceptibility to generalized hypothermia?

    (a) Generalized infections.
    (b) Diabetes and hypoglycemia.
    (c) Injuries to the spinal cord.
    (d) Only answers (a) and (b).
    (e) Answers (a), (b), and (c).

216. Which of the following conditions may increase any patient's susceptibility to generalized hypothermia?

    (a) Alcohol ingestion.
    (b) Overdose or poisoning.
    (c) Any major trauma.
    (d) Only answers (a) and (b).
    (e) Answers (a), (b), and (c).

217. Which of the following conditions may increase any patient's susceptibility to generalized hypothermia?

    (a) Outdoor resuscitation.
    (b) Water immersion.
    (c) Presence of high winds.
    (d) Only answers (b) and (c).
    (e) Answers (a), (b), and (c).

218. One of the signs and symptoms of generalized hypothermia is cool or cold skin temperature. The best method of assessing skin temperature (as it relates to the patient's internal body temperature) is by placing

    (a) your palm on the patient's forehead.
    (b) the back of your hand on the patient's forehead.
    (c) your palm on the patient's abdomen (beneath his clothing).
    (d) the back of your hand on the patient's abdomen (beneath his clothing).
    (e) the back of your hand on the patient's cheeks.

219. Which of the following statements regarding the signs and symptoms of increasing degrees of hypothermia is false?

(a) Mental status progressively deteriorates as a patient develops a lower body temperature. Poor judgment actually may lead the hypothermic patient to remove her/his clothes.

(b) Motor function progressively deteriorates as a patient develops a lower body temperature.

(c) In the early stages of hypothermia, a patient's pulse may be normal to slow. As the patient develops a lower body temperature, her/his pulse gradually increases (in an effort to generate heat) until becoming so fast that her/his heart stops.

(d) Muscular rigidity becomes progressively worse as a patient develops a lower body temperature. Stiff or rigid postures may develop.

(e) The lower the patient's body temperature, the less able she/he is to attempt generation of heat by shivering. Thus, the absence of shivering is a dire sign in hypothermia cases.

220. Which of the following statements regarding the signs and symptoms of increasing degrees of hypothermia is true?

(a) In the early stages of hypothermia, a patient's respiratory rate will usually be slow and shallow (in an effort to retain body heat). As the patient develops a lower body temperature, her/his rate and depth of breathing gradually increases, hyperventilating until just before respiratory arrest occurs.

(b) In the early stages of hypothermia, a patient's skin may appear red. It is only in later stages of hypothermia that the patient's skin may become pale or cyanotic.

(c) In the most extreme cases of hypothermia, some of a patient's body parts may feel stiff or hard, as though the patient is almost completely frozen.

(d) Both answers (a) and (c) are true.

(e) Both answers (b) and (c) are true.

221. Which of the following statements regarding emergency medical care for a victim of generalized hypothermia is false?

(a) Immediately remove the patient from the environment and protect the patient from further heat loss.

(b) Remove all of the patient's wet clothing and wrap her/him with blankets.

TEST SECTION FOUR

(c) Handle the patient gently. Rough handling may cause the patient's heart to go into ventricular fibrillation.
(d) If the patient is conscious, assist her/him to her/his feet and begin forced exercise (walk the patient for at least 5 minutes prior to transportation). This activity will increase circulation of warm body-core blood to the patient's near-frozen extremities and will help the patient begin to generate heat again.
(e) Administer oxygen, preferably warmed and humidified oxygen.

222. Which of the following statements regarding the pulse assessment for a victim of extreme generalized hypothermia is true?

(a) Carotid pulse assessment should be performed for as long as 30 to 45 seconds. If any pulse is felt during that time (even a heart rate as low as 10 per minute), chest compressions should not be performed.
(b) Carotid pulse assessment should be performed for no longer than 30 seconds. If the patient's detectable pulse rate is slower than 60 beats per minute, begin chest compressions.
(c) If a radial pulse is not present, begin CPR.
(d) Carotid pulse assessment should be performed for no longer than 15 seconds. If the patient's detectable pulse rate is slower than 60 beats per minute, begin chest compressions.
(e) If a radial pulse is present, but less than 60 beats per minute, begin chest compressions.

223. Which of the following statements describe *passive rewarming* techniques?

(a) Apply warm blankets.
(b) Turn the ambulance patient compartment heater to a high setting.
(c) Apply heat packs or hot water bottles to the patient's groin, axillary, and cervical regions.
(d) Only answers (a) and (b).
(e) Answers (a), (b), and (c).

224. Which of the following statements describe *active rewarming* techniques?

(a) Apply warm blankets.
(b) Turn the ambulance patient compartment heater to a high setting.
(c) Apply heat packs or hot water bottles to the patient's groin, axillary, and cervical regions.
(d) Only answers (a) and (b).
(e) Answers (a), (b), and (c).

225. If allowed by local protocols, active rewarming techniques are indicated for patients who are

   (a) alert and responding appropriately.
   (b) alert but not responding appropriately.
   (c) unconscious.
   (d) Either answer (a) or (b) only.
   (e) Either answer (b) or (c) only.

226. Even when active rewarming techniques are allowed by local protocols, only passive rewarming techniques are indicated for patients who are

   (a) alert and responding appropriately.
   (b) alert but not responding appropriately.
   (c) unconscious.
   (d) Both answers (a) and (b).
   (e) Both answers (b) and (c).

227. Local cold injuries are now classified as early (or superficial) and late (or deep) local cold injuries. Early or superficial local cold injuries were once called

   (a) frostbite.
   (b) frost nip.
   (c) first-degree frost nip.
   (d) second-degree frost nip.
   (e) third-degree frostbite.

228. Late or deep local cold injuries were once called

   (a) frostbite.
   (b) frost nip.
   (c) first-degree frost nip.
   (d) second-degree frost nip.
   (e) third-degree frostbite.

229. Signs and symptoms of early or superficial local cold injuries include any of the following, except

   (a) blanching of the skin.
   (b) loss of feeling and sensation in the injured area.
   (c) swelling is almost always present.
   (d) the skin remains soft.
   (e) if the part has been rewarmed, the patient may complain of a tingling or burning sensation.

230. Signs and symptoms of late or deep local cold injuries include any of the following, except

   (a) red, icy-looking skin.
   (b) a firm or frozen feeling upon palpation.

(c) the presence of swelling.
(d) the presence of blisters.
(e) the patient complaining of moderate to severe pain in a part that has been partially or completely thawed.

231. Which of the following statements regarding general emergency care measures for all local cold injuries is false?

(a) Remove the patient from the cold environment.
(b) Remove all wet or restrictive clothing.
(c) Protect the cold injured extremity from further injury.
(d) Administer oxygen.
(e) If transportation will require re-exposure of the patient to the cold, perform active rewarming (thawing) measures before re-exposure.

232. Which of the following statements regarding emergency care measures for early or superficial local cold injuries is true?

(a) Encourage the patient to vigorously exercise her/his superficially cold injured hands and fingers to stimulate circulation of warm blood to those parts.
(b) Encourage the patient to gently massage her/his superficially cold injured nose and/or ears (or massage them for the patient) to stimulate circulation of warm blood to those parts.
(c) Encourage the patient to gently massage her/his superficially cold injured toes and/or feet (or massage them for the patient) to stimulate circulation of warm blood to those parts.
(d) If in a warm environment and dry socks or slippers are available, put them on the patient and encourage gentle pacing to stimulate circulation of warm blood to her/his superficially cold injured toes and/or feet.
(e) If any extremity is involved, splint and cover it after passive warming.

233. Which of the following statements regarding emergency care measures for late or deep local cold injuries is true?

(a) Cover the injured area with dry clothing or dressings (if any jewelry is present, remove it from the affected part before dressing).
(b) Since the patient is unlikely to be able to exercise or massage the part herself/himself, gently massage the part for her/him to stimulate circulation of warm blood to the injured areas.
(c) Apply hot packs to all deeply cold injured parts as soon as possible (especially if re-exposure to cold will occur before or during transport).
(d) Both answers (a) and (b) are true.
(e) Both answers (a) and (c) are true.

234. Active, rapid rewarming of late or deep local cold injuries is

  (a) never recommended, for any reason.
  (b) recommended only when an extremely long or delayed transport is inevitable.
  (c) important to accomplish prior to re-exposure to cold.
  (d) a primary recommended treatment for any local cold injury.
  (e) a procedure that should be performed only if transport time is less than 30 minutes.

AUTHORS' NOTE: Questions 235 through 238 and 242 through 245 may require an unusual amount of time to answer. If you are timing your test performance, stop timing now. If you could use a break, take a break now. Then return to the test without timing your performance until cued to resume doing so.

AUTHORS' TIP: Remember, rather than trying to compare the presented activities or statements with the provided answer options, just read through the activities and statements first. Then, on lined paper, write out your choices of the true activities or statements. When you are done, compare your number sequence with the available answers. If none of them match, you have a problem. Otherwise, select the answer option that matches your own numbers.

235. Of the following activities and statements regarding the performance of active, rapid rewarming of a late or deep local cold injury, which activities and statements are true?

  1. Immerse the affected part in a warm-water bath (100° to 105° F).
  2. Immerse the affected part in a tepid-water bath (no warmer than body temperature).
  3. Immerse the affected part in a hot-water bath (105° to 110° F).
  4. The water bath container must be large enough to allow the injured area to be fully immersed without touching the bottom or sides of the container.
  5. Continuously stir the water, replacing it when it cools below the desired water bath temperature.
  6. Expect the patient to complain of moderate to severe pain throughout the thawing process.
  7. Continue the water bath until the part is soft, with return of color and sensation.
  8. After thawing, gently dry the area and dress with dry, sterile dressings.

9. After thawing, keep the part moist by covering with sterile saline-soaked dressings.
10. If the hands and/or feet are involved, place dressings between fingers and toes.
11. Protect against refreezing of the injured part.

(a) 2, 4, 5, 6, 7, 9, 10, and 11
(b) 2, 4, 5, 6, 7, 8, 10, and 11
(c) 1, 4, 5, 6, 7, 8, 10, and 11
(d) 1, 4, 5, 6, 7, 9, 10, and 11
(e) 3, 4, 5, 6, 7, 9, 10, and 11

236. Of the following list of statements regarding patients with special susceptibility to heat injuries, which statements are true about elderly patients?

1. These patients always cause their own heat injuries, because they are always turning up the furnace thermostat.
2. These patients cannot remove their own clothing to compensate for increased heat.
3. These patients are always complaining of being too hot, when (in reality) they do *not* have a heat-related problem or injury. They simply cannot feel any temperature sensation other than that of being "too hot," even when they are in a cool environment. They are actually much more susceptible to hy**po**thermia than they are to hy**per**thermia.
4. These patients have poor thermoregulation abilities.
5. These patients may be on medications that inhibit their ability to respond to temperature regulation needs.
6. These patients may lack mobility and may not be able to escape from a hot environment.
7. These patients always should be considered more susceptible to heat injury.

(a) 1, 4, 5, 6, and 7 only.
(b) 1, 2, 3, 5, and 6 only.
(c) 4, 5, 6, and 7 only.
(d) 1, 5, 6, and 7 only.
(e) 1, 3, and 5 only.

237. Of the following statements regarding heat injuries, which statements are true?

1. High ambient temperature reduces the body's ability to lose heat by radiation.
2. High ambient temperature increases the body's ability to lose heat by conduction.
3. In a still environment, high relative humidity reduces the body's ability to lose heat through evaporation.
4. In a still environment, high relative humidity increases the body's ability to lose heat through convection.
5. Exercise and activity can cause the loss of more than 1 liter of sweat per hour, which may result in a form of hypovolemic shock.
6. Exercise and activity can cause the loss of fluid but protects the body from heat injury because of rapid movement.

   (a) 1, 2, 3, 4, and 6.
   (b) 1, 4, and 6.
   (c) 2, 3, and 6.
   (d) 1, 3, and 5.
   (e) 1, 4, and 5.

238. From the same list of statements regarding patients with special susceptibility to heat injuries that accompanies question 237, which statements are true about newborns and infants?

   (a) 2, 6, and 7 only.
   (b) 2, 4, 6, and 7 only.
   (c) 2, 5, 6, and 7 only.
   (d) 1, 3, and 5 only.
   (e) 2, 3, 6, and 7 only.

239. Once upon a time, heat emergencies were divided into three categories: Heat Cramps, Heat Exhaustion, and Heat Stroke. The signs and symptoms that accompany the condition sometimes called "Heat Cramps" are now classified as the heat emergency called

   (a) Patient with Warm, Dry, Pink Skin.
   (b) Patient with Moist, Pale, Normal to Cool Skin temperature.
   (c) Patient with Hot, Dry, or Moist Skin.
   (d) Either answer (a) or (c).
   (e) Either answer (b) or (c).

240. The signs and symptoms that accompany the condition sometimes called "Heat Exhaustion" are now classified as the heat emergency called

   (a) Patient with Warm, Dry, Pink Skin.
   (b) Patient with Moist, Pale, Normal to Cool Skin temperature.

(c) Patient with Hot, Dry, or Moist Skin.
(d) Either answer (a) or (c).
(e) Either answer (b) or (c).

241. The signs and symptoms that accompany the condition sometimes called "Heat Stroke" are now classified as the heat emergency called

(a) Patient with Warm, Dry, Pink Skin.
(b) Patient with Moist, Pale, Normal to Cool Skin temperature.
(c) Patient with Hot, Dry, or Moist Skin.
(d) Either answer (a) or (c).
(e) Either answer (b) or (c).

242. Which of the following signs and symptoms may be exhibited by a patient suffering from the condition sometimes called "Heat Exhaustion"?

1. Altered mental status
2. Dizziness or faintness
3. Excitement and euphoria
4. Heavy perspiration (called *diaphoresis*)
5. Hot, dry, or moist skin
6. Little or no perspiration
7. Moist, pale skin of normal to cool temperature
8. Muscular cramping (most often in the legs or abdomen)
9. Rapid pulse
10. Rapid, shallow respirations
11. Seizure activity
12. Shivering
13. Unconsciousness
14. Warm, dry, and pink skin
15. Weakness or exhaustion

(a) 1, 2, 3, 5, 6, 9, 12, and 15 only.
(b) 1, 2, 5, 6, 9, 10, 11, 13, and 15 only.
(c) 3, 7, 8, 12, 14, and 15 only.
(d) 1, 2, 4, 7, 8, 9, 10, 13, and 15 only.
(e) 2, 5, 6, 8, 9, and 10 only.

243. Which of the signs and symptoms listed for question 242 would most commonly be exhibited by a patient suffering from the condition sometimes called "Heat Stroke"?

(a) 1, 2, 3, 5, 6, 9, 12, and 15 only.
(b) 1, 2, 5, 6, 9, 10, 11, 13, and 15 only.
(c) 3, 7, 8, 12, 14, and 15 only.
(d) 2, 4, 7, 8, 9, 10, and 15 only.
(e) 2, 5, 6, 8, 9, and 10 only.

244. Which of the following methods of emergency care should be employed for the patient suffering from the condition sometimes called "Heat Exhaustion"?

1. Administer oxygen by nonrebreather mask at 15 liters per minute.
2. Withhold oxygen administration; none is needed.
3. Apply cold packs to the patient's forehead, but keep the patient lightly covered with warm blankets to prevent a rebound hypothermic reaction.
4. Apply cold packs to the patient's neck, groin, and armpits.
5. Cool the patient by light fanning only.
6. Cool the patient by aggressive fanning.
7. Delay transport to immerse the patient in water containing several bags of ice (keeping head and neck above the water line). Rapid cooling is more important than rapid transport.
8. If transport cannot be immediately arranged, find a tub or similar container and immerse the patient in cool water (keeping head and neck above the water line).
9. Even when the patient's mechanism of injury does **not** suggest spinal trauma, immobilize the patient on a long backboard for spinal injury precautions.
10. If the patient is responsive and not nauseated, have the patient drink water.
11. If the patient is unresponsive or nauseated, trickle only small amounts of water under her/his tongue.
12. If the patient is nauseated or unresponsive, withhold oral fluids and transport with the patient on her/his left side.
13. Keep the patient's skin wet by sponging with water or applying wet towels to her/his entire body.
14. Loosen or remove only constrictive or warm clothing.
15. Place patient in supine position with feet elevated and keep her/him at rest.
16. Remove the patient from the hot environment and place in a cool environment (such as an air-conditioned ambulance).
17. Remove all of the patient's clothing.
18. Transport the patient without any delay.

   (a) 1, 4, 6, 8, 12, 13, 15, 16, 17, and 18 only.
   (b) 2, 3, 6, 9, 13, 16, and 18 only.
   (c) 2, 3, 10, 12, 14, 15, 16, and 18 only.
   (d) 1, 4, 6, 7, 9, 12, 16, and 18 only.
   (e) 1, 5, 10, 12, 14, 15, 16, and 18 only.

245. Which of the methods of emergency care listed for question 244 should be employed for the patient suffering from the condition sometimes called "Heat Stroke"?

    (a) 1, 4, 6, 8, 12, 13, 15, 16, 17, and 18 only.
    (b) 2, 3, 6, 9, 13, 16, and 18 only.
    (c) 2, 3, 10, 12, 14, 15, 16, and 18 only.
    (d) 1, 4, 6, 7, 9, 12, 16, and 18 only.
    (e) 1, 5, 10, 12, 14, 15, 16, and 18 only.

AUTHORS' NOTE: You may resume timing your performance now.

246. The term **near-drowning** can be applied to any patient who was submerged in water,

    (a) but did not lose consciousness.
    (b) lost consciousness, but had a pulse when removed from the water.
    (c) was unconscious, was not breathing, and was pulseless when removed from the water, but was resuscitated after removal.
    (d) Answer (b) or (c) only.
    (e) Answers (a), (b), and/or (c).

247. Which of the following statements regarding drowning and near-drowning emergencies is false?

    (a) If you have not been trained in (and/or are not equipped for) deep water rescue, do not, under **any** circumstances, attempt a deep water rescue.
    (b) To rescue a victim, untrained personnel may enter shallow ponds or pools (for example, rescuer-waist-deep only) that have a known depth and a uniform bottom.
    (c) Any pulseless, nonbreathing patient who has been submerged in cold water should receive all resuscitation efforts.
    (d) Both answers (b) and (c) are false.
    (e) None of the above are false.

248. Which of the following statements regarding emergency medical care of drowning and near-drowning victims is true?

    (a) Every unconscious drowning or near-drowning patient should be considered to have a spinal injury (even one retrieved from only a shallow pond or pool).
    (b) If a diving or boating accident is involved, the conscious victim should be considered to have a spinal injury.
    (c) In-line immobilization and use of a long backboard (or the like) are required for removing all unconscious patients from the water.
    (d) Only answers (b) and (c) are true.
    (e) All of the above are true.

249. An unconscious near-drowning victim

(a) may have only a small amount of water in her/his lungs.
(b) will always have a large amount of water in her/his lungs.
(c) may or may not have a large amount of water in her/his stomach.
(d) Both answers (a) and (c).
(e) Both answers (b) and (c).

250. Which of the following statements regarding emergency medical care of drowning and near-drowning victims is false?

(a) If there is no suspected spine injury, the EMT should place the conscious patient on her/his left side to allow water, vomitus, and secretions to drain away from the upper airway.
(b) The EMT should administer oxygen in high concentrations and suction the patient as needed.
(c) Abdominal pressure to manually relieve gastric distention is always contraindicated (forcing evacuation of stomach contents will result in aspiration of the contents and cause death).
(d) If gastric distention interferes with artificial ventilation, the patient should be logrolled to her/his left side. With suction immediately available, the EMT should place her/his hand over the epigastric area of the patient's abdomen and apply firm pressure to relieve the distention.
(e) Rescue breathing may be performed in the water, but chest compressions are effective only after removal from the water.

251. A patient who has become apneic (nonbreathing) and pulseless while submerged in

(a) cold water also will have severe hypothermia. Thus, it is highly unlikely that the patient can be successfully resuscitated.
(b) cold water has a better chance of successfully responding to resuscitation efforts than a victim from a warm water submersion of equal time (even when in respiratory and cardiac arrest for up to 30 minutes of cold water submersion).
(c) warm water has a much better chance of successfully responding to resuscitation efforts than a cold water submersion victim, because severe hypothermia will not have occurred.
(d) Either answer (a) or (c).
(e) None of the above.

252. Which of the following signs and symptoms are common to most bites or stings from poisonous animals or insects?

(a) Bite marks or stinger puncture sites with pain, redness, and/or swelling at the site.
(b) Chills and/or fever.
(c) Nausea and vomiting, weakness, and/or dizziness.
(d) Only answers (a) and (c).
(e) Answers (a), (b), and (c).

TEST SECTION FOUR

253. Which of the following statements regarding emergency care of an insect sting, with the stinger still present, is true?

(a) Use tweezers or forceps to grasp and remove the stinger as soon as possible (before additional poison is injected).
(b) With gloves on, use your thumb and forefinger to squeeze the site from either side and expel the stinger. Wipe the loosened stinger from the site with a sterile 4 X 4 (do not pinch the stinger to pick it up because it may penetrate your glove!).
(c) Scrape the stinger from the site using the edge of a plastic card (credit cards or automated teller machine cards work nicely).
(d) Both answers (a) and (b) are true.
(e) None of the above are true. The stinger should be left in place (and the site dressed) until a physician can determine the appropriate removal technique.

254. From the following selection of emergency care measures, select those that are appropriate (true) for the treatment of snake or insect bites and stings.

1. Apply constricting bands above and below the bite/sting site.
2. Apply a cold pack to the site (especially if it is a snake bite).
3. Consult the medical director regarding the use of constricting bands for extremity injury sites.
4. Splint and elevate the injured extremity (above the level of the patient's heart) to prevent excessive swelling.
5. Gently cleanse the bite or sting area with soap and water (or the like).
6. If constricting bands are authorized, they should be applied tightly enough to stop the patient's pulse in that limb (if a pulse is still present beyond the band, the blood is still circulating the poison to the heart—increase the band's tightness).
7. Observe for signs and symptoms of allergic reaction (or anaphylaxis) and treat as directed.
8. Oxygen should be administered only if the patient is complaining of shortness of breath.
9. Splint and place the wounded extremity slightly below the level of the patient's heart.
10. Remove jewelry from beyond the injured area.
11. Treat the patient for shock (including oxygen administration), even if "shock" signs and symptoms are not present.

(a) 3, 5, 7, 9, 10, and 11 only.
(b) 3, 4, 6, 7, 8, and 9 only.
(c) 2, 4, 5, 7, and 10 only.
(d) 2, 4, 5, 7, 10, and 11 only.
(e) 1, 5, 6, 7, 8, 9, and 10 only.

255. Which of the following statements best describes a ***behavioral emergency***?

(a) When the patient is acting in a manner that she/he (the patient) considers to be abnormal, unacceptable, intolerable or dangerous (to herself/himself or others).
(b) When the patient is acting in a manner that the patient's family considers to be abnormal, unacceptable, intolerable, or dangerous (to the patient or others).
(c) When the patient is acting in a manner that community members consider to be abnormal, unacceptable, intolerable, or dangerous (to the patient or others).
(d) Only answers (b) and (c).
(e) Answers (a), (b), and (c).

256. Common medical (nonpsychiatric) causes for abnormal behavior changes include all of the following, except

(a) low blood sugar and/or lack of oxygen.
(b) psychosis (hallucinations and/or delusions), mania, and/or severe depression.
(c) head trauma and/or inadequate blood flow to the brain.
(d) drug or alcohol use (use of any mind-altering substances).
(e) excessive cold or excessive heat.

257. Which of the following signs and symptoms is least likely to be exhibited by a patient who does not have any medical problems but is experiencing a psychological crisis?

(a) A slow heart rate and/or low blood pressure.
(b) Panic and/or agitation.
(c) Bizarre thinking (delusions) and/or bizarre behavior.
(d) Comments or activities suggesting suicidal or self-destructive thinking.
(e) Comments or activities suggesting dangerousness or homicidal thinking.

258. Which of the following factors (or situations) may be considered risk factors for developing self-destructive behavior or suicidal ideas?

1. An individual over the age of 40.
2. An unmarried individual.
3. Persons who have lost their spouse through divorce or death.
4. A person with an alcohol-abuse problem.
5. A person who can verbalize a specific, lethal plan of action.

TEST SECTION FOUR

6. A person who gathers articles such as guns or large volumes of pills.
7. A patient with a previous history of self-destructive behavior.
8. A patient who recently has been diagnosed with a serious illness.
9. A person who recently has lost a loved one.
10. Someone who recently has lost her/his job.
11. A person placed under arrest and/or imprisoned.

   (a) 3, 4, 5, 6, 7, 8, 9, and 10 only.
   (b) 3, 5, 6, 7, 8, 9, and 11 only.
   (c) 1, 2, 3, 4, 5, 6, 7, 8, 9, 10, and 11.
   (d) 1, 3, 5, 6, 7, 8, 9, and 11 only.
   (e) 2, 3, 5, 6, 7, 8, 9, and 11 only.

259. When initially assessing a patient who appears to be having a behavioral emergency, the EMT should ask all except which of the following questions?

   (a) Could the patient's behavior be the result of a medical problem?
   (b) Is it safe for me to be here with this patient, or should I leave?
   (c) What is the quickest way to restrain this patient so that we can get back in service?
   (d) Is the patient a threat to herself/himself or others?
   (e) How does this patient feel?

260. Which of the following statements regarding behavioral emergency medical and legal considerations is false?

   (a) Any person acting in any type of unusual manner can easily be legally arrested by the police and treated against her/his will. If in doubt, have the police arrest the patient.
   (b) If you can convince an emotionally disturbed patient to consent to treatment, the risk of legal difficulties will be greatly reduced.
   (c) To provide care against a patient's will, you must show a reasonable belief that the patient would harm herself/himself or others if treatment were not rendered.
   (d) A patient who is acting in a manner that suggests a threat to herself/himself and/or others may be transported and treated against her/his will after contacting the medical director and/or after obtaining law enforcement's assistance.
   (e) Emotionally disturbed patients often resist treatment and frequently pose a threat to the safety of EMTs and others.

261. Which of the following statements regarding the use of force when restraining a patient for the purpose of treatment against the patient's consent is false?

(a) EMS personnel may use any reasonable force to defend against an attack by emotionally disturbed patients.
(b) EMS personnel should make every effort to avoid the use of physical force that may result in patient injury.
(c) Once a restrained patient is calm and acting rationally, there is no longer a risk of danger to herself/himself or others, so restraints must be removed. Additionally, it is unlawful to continue the use of restraints after a patient has become calm and cooperative.
(d) An EMT should seek medical direction and/or police assistance when considering the use of restraints on a patient.
(e) None of the above are false.

262. Which of the following methods for calming behavioral emergency patients are rarely ever helpful (false)?

(a) Specifically verbalize your observations to the patient and repeatedly assure her/him that you are there to help. For example, if the patient appears upset, you should say something to the effect of "I can hear (or see) that you are upset. How can I help you?"
(b) Avoid saying anything that you believe might upset and/or further agitate the patient. If this means having to lie to the patient, then a small amount of lying is acceptable (but only to avoid conflict).
(c) Always inform the patient of what you intend to do before you do it.
(d) Maintain a comfortable distance from the patient.
(e) Do not make any rapid or quick moves.

263. Which of the following methods for calming behavioral emergency patients are rarely ever helpful (false)?

(a) Do not threaten, challenge, or argue with emotionally disturbed patients.
(b) Tell the truth at all times. Never lie to a patient.
(c) If the patient is experiencing visual or auditory hallucinations, "play along" with the patient's abnormal perceptions (this provides a sense of "agreement" on your part and quickly wins the patient's confidence and cooperation).
(d) When family members or friends are present (and are calm and in control of their own emotions), encourage their participation in convincing the patient to consent to treatment and transport.
(e) Be prepared to remain on the scene for an extended length of time. Unless your safety is threatened, you should always remain with the patient.

264. Which of the following statements regarding restraint of patients is false?

(a) Restraint should be avoided unless the patient's behavior represents a danger to herself/himself and/or others.
(b) Before initiating restraints, get approval from the medical director and/or have the police present to assist.
(c) Even if you don't have an adequate number of people available to safely restrain the patient, you have no choice but to risk proceeding with inadequate assistance (you cannot allow the patient to continue her/his abnormal behavior).
(d) Use only the amount of force necessary to apply the restraints safely.
(e) Only one EMT should talk to the patient throughout the entire restraining procedure, reassuring the patient of safety, and encouraging the patient to understand that the restraints are for the patient's safety and care.

265. There are general rules for appropriate and successful communication with emotionally disturbed patients. Which of the following statements does not represent one of these generally accepted and appropriate communication rules?

(a) Always make every effort to convince the patient to willingly allow treatment.
(b) Maintain a calm, nonthreatening attitude and treat the patient with respect.
(c) Avoid arguing with irrational patients, but do not agree with any of the patient's disturbed thinking or perceptions.
(d) Threaten the patient with arrest and/or restraint. This may obtain the patient's cooperation without force. But this should be done only if you have sufficient force to support the threat.
(e) Reassure the patient and remove or diminish any potentially distressing external stimuli (such as large numbers of people or extraneous noise).

266. The term _____ is the medical term for the developing unborn baby.

(a) zygote
(b) fetus
(c) ovum
(d) spermatozoa
(e) uterus

267. The term _____ is the medical term for the organ in which the developing unborn baby grows. It is also responsible for labor and expulsion of the infant.

  (a) placenta
  (b) vagina
  (c) cervix
  (d) abdomen
  (e) uterus

268. The actual **birth canal** consists of the lower part of the uterus and

  (a) the vagina.
  (b) the cervix.
  (c) the placenta.
  (d) Both answers (b) and (c).
  (e) None of the above (the birth canal is a completely separate organ).

269. The **placenta** is best defined as

  (a) the organ in which the developing unborn baby grows.
  (b) the bag of waters in which a baby develops.
  (c) the organ through which the unborn baby exchanges nourishment and waste products during pregnancy.
  (d) the cushion that protects the unborn baby from harm.
  (e) the organ that seals the bottom of the womb, to prevent premature expulsion of the developing baby.

270. The **umbilical cord** is best defined as

  (a) the "anchor" that attaches the developing baby to the mother's abdomen (preventing premature expulsion).
  (b) the "anchor" that attaches the developing baby to the mother's placenta (preventing premature expulsion).
  (c) an organ that creates its own oxygenated blood cells to "ventilate" the developing baby until its lungs are functional.
  (d) a cord that acts as an extension of the placenta, through which the developing baby receives nourishment while in the womb.
  (e) None of the above.

271. The _____ is the medical term for a container, within the womb, that surrounds the developing baby. This container floats the baby in about one to two quarts of fluid, cushioning the baby against trauma. The common term for this container is the "bag of waters."

  (a) amniotic sac
  (b) placental sac

(c) vaginal sack
(d) uterine sack
(e) cervical sac

272. The lower part of the birth canal is called the

(a) uterus.
(b) placenta.
(c) hymen.
(d) fallopian tube.
(e) vagina.

273. The area of skin between the vaginal opening and the anus is often torn during delivery. This area of skin is called the

(a) hymen.
(b) perineum.
(c) cervix.
(d) genitalia.
(e) "no man's land" (because the EMT is not to touch it).

274. The term (or phrase) _____ refers to when the vagina appears to "bulge out," because the first portion of the infant is pressing against the opening.

(a) breech presentation
(b) pushing phase
(c) bloody show
(d) crowning
(e) caudal presentation

275. Technically, labor is divided into three (sometimes four) stages. As a whole, however, the entire process of *labor* is best defined as beginning when

(a) contractions are three minutes apart.
(b) the first uterine contraction is felt.
(c) the vagina begins to bulge out.
(d) "bloody show" is controlled.
(e) the uterus begins to bulge out.

276. The entire process of *labor* is best defined as ending when the

(a) baby is delivered.
(b) amniotic sac is broken.
(c) placenta is delivered.
(d) hymen is perforated or torn.
(e) postpartum bleeding is controlled.

277. The medical phrase **presenting part** is best defined as

    (a) the delivery of the placenta.
    (b) the appearance of the infant's head in the vaginal opening.
    (c) the part of the infant that first appears in the vaginal opening.
    (d) Either answer (a) or (b).
    (e) Either answer (a) or (c).

278. The medical term **crowning** is best defined as

    (a) the breaking of the bag of waters.
    (b) the bulging caused at the vaginal opening by the infant's presenting part.
    (c) the stage of labor when the mother needs to push.
    (d) Either answer (a) or (c).
    (e) None of the above.

279. The phrase **bloody show** refers to

    (a) the excessive amount of bleeding that accompanies normal childbirth (up to four liters of blood).
    (b) the breaking of the bag of waters.
    (c) the stage of labor when the mother needs to push and begins to bleed heavily.
    (d) a small vaginal discharge of blood-tinged, watery mucus that may occur as labor begins.
    (e) the delivery of the placenta.

280. The medical term **miscarriage** is best defined as

    (a) the delivery of products of conception early in a pregnancy.
    (b) the spontaneous termination of a pregnancy.
    (c) the induced termination of a pregnancy.
    (d) Either answer (a) or (b).
    (e) Either answer (a), (b), or (c).

281. The medical term **abortion** is best defined as

    (a) the delivery of products of conception early in a pregnancy.
    (b) the spontaneous termination of a pregnancy.
    (c) the induced termination of a pregnancy.
    (d) Either answer (a) or (b).
    (e) Either answer (a), (b), or (c).

282. Emergency care for a miscarriage includes all of the following, except

    (a) obtaining baseline vital signs.
    (b) treatment based on signs and symptoms.

(c) application of an external vaginal pad (the EMT must not actually pack the vagina).
(d) close inspection of conception or fetal tissues passed into the toilet prior to flushing them (the EMT must be able to clearly describe the tissues observed).
(e) emotional support of the mother.

283. Which of the following statements regarding seizures in pregnancy are true?

(a) Seizures are not related to any aspect of pregnancy. Only a patient who already has a seizure disorder may have seizures when pregnant.
(b) Low blood pressure is associated with seizures in pregnancy.
(c) Seizures cause a serious life-threat only to the unborn baby.
(d) Both answers (a) and (c) are true.
(e) None of the above are true.

284. Emergency care for the seizing pregnant woman includes

(a) airway maintenance and high-flow oxygen.
(b) positioning the patient on her right side.
(c) assisting the patient to take her prescribed seizure medication.
(d) Only answers (a) and (c).
(e) Answers (a), (b), and (c).

285. Vaginal bleeding

(a) may occur early or late in pregnancy.
(b) will always be accompanied by pain if an emergency exists.
(c) may not be accompanied by pain, even if an emergency exists.
(d) Both answers (a) and (b).
(e) Both answers (a) and (c).

286. Emergency care for vaginal bleeding includes

(a) obtaining the patient's medical and gynecological history, performing a physical examination, and obtaining baseline vital signs.
(b) treatment based on signs and symptoms of shock, high-flow oxygen, and transportation to an emergency department.
(c) devising a direct-pressure bandage for the vagina, to include "packing" the vagina with vaginal pads to occlude bleeding. Packing is often required because the bleeding must be stopped.
(d) Only answers (a) and (b).
(e) Answers (a), (b), and (c).

287. Which of the following statements regarding emergency medical care for the pregnant trauma patient is false?

(a) Trauma care for pregnant patients is basically the same as for any other patients.
(b) Perform a standard initial assessment and physical examination; obtain the patient's history and baseline vital signs.
(c) Transport the patient on her right side. If the patient requires spinal immobilization, secure the patient to a long backboard, then elevate the left side of the board to cause the patient's abdomen to shift its weight to the right side.
(d) Both answers (a) and (c) are false.
(e) None of the above are false.

288. Timing of contraction duration and frequency is important. Contraction duration is measured from the time of a contraction's beginning to the time of that contraction's end (when the uterus relaxes). The frequency (or interval) of contractions is measured by timing from

(a) the end of one contraction to the beginning of the next contraction (from end to beginning).
(b) the beginning of one contraction to the beginning of the next contraction (from start to start).
(c) the beginning of one contraction to the end of that contraction (from start to finish).
(d) Any of the above timing methods are acceptable.
(e) None of the above timing methods are correct.

289. Which of the following signs, symptoms, and patient history factors may be noted at any time during labor and are of little value when assessing the likelihood of imminent delivery (delivery within the next 10 minutes)?

1. A patient who previously has delivered 3 children.
2. A patient who insists that "the baby is coming now!"
3. A patient with no previous pregnancies or deliveries.
4. Contractions are lasting 30 seconds to 1 minute in duration and are occurring every 2 to 3 minutes.
5. Contractions have just started, last less than 20 seconds, and are 5 to 10 minutes apart.
6. The "bag of waters" has already broken.
7. The "bag of waters" has not broken yet.
8. The infant is crowning.
9. The infant is not crowning.
10. The patient complains of needing to move her bowels.

11. The patient describes having had a small, watery vaginal discharge soon after the onset of contractions.
12. The patient strongly feels the need to push.

   (a) 6, 7, and 11.
   (b) 1, 2, 4, 8, 10, and 12.
   (c) 3, 5, and 9.
   (d) 3, 5, 7, and 11.
   (e) 2, 7, and 11.

290. Which of question number 289's signs, symptoms, and patient history factors indicate a patient who is unlikely to be delivering her baby within the next 10 minutes?

   (a) 6, 7, and 11.
   (b) 1, 2, 4, 8, 10, and 12.
   (c) 3, 5, and 9.
   (d) 3, 5, 7, and 11.
   (e) 2, 7, and 11.

291. Which of question number 289's signs, symptoms, and patient history factors indicate a patient who is highly likely to be delivering her baby within the next 10 minutes?

   (a) 6, 7, and 11.
   (b) 1, 2, 4, 8, 10, and 12.
   (c) 3, 5, and 9.
   (d) 3, 5, 7, and 11.
   (e) 2, 7, and 11.

292. Which of the following statements regarding the decision to remain on scene to assist with the delivery of a baby is true?

   (a) If the mother absolutely insists on going to the bathroom before delivery, escort her.
   (b) Delivery should never be allowed to occur at home, even when it appears imminent. Carry the patient to the ambulance and, if necessary, assist with the delivery while continuing to drive to the hospital.
   (c) If the decision is made to delay transport and assist with a home delivery, be prepared for a long stay. You may be required to remain on scene for up to 30 or 40 minutes before being able to transport the mother and newborn.
   (d) Both answers (a) and (c) are true.
   (e) None of the above are true.

293. When the infant's head begins to emerge, place your fingers

   (a) within the vaginal opening on either side of the infant's head so that you may gently grasp the infant's jaws (as in the jaw-thrust airway maneuver). Apply gentle traction to speed the delivery in a controlled manner.
   (b) around the bony parts of the infant's exposed skull (avoiding the face and the skull's soft spot) and apply evenly distributed, gentle traction to speed the delivery in a controlled manner.
   (c) at a distance from the infant's skull and the mother's vaginal area, forming a "cup" with which to "catch" the infant's head and prevent trauma.
   (d) on the bony parts of the infant's exposed skull (avoiding the face and the skull's soft spot), applying evenly distributed, gentle pressure to prevent an explosive delivery.
   (e) at your sides! Mothers have been delivering babies without assistance since time began. Occupy yourself by recording this moment as the official time of birth.

294. If the "bag of waters" has not already broken by the time the infant's head is being delivered,

   (a) instruct the mother to stop pushing and to hold her legs together. Immediately remove her to the ambulance for rapid transport to the emergency department.
   (b) use a sterile scalpel to carefully puncture the sac and pull all of the sac tissues away from the baby's face and head.
   (c) use your fingers to pinch and puncture the sac, pulling the sac tissues away from the baby's mouth and nose.
   (d) do not attempt to break it. The membrane will break on its own, at the appropriate time. Simply continue with the delivery.
   (e) have the mother reach down and break the sac. (EMTs who break membranes are often charged with negligence.)

295. As the infant's head completes its delivery, determine if the umbilical cord is around the infant's neck. If the cord is around the infant's neck,

   (a) gently loosen it before sliding it over the infant's upper shoulder and head. If the cord will not loosen, securely clamp it in two places, carefully cut the cord between the clamps, and then gently remove the cord from around the infant's neck.
   (b) instruct the mother to stop pushing and to hold her legs together. Immediately remove her to the ambulance for rapid transport to the emergency department.

(c) immediately sever the cord using a sterile scalpel; then continue with the delivery. Blood loss from the severed cord will not affect the mother or the infant.
(d) suction the infant at once and stimulate the infant to begin breathing. Leave the cord in place and continue the delivery.
(e) immediately clamp the cord and then suction the infant to stimulate breathing. Leave the clamped cord in place and continue the delivery.

296. After the infant's head is born, support the head and suction the infant's

(a) nose, once or twice in each nostril. Then suction the mouth two or three times.
(b) nose, once in each nostril, before suctioning the mouth once. Repeat this process, in this order, as needed until the infant's airway is clear.
(c) mouth two or three times. Then suction the nose, once or twice for each nostril.
(d) nose only (infants are "nose breathers").
(e) mouth only (infants are "mouth breathers").

297. After the infant is completely delivered,

(a) perform the time-honored "smack on the bottom" to initiate breathing. Invert the baby, holding it firmly by the feet (infants are slippery; be careful), and slap the baby's buttocks once or twice.
(b) wrap the infant in a warm blanket and place it on its side with the head slightly lower than the trunk to allow for drainage.
(c) if the umbilical cord has not been cut, keep the baby level with the vagina.
(d) Only answers (b) and (c).
(e) Answers (a), (b), and (c).

298. The procedure for severing the umbilical cord for a normally delivered baby includes

(a) waiting until the baby is breathing on its own and the cord no longer has a pulse.
(b) placing the farthest clamp approximately 3 inches beyond the closest clamp, which should be about 4 finger widths away from the baby.
(c) placing the farthest clamp approximately 3 inches beyond the closest clamp, which should be about 10 inches away from the baby.
(d) Both answers (a) and (b).
(e) Both answers (a) and (c).

299. The umbilical cord normally should be severed

   (a) beyond the farthest clamp (blood samples will be obtained using the section of cord between the clamps).
   (b) in between the two clamps (thus, the closest clamp must be far enough away from the baby to allow for blood sample work or IV access to be performed on the section that remains with the baby).
   (c) in the emergency department. Do not cut the cord in the field.
   (d) before the baby is wrapped in a dry blanket (bleeding from the cut end may soil the blanket).
   (e) by the mother (EMTs who cut cords are often charged with negligence).

300. Bleeding from the umbilical cord beyond the clamp nearest to the baby

   (a) is normal and may continue for 30 to 45 minutes.
   (b) is a serious emergency and is the reason EMTs are not allowed to cut the umbilical cord in the field.
   (c) should be controlled by immediately removing the clamp (or umbilical tape tie) and reapplying it closer to the baby, in a slightly tighter manner.
   (d) should be controlled by immediately applying an additional clamp (or umbilical tape tie) as close to the first one as possible, in a slightly tighter manner.
   (e) should be controlled by removing the clamp, squeezing the excess blood out of the cord (beginning at the baby's end), and reapplying the clamp at the cord end.

301. Delivery of the placenta

   (a) is not an EMT function for field deliveries. Transport the patient to the emergency department prior to placenta delivery. Have the mother keep her legs together, and use transport with "lights and sirens" if placental delivery appears imminent.
   (b) may occur soon after delivery of the infant. EMTs may wait on scene for up to 20 minutes for placental delivery. If placental delivery doesn't occur by then, transport the patient. Placental delivery may or may not occur en route to the emergency department.

(c) must occur, but will not occur unless the EMT applies aggressive pressure to the uterus (over the abdomen). This pressure should be provided immediately after the baby's delivery and continued in an aggressive manner until the placenta is delivered.
(d) is a natural occurrence that always immediately follows childbirth. Closely observe the delivered placenta before disposing of it, and then transport mother and child to the emergency department.
(e) is required before transportation of the mother can be accomplished. Until the placenta delivers, do not, for any reason, move the mother. Doing so may increase the mother's blood loss and pose a significant risk of death. If necessary, summon another vehicle to transport the newborn infant, while waiting on scene with the mother for placental delivery.

302. Once the placenta is delivered,
(a) place it in a container or towel and put both in a plastic bag (or paper bag, if plastic is not readily available) for transport to the hospital with the mother and child. All placental tissues must accompany the mother to the hospital.
(b) the patient may finally be transported to the emergency department. Closely observe the amount of tissue passed and record your findings, prior to proper disposal of the placenta (flushing it down the toilet) and leaving the scene.
(c) the patient may finally be transported. If the infant was not transported earlier than the mother, have the mother begin breast-feeding the baby while you dispose of the placenta. Then transport mother and baby.
(d) it should be discarded immediately (avoid allowing the mother to observe the placenta, as this sight is often disturbing).
(e) the EMT is subject to charges of negligence.

303. After delivery of the baby and/or the placenta, emergency care for the mother includes all of the following, except
(a) vigorous soap and water cleansing of the vaginal opening to prevent infection (especially if any tearing of the mother's genitalia occurred during delivery).
(b) placing a sterile pad over the vaginal opening.
(c) lowering the mother's legs and helping her keep them together ("squeezing" the legs together is not necessary).
(d) assisting with control of postdelivery bleeding by massaging the mother's uterus (massaging the mother's abdomen).
(e) assisting control of postdelivery bleeding by allowing the mother to nurse the baby (only if she desires to do so).

304. Which of the following statements regarding vaginal bleeding following delivery is false?

(a) Blood loss after delivery is common and does not threaten the mother's well-being. Up to 500 cc of blood loss is well tolerated and should not cause undue psychological stress to the EMT or mother.
(b) Blood loss after delivery is common and does not threaten the mother's well-being. Up to 2,000 cc (2 liters) of blood loss is well tolerated and should not cause undue psychological stress to the EMT or mother.
(c) If blood loss is excessive, the EMT should massage the uterus (massage the abdomen).
(d) Regardless of estimated blood loss, if the mother appears to be in shock (hypoperfusion), the EMT should treat her for shock and transport her to a hospital prior to uterine massage. Massage may occur en route.
(e) If bleeding continues despite uterine massage, check the massage technique and transport the patient immediately, providing oxygen and treatment for shock, in addition to ongoing assessments.

305. Initial care of the newborn includes all of the following, except

(a) wrapping in a warm, dry blanket and covering the infant's head to conserve heat.
(b) positioning the infant on its side, level with the vagina, until the umbilical cord is cut.
(c) repeated suctioning as needed.
(d) the traditional inverted-buttocks spanking (tactile stimulation) to encourage the baby to breathe.
(e) flicking the soles of the infant's feet or rubbing the infant's back (tactile stimulation) to encourage breathing if the baby doesn't spontaneously breath or cry.

306. Place all of the following emergency care measures in their preferred order of performance, as specified by the **inverted pyramid** of newborn resuscitation.

1. Application of oxygen
2. Bag-valve-mask ventilation
3. Chest compressions
4. Drying, warming, positioning, suction, and tactile stimulation
5. Endotracheal intubation
6. Medications

(a) 1, 2, 3, 5, 6, and 4.
(b) 4, 1, 2, 3, 5, and 6.
(c) 1, 4, 2, 3, 5, and 5.
(d) 6, 1, 2, 3, 5, and 4.
(e) 5, 1, 2, 3, 6, and 4.

307. A newborn infant should begin breathing spontaneously within _____ second(s) of delivery. If it does not, tactile stimulation of breathing should be performed.

(a) 1
(b) 5
(c) 7
(d) 30
(e) 60

308. A newborn infant's breathing is considered to be "slow" only if it is below _____ times per minute.

(a) 12
(b) 12 to 20
(c) 40 to 60
(d) 60 to 100
(e) 100 to 120

309. If a newborn infant's breathing is slow, the EMT should ventilate the infant at a rate of _____ times per minute.

(a) 12
(b) 20
(c) 60
(d) 100
(e) 120

310. If artificial ventilation of a newborn infant is required, the EMT should reassess the infant's natural breathing after

(a) 30 seconds.
(b) 2 minutes.
(c) 3 minutes.
(d) 5 minutes.
(e) 10 minutes.

311. A newborn infant's heart rate is considered to be "slow" only if it is below _____ times per minute.

(a) 60
(b) 80
(c) 100
(d) 110
(e) 120

312. If a newborn infant's heart rate is slow, the EMT should
  (a) immediately begin chest compressions, with artificial ventilations.
  (b) artificially ventilate the infant for 30 seconds and then re-evaluate the infant's heart rate.
  (c) begin chest compressions only if 30 seconds of artificial ventilation has failed to encourage a heart rate above 80 beats per minute.
  (d) Both answers (b) and (c).
  (e) Do none of the above. A slow heart rate is normal for the newborn infant.

313. If the newborn infant has adequate respiration and pulse, but cyanotic feet and arms are noted, the EMT should
  (a) immediately begin chest compressions, with artificial ventilations.
  (b) artificially ventilate the infant for 30 seconds and then re-evaluate the infant's skin color.
  (c) begin chest compressions.
  (d) Both answers (b) and (c).
  (e) Do none of the above. The presence of cyanotic feet and arms is not abnormal for the newborn infant. This condition should be quickly improved by external application of passive, "blow-by," oxygenation.

314. If the newborn infant has adequate respiration and pulse, but central cyanosis (trunk, head, and extremities) is present, the EMT should
  (a) immediately begin chest compressions, with artificial ventilations.
  (b) artificially ventilate the infant for 30 seconds and then re-evaluate the infant's skin color.
  (c) begin chest compressions only if 30 seconds of artificial ventilation has failed to improve the patient's skin color.
  (d) Both answers (b) and (c).
  (e) Do none of the above. Central cyanosis, although not an optimal finding, may not be abnormal for the newborn infant. This condition should be quickly improved by external application of high-flow oxygen, administered at 10 to 15 liters per minute, using oxygen tubing held as close as possible to (but not directly aimed at) the newborn's face.

315. The condition where the umbilical cord is visible, protruding from the vaginal opening prior to the infant's delivery, is called

   (a) umbilical crowning. This condition is not unusual and does not present a concern for the normal EMT-assisted delivery.
   (b) cord crowning. This condition is not unusual and does not present a concern for the normal EMT-assisted delivery.
   (c) a prolapsed cord. This condition presents a serious emergency that endangers the life of the unborn fetus; delivery absolutely cannot be accomplished in the field. Transport the patient immediately, using lights and sirens.
   (d) a prolapsed cord. This condition, although unusual, is easily rectified in the field. If necessary, contact medical control for special delivery directions.
   (e) a prolapsed cord. Clamp the cord in two places, sever the cord between the clamps, and proceed with delivery as normal.

316. Treatment for the condition where the umbilical cord is visible, protruding from the vaginal opening prior to the infant's delivery, includes all of the following emergency care steps, except

   (a) high-flow oxygenation of the mother.
   (b) positioning the mother on her left side with her legs tightly squeezed together.
   (c) insertion of the EMT's sterile-gloved hand into the mother's vagina, to push the infant's presenting part away from the pulsating umbilical cord.
   (d) assessment of the mother's baseline vital signs.
   (e) gentle but rapid transport to the emergency department.

317. A ***breech birth*** presentation is best defined as when

   (a) the infant's head is crowning.
   (b) one of the infant's limbs protrudes from the vaginal opening.
   (c) the buttocks or both lower extremities of the infant are the first portions to present at the vaginal opening.
   (d) only when the buttocks of the infant appears as the first presenting part at the vaginal opening.
   (e) when the infant explosively delivers, head first, from the vaginal opening (accompanied by tearing or "breeching" of the mother's vaginal tissues).

318. Which of the following statements regarding a single **limb presentation** is true?

   (a) A single limb presentation birth is most commonly a foot presentation, with the infant in a breech position within the womb.
   (b) A single limb presentation birth cannot be delivered in the field. Rapidly transport the patient with her head down and her pelvis (buttocks) elevated to the emergency department.
   (c) A single limb presentation birth is most commonly an arm presentation, and can be delivered easily in the field with on-line medical direction.
   (d) Both answers (a) and (b) are true.
   (e) None of the above are true.

319. Which of the following statements regarding multiple births (twins, triplets) is true?

   (a) A multiple birth delivery cannot be accomplished in the field. If the mother knows that there is more than one fetus to be delivered, have her hold her legs together and transport her with lights and sirens to the emergency department. Do not attempt a multiple birth delivery in the field.
   (b) Multiple birth deliveries may require more than one infant resuscitation. Call for additional assistance as soon as you are aware that more than one fetus may be delivered.
   (c) Multiple birth deliveries, although more time-consuming, are no different than single birth deliveries. Simply coach the mother through both births and proceed normally.
   (d) All multiple birth deliveries in the field will involve the death of at least one of the infants. Do not be upset by this, and be prepared to counsel and support the mother when one (or more) of the infants is born dead.
   (e) None of the above are true.

320. Amniotic fluid is supposed to be clear. If it is greenish or brownish-yellow, this indicates that the fetus has expelled stool into the fluid prior to birth. It also indicates that fetal distress (or maternal distress) may have occurred during labor. The medical term for amniotic fluid that is greenish or brownish-yellow is

   (a) mercronium.
   (b) bile.
   (c) meconium.
   (d) lymph.
   (e) cronium.

321. A premature birth is defined as any infant that weighs less than 5½ pounds at birth or any infant born before the 37th week of pregnancy. Which of the following statements regarding premature newborns is false?

(a) Premature infants are always at risk for profound hypothermia (even in an environment that feels warm to the EMT).
(b) Suctioning of the premature infant's airway is particularly important. Keep the airway clear and provide oxygen without "blowing" it directly at the infant's face.
(c) Resuscitation is often required for premature infants and may be unsuccessful.
(d) All of the above are false.
(e) None of the above are false.

322. When treating a patient who has allegedly been sexually assaulted, the EMT should

(a) question the patient extensively about the assailant's description and all activities her assailant is accused of. Document these criminal information findings on the patient's official prehospital medical report.
(b) provide basic medical interventions only if the patient appears to be in serious physical shock. Otherwise, transport the patient without conversation or treatment to the closest emergency department. Avoid eye contact with the patient and never, ever document a patient as having been "sexually assaulted." This is always a patient-initiated responsibility.
(c) closely examine every allegedly sexually assaulted patient's genitals to determine if any trauma or bleeding is present or requires treatment.
(d) allow the patient time to bathe and use the toilet before requiring transportation to the emergency department for a rape examination. (This is the least you can do to provide emotional support for the physically and emotionally traumatized patient.)
(e) not allow the patient to bathe, urinate, or change clothing. In addition to all standard medical assessments, interventions, and treatment, the EMT should provide kind and nonjudgmental emotional support to the patient, regardless of any personal suspicions regarding the patient's situation.

The following 8 questions (323 through 330) are an elective group of questions about gynecological and/or obstetrical conditions, emergencies, and/or medical terminology. These questions represent information that is not DOT-required knowledge for the EMT-Basic but may be included in local or state examinations. Page numbers keyed to Brady's Emergency Care, 7th ed., are provided for these questions in the answer key.

323. The **stillborn** infant is best defined as a baby that

    (a) is delivered alive but dies within 24 hours of birth.
    (b) dies within the mother's womb several hours before delivery.
    (c) dies within the mother's womb several weeks before delivery.
    (d) Either answer (a) or (b).
    (e) Either answer (b) or (c).

324. The condition called **placenta previa** may produce vaginal bleeding without abdominal pain and is best defined as when the placenta

    (a) separates (partially or fully) from the wall of the uterus.
    (b) develops abnormally low in the uterus, partially or completely covering the opening to the uterus.
    (c) is undeveloped and unable to perform its functions.
    (d) Either answer (a) or (c).
    (e) Either answer (b) or (c).

325. The condition called **abruptio placentae** may produce abdominal pain without external (vaginal) bleeding and is best defined as when the placenta

    (a) separates (partially or fully) from the wall of the uterus.
    (b) develops abnormally low in the uterus, partially or completely covering the opening to the uterus.
    (c) is undeveloped and unable to perform its functions.
    (d) Either answer (a) or (c).
    (e) Either answer (b) or (c).

326. Which of the following statements regarding trauma and pregnancy is false?

    (a) A pregnant woman normally has a pulse rate that is 10 to 15 beats per minute slower than a nonpregnant woman.
    (b) In the late stages of pregnancy, a woman may have a blood volume that is up to 48 percent greater than a nonpregnant woman. Thus, a greater blood loss may be required before a pregnant woman shows signs of blood loss.

(c) Because pregnant women have a slower digestive tract and delayed gastric emptying, they are at greater risk for vomiting and aspiration of emesis.

(d) In the late stages of pregnancy, a woman requires 10 to 20 percent more oxygen than a nonpregnant woman.

(e) A pregnant patient should be transported on her left side. If the patient requires spinal immobilization, secure the patient to a long backboard, then elevate the right side of the board to cause the patient's abdomen to shift its weight to the left side.

327. When a pregnant woman is transported on her back, the weight of her enlarged uterus (containing the developing baby, the placenta, and the amniotic fluid) may compress the inferior vena cava and obstruct blood return to her heart. This obstruction causes classic signs and symptoms which include

(a) a severe headache.
(b) low blood pressure.
(c) the sensation of dizziness or lightheadedness.
(d) Answers (a) and (b) only.
(e) Answers (b) and (c) only.

328. Because the inferior vena cava lies behind the uterus, on the _____ side of midline, pregnant women always should be transported with the weight of the uterus shifted to the _____ side.

(a) right/left
(b) left/right
(c) right or left/left or right (the location differs in some women)
(d) Any of the above.
(e) None of the above.

329. The condition that produces signs and symptoms if a pregnant woman is not transported on her side is called

(a) migraine positioning disorder.
(b) supine hypotensive syndrome.
(c) supine positioning disorder.
(d) migraine positioning syndrome.
(e) prebirth positioning syndrome.

330. For the majority of births, the baby's head is the first part to emerge from the birth canal. This head-first presentation is called a

(a) dorsal presentation.
(b) breech presentation.
(c) cephalic presentation.
(d) caudal presentation.
(e) ventral presentation.

The answer key for Test Section Four is on pages 361 through 368.

Test Section Five

This test section covers the following subjects:

* Bleeding and Shock
* Soft-tissue Injuries
* Musculoskeletal Injuries
* Injuries to the Head and Spine

1994 Revised EMT-Basic National Standards Review Self-Test

1. The heart is the circulatory pump of the body. The right side of the heart pumps _____ blood through the _____ circulation.

    (a) oxygen rich/systemic
    (b) oxygen poor/systemic
    (c) oxygen rich/pulmonary
    (d) oxygen poor/pulmonary
    (e) either oxygenated or deoxygenated/systemic or pulmonary

2. The _____ receives blood from the veins of the body and the heart.

    (a) left ventricle
    (b) right ventricle
    (c) ventricular septum
    (d) right atrium
    (e) left atrium

3. The _____ receives blood from the lungs (via pulmonary veins).

    (a) left ventricle
    (b) right ventricle
    (c) ventricular septum
    (d) right atrium
    (e) left atrium

4. The _____ pumps blood to the lungs.

    (a) left ventricle
    (b) right ventricle
    (c) ventricular septum
    (d) right atrium
    (e) left atrium

5. The _____ pumps blood to the body.

    (a) left ventricle
    (b) right ventricle
    (c) ventricular septum
    (d) right atrium
    (e) left atrium

6. The cardiac valves
    (a) propel blood from one chamber of the heart to another.
    (b) propel blood from heart chambers into blood vessels.
    (c) prevent backflow of blood.
    (d) Both answers (a) and (b).
    (e) Both answers (a) and (c).

7. All arteries
    (a) carry blood away from the heart.
    (b) carry blood back to the heart.
    (c) carry only oxygenated blood.
    (d) Both answers (a) and (c).
    (e) Both answers (b) and (c).

8. All veins
    (a) carry blood away from the heart.
    (b) carry blood back to the heart.
    (c) carry only deoxygenated blood.
    (d) Both answers (a) and (c).
    (e) Both answers (b) and (c).

9. Pulmonary arteries
    (a) carry blood away from the heart.
    (b) carry blood back to the heart.
    (c) carry only deoxygenated blood.
    (d) Both answers (a) and (c).
    (e) Both answers (b) and (c).

10. Pulmonary veins
    (a) carry blood away from the heart.
    (b) carry blood back to the heart.
    (c) carry only oxygenated blood.
    (d) Both answers (a) and (c).
    (e) Both answers (b) and (c).

11. The major blood vessel that originates from the heart, then descends through the thoracic and abdominal cavities (in front of the spine), is the
    (a) superior vena cava.
    (b) inferior vena cava.
    (c) aorta.
    (d) Either answer (a) or (b).
    (e) Either answer (b) or (c).

12. A major blood vessel that returns blood to the heart is the

   (a) superior vena cava.
   (b) inferior vena cava.
   (c) aorta.
   (d) Either answer (a) or (b).
   (e) Either answer (b) or (c).

13. The heart muscle is supplied with blood by the _____, which branch off from the aorta.

   (a) femoral arteries
   (b) radial arteries
   (c) carotid arteries
   (d) coronary arteries
   (e) brachial arteries

14. The head is supplied with blood by the _____, producing a pulse that can be palpated on either side of the neck.

   (a) femoral arteries
   (b) radial arteries
   (c) carotid arteries
   (d) coronary arteries
   (e) brachial arteries

15. Major arteries of each thigh, the _____ supply the groin and lower extremities with blood. Their pulse can be palpated in the groin area.

   (a) femoral arteries
   (b) radial arteries
   (c) carotid arteries
   (d) coronary arteries
   (e) brachial arteries

16. The _____ produce a pulse that can be palpated between the elbow and the shoulder on the inside of the arm.

   (a) femoral arteries
   (b) radial arteries
   (c) carotid arteries
   (d) coronary arteries
   (e) brachial arteries

17. The _____ produce a pulse that can be palpated on the _____ side of either wrist.

   (a) radial arteries/small finger (medial)
   (b) radial arteries/thumb (lateral)

(c) pulsating arteries/small finger (lateral)
(d) brachial arteries/thumb (lateral)
(e) brachial arteries/small finger (medial)

18. The pulse produced by the _____ is auscultated when using a sphygmomanometer and stethoscope to determine the blood pressure.

    (a) femoral artery
    (b) radial artery
    (c) carotid artery
    (d) coronary artery
    (e) brachial artery

19. An artery on the posterior surface of the medial malleolus that can be palpated for a pulse is the

    (a) anterior tibial artery.
    (b) posterior tibial artery.
    (c) dorsalis pedis artery.
    (d) superior pedal artery.
    (e) posterior pedal artery.

20. An artery on the anterior surface of the foot that can be palpated for a pulse is the

    (a) anterior tibial artery.
    (b) posterior tibial artery.
    (c) dorsalis pedis artery.
    (d) superior pedal artery.
    (e) posterior pedal artery.

21. Capillaries are found in all parts of the body. They are tiny blood vessels that

    (a) receive blood from the smallest arteries and send it to the smallest veins.
    (b) receive blood from the smallest veins and send it to the smallest arteries.
    (c) are responsible for the exchange of nutrients and waste, oxygen and carbon dioxide, at the cellular level of the body.
    (d) Both answers (a) and (c).
    (e) Both answers (b) and (c).

22. The smallest branch of an artery is called

    (a) a capillary.
    (b) an arteriette.
    (c) an arteriole.
    (d) Any of the above.
    (e) None of the above.

23. The smallest branch of a vein is called

  (a) a capillary.
  (b) a veinette.
  (c) a venule.
  (d) Either answer (a) or (b).
  (e) None of the above.

24. Blood is made up of several components. Red blood cells (RBCs, or red corpuscles) carry oxygen to the tissues and carbon dioxide away from the tissues. Another medical term for RBCs is

  (a) leukocytes.
  (b) platelets.
  (c) erythrocytes.
  (d) plasma.
  (e) packed cells.

25. White blood cells (WBCs, or white corpuscles) are the body's immune defense against infections. Another medical term for WBCs is

  (a) leukocytes.
  (b) platelets.
  (c) erythrocytes.
  (d) plasma.
  (e) packed cells.

26. The formation of blood clots is largely dependent on the _____ found in blood.

  (a) leukocytes
  (b) platelets
  (c) erythrocytes
  (d) plasma
  (e) packed cells

27. The fluid that carries the blood cells and nutrients is called

  (a) whole blood.
  (b) platelets.
  (c) erythroliquid.
  (d) plasma.
  (e) packed cells.

28. A pulse is formed when the _____ contracts, sending a wave of blood through the arteries.

  (a) left atrium
  (b) right atrium

(c) left ventricle
(d) right ventricle
(e) ventricular septum

29. A pulse can be palpated
   (a) only at the neck, inner arm, and wrist.
   (b) anywhere an artery simultaneously passes near the skin surface and over a bone.
   (c) anywhere a vein simultaneously passes near the skin surface and over a bone.
   (d) anywhere a vein or artery simultaneously passes near the skin surface and over a large muscle.
   (e) only at the neck, inner arm, wrist, and foot.

30. *Peripheral* pulses include all of the following except the _____ pulse.
   (a) carotid
   (b) brachial
   (c) radial
   (d) dorsalis pedis
   (e) posterior tibial

31. *Central* pulses consist of the carotid pulse and the _____ pulse.
   (a) femoral
   (b) brachial
   (c) radial
   (d) dorsalis pedis
   (e) posterior tibial

32. The medical term *perfusion* is best defined as
   (a) the circulation of blood through an organ structure or tissues.
   (b) delivery of oxygen and other nutrients to the cells of all organ systems and tissues.
   (c) the removal of waste products from all organ systems and tissues.
   (d) Only answers (a) and (b).
   (e) Answers (a), (b), and (c).

33. The medical term _____ means bleeding, or losing blood.
   (a) exsanguine
   (b) hemorrhage
   (c) perfusion
   (d) anemia
   (e) hemoptysis

34. Bleeding is separated into three types, each with specific qualities. _____ bleeding is usually oxygen rich, bright and red in color.

  (a) Capillary
  (b) Venous
  (c) Arterial
  (d) Both answers (a) and (b).
  (e) Both answers (b) and (c).

35. _____ bleeding is usually oxygen poor and dark red in color.

  (a) Capillary
  (b) Venous
  (c) Arterial
  (d) Both answers (a) and (b).
  (e) Both answers (b) and (c).

36. _____ bleeding is the most difficult to control.

  (a) Capillary
  (b) Venous
  (c) Arterial
  (d) Both answers (a) and (b).
  (e) Both answers (b) and (c).

37. _____ bleeding can be profuse; however, it is usually easy to control.

  (a) Capillary
  (b) Venous
  (c) Arterial
  (d) Both answers (a) and (c).
  (e) Both answers (b) and (c).

38. _____ bleeding oozes from a wound and often clots, or stops bleeding, spontaneously. Bleeding control measures usually are not needed.

  (a) Capillary
  (b) Venous
  (c) Arterial
  (d) Both answers (a) and (c).
  (e) Both answers (b) and (c).

39. _____ bleeding may rhythmically spurt from a wound.

  (a) Capillary
  (b) Venous
  (c) Arterial
  (d) Both answers (a) and (b).
  (e) Both answers (b) and (c).

TEST SECTION FIVE

40. _____ bleeding usually flows from a wound in a steady stream.

   (a) Capillary
   (b) Venous
   (c) Arterial
   (d) Both answers (a) and (b).
   (e) Both answers (b) and (c).

41. The sudden loss of _____ of blood from the adult patient is considered serious blood loss.

   (a) 100 to 200 cc
   (b) 500 cc
   (c) 1 liter (1,000 cc)
   (d) Either answer (a) or (b).
   (e) None of the above (an adult does not have a serious blood loss until at least 2 liters of blood are lost).

42. The sudden loss of as little as _____ of blood from a child is considered serious blood loss.

   (a) 10 to 20 cc
   (b) 100 to 200 cc
   (c) 500 cc
   (d) Either answer (a) or (b).
   (e) None of the above (a child does not have a serious blood loss until at least 1 liter [1,000 cc] of blood is lost).

43. The sudden loss of as little as _____ of blood from an infant is considered serious blood loss.

   (a) 10 to 20 cc
   (b) 100 to 200 cc
   (c) 500 cc
   (d) Any of the above amounts (any bleeding from an infant is life-threatening).
   (e) None of the above (an infant does not have a serious blood loss until at least 1 liter [1,000 cc] of blood is lost).

44. Determination of blood loss severity is based on

   (a) the patient's signs and symptoms.
   (b) an exact measurement of blood loss.
   (c) the patient's blood pressure.
   (d) Answers (a) and (b) only.
   (e) Answers (b) and (c) only.

45. Uncontrolled bleeding or significant blood loss leads to shock from _____, and possibly death.

    (a) low blood pressure
    (b) hypoperfusion
    (c) a slow pulse
    (d) hyperperfusion
    (e) Either answer (a) or (c).

46. Which of the following statements regarding bleeding control methods is false?

    (a) Direct pressure to the site of bleeding is the first method of bleeding control.
    (b) Large, gaping wounds may require packing with sterile gauze and direct hand pressure.
    (c) An injured extremity should be kept at or below the level of the patient's heart. Elevation will increase the bleeding.
    (d) Pressure points may be used to control bleeding in the extremities.
    (e) Splinting may assist in bleeding control when associated with a fracture.

47. Which of the following statements regarding pressure points is false?

    (a) Pressure points are a last resort, used only when all other methods of bleeding control have failed.
    (b) The pressure point for upper extremities is at the brachial artery.
    (c) The pressure point for lower extremities is at the femoral artery.
    (d) All of the above are false.
    (e) None of the above are false.

48. Which of the following statements regarding the use of a tourniquet to control bleeding is false?

    (a) A tourniquet is a last resort, used only when all other methods of bleeding control have failed.
    (b) Application of a tourniquet can cause permanent damage to nerves, muscles, and blood vessels, resulting in the loss of the extremity.
    (c) A tourniquet should be applied only tightly enough to stop the bleeding.
    (d) All of the above are false.
    (e) None of the above are false.

49. Which of the following statements regarding the use of a tourniquet to control bleeding is false?

  (a) Do not remove a tourniquet once it has been applied, unless ordered to do so by the medical director.
  (b) Do not loosen a tourniquet once it has been applied, unless ordered to do so by the medical director.
  (c) The width of the tourniquet should be as thin as possible (to minimize the amount of tissue, nerve, or blood vessel damage beneath it). A rope or the patient's thin belt may be used.
  (d) Do not cover a tourniquet. It should remain in open view.
  (e) Do not apply a tourniquet directly over any joint, but do apply it as close to the injury as possible.

50. Bleeding from the nose may be caused by any of the following, except

  (a) internal abdominal hemorrhage.
  (b) hypertension.
  (c) digital trauma (nose picking).
  (d) skull or facial fractures.
  (e) sinusitis and/or upper respiratory tract infections.

51. The medical term for nose bleeding is

  (a) rhinorrhea.
  (b) epistaxis.
  (c) rhinitis.
  (d) sinusitis.
  (e) hemoptysis.

52. Which of the following statements regarding bleeding from the ears or nose is true?

  (a) Bleeding from the ears or nose may occur because of a skull fracture.
  (b) If the bleeding is the result of trauma, do not attempt to stop the blood flow.
  (c) Collect the blood with a loose, sterile dressing. This may also limit exposure to sources of infection.
  (d) All of the above are true.
  (e) None of the above are true.

53. Which of the following statements regarding emergency medical care for a nosebleed is false?

   (a) Have the patient lie flat, or (if she/he will not) remain seated with her/his head tilted backward.
   (b) Apply direct pressure by pinching the fleshy portion of the nostrils together.
   (c) Keep the patient calm and quiet.
   (d) If the patient becomes unconscious, place her/him on her/his side and employ suction and airway management techniques.
   (e) None of the above are false.

54. Which of the following statements regarding internal bleeding is false?

   (a) Internal bleeding can result in severe blood loss, shock, and subsequent death.
   (b) Injured or damaged internal organs commonly lead to extensive bleeding that is concealed (hidden) from emergency care providers.
   (c) Closed extremity injuries, even when painful, swollen, and/or deformed, are never the cause of shock from internal bleeding. Look elsewhere for sites of internal bleeding.
   (d) Suspicion of internal bleeding should be based on the mechanism of injury.
   (e) Severity of internal bleeding should be determined by the patient's clinical signs and symptoms and the mechanism of injury.

55. Mechanisms of injury that may produce serious internal bleeding include all of the following, except

   (a) blast injuries.
   (b) any penetrating trauma to the chest, abdomen, or pelvis.
   (c) any blunt trauma to the chest, abdomen, or pelvis.
   (d) falls.
   (e) a crush injury of the forearm.

56. Signs and symptoms of internal bleeding include all of the following, except

   (a) external bleeding from the mouth, rectum, vagina, or any other orifice.
   (b) external bleeding from the metacarpal area.
   (c) vomiting dark-colored, coffee-ground-like, emesis.
   (d) dark, tar-colored stools.
   (e) a tender, rigid, and/or distended abdomen.

57. Signs and symptoms of hypovolemic shock include all of the following, except

  (a) anxiety and restlessness.
  (b) shallow, rapid breathing.
  (c) a slow, bounding pulse.
  (d) pale, cool, clammy skin.
  (e) thirst.

58. Which of the following represents late signs and symptoms of shock?

  (a) Combativeness or altered mental status.
  (b) A rapid and bounding radial pulse.
  (c) Decreased blood pressure.
  (d) Answers (a) and (c) only.
  (e) Answers (a), (b), and (c).

59. Which of the following signs and symptoms of shock is usually the earliest to develop?

  (a) Anxiety and restlessness.
  (b) Nausea and vomiting.
  (c) Decreasing blood pressure.
  (d) Increasing pulse rate.
  (e) Increasing respiratory rate.

60. Which of the following signs and symptoms of shock is usually the latest to develop?

  (a) Anxiety and restlessness.
  (b) Nausea and vomiting.
  (c) Decreasing blood pressure.
  (d) Increasing pulse rate.
  (e) Increasing respiratory rate.

61. _____ is the medical term for shock of any kind.

  (a) Hypovolemia or hypovolemic shock
  (b) Hypoperfusion syndrome
  (c) Hemorrhagic shock
  (d) Cushing's syndrome
  (e) Hyperperfusion syndrome

62. _____ is the medical term specifically for shock from blood loss.

  (a) Hypovolemia or hypovolemic shock
  (b) Hyperperfusion syndrome or hypervolemic shock
  (c) Hemorrhagic shock
  (d) Either answer (a) or (b).
  (e) Either answer (a) or (c).

63. Shock is caused by

    (a) the heart failing to adequately pump blood (heart failure).
    (b) inadequate blood volume (dehydration or actual blood loss).
    (c) dilation of the body's blood vessels (a vascular container that is too large).
    (d) Answers (a) and/or (b) only.
    (e) Answers (a), (b), and/or (c).

64. Which of the following statements regarding shock in infants or children is true?

    (a) Infants and children can maintain their blood pressure until more than 50 percent of their blood volume is lost.
    (b) The blood pressure of infants and children drops as soon as any bleeding occurs (unlike adults).
    (c) Infants and children have less reserve blood volume than adults.
    (d) Both answers (a) and (c) are true.
    (e) Both answers (b) and (c) are true.

65. From the following list of activities, select all that suggest appropriate emergency medical treatment of patients in shock.

1. Administer high-flow oxygen.
2. Control any external bleeding.
3. Elevate the lower extremities (or lower end of the backboard) approximately 8 to 12 inches, only if the patient does not have serious injuries to the pelvis, lower extremities, head, chest, abdomen, neck, or spine.
4. Elevate the lower extremities (or lower end of the backboard) approximately 8 to 12 inches, especially if the patient has serious injuries to the pelvis, lower extremities, head, chest, abdomen, neck, or spine.
5. If your protocol allows pneumatic antishock garment (PASG) use, request orders to apply the garment to all abdominal-injury patients who have no chest injuries, but have shock signs and symptoms.
6. If your protocol allows pneumatic antishock garment (PASG) use, request orders to apply the garment to all pelvic-injury patients who have no chest injuries, but have shock signs and symptoms.
7. If your protocol allows pneumatic antishock garment (PASG) use, request orders to apply the garment to all chest-injury patients who have no abdominal or pelvic injuries, but have shock signs and symptoms.
8. Maintain the patient's airway; provide artificial ventilation or CPR if needed.

9. Prevent loss of body heat by covering the patient with a blanket when in cool or cold environments.
10. Splint any suspected bone or joint injuries.

   (a) 1, 2, 3, 5, 6, 7, 8, 9, and 10 only.
   (b) 1, 2, 4, 5, 6, 7, 8, 9, and 10 only.
   (c) 1, 2, 3, 7, 8, 9, and 10 only.
   (d) 1, 2, 4, 7, 8, 9, and 10 only.
   (e) 1, 2, 3, 5, 6, 8, 9, and 10 only.

66. All of the following functions are performed by the skin, except for

   (a) protection of the body from the environment and provision of a barrier to keep out bacteria and other organisms.
   (b) prevention of body water loss and provision of a barrier to keep out environmental water.
   (c) production of WBCs to combat infection.
   (d) body temperature regulation.
   (e) reception and transmission of environmental information to the brain.

67. The outermost layer of skin, composed primarily of dead cells that constantly are being rubbed or sloughed off and replaced, is called the

   (a) endodermis.
   (b) epidermis.
   (c) dermis.
   (d) subcutaneous layer.
   (e) sebaceous layer.

68. The layer of skin containing sweat and sebaceous glands is called the

   (a) endodermis.
   (b) epidermis.
   (c) dermis.
   (d) subcutaneous layer.
   (e) sebaceous layer.

69. The layer of skin containing hair follicles, blood vessels, and nerve endings is called the

   (a) endodermis.
   (b) epidermis.
   (c) dermis.
   (d) subcutaneous layer.
   (e) sebaceous layer.

70. The layer of skin containing fat and soft tissue is largely responsible for temperature insulation and shock absorption (protection from impact injuries to the body organs). This layer is called the

    (a) endodermis.
    (b) epidermis.
    (c) dermis.
    (d) subcutaneous layer.
    (e) sebaceous layer.

71. A bruise is an example of

    (a) a closed injury.
    (b) an open injury.
    (c) an open or closed injury.
    (d) an insignificant injury that never requires emergency medical attention.
    (e) None of the above.

72. A crush injury is an example of

    (a) a closed injury.
    (b) an open injury.
    (c) an open or closed injury.
    (d) an insignificant injury that never requires emergency medical attention.
    (e) None of the above.

73. A laceration is an example of

    (a) a closed injury.
    (b) an open injury.
    (c) an open or closed injury.
    (d) a serious injury that always results in loss of life or limb.
    (e) None of the above.

74. A puncture wound is an example of

    (a) a closed injury.
    (b) an open injury.
    (c) an open or closed injury.
    (d) an insignificant injury that never requires emergency medical attention.
    (e) None of the above.

75. An abrasion is an example of

    (a) a closed injury.
    (b) an open injury.

(c) an open or closed injury.
(d) an insignificant injury that never requires emergency medical attention.
(e) None of the above.

76. _____ is the medical term for a "goose egg."

(a) Abrasion
(b) Avulsion
(c) Contusion
(d) Hematoma
(e) Laceration

77. _____ is the medical term for a bruise.

(a) Abrasion
(b) Avulsion
(c) Contusion
(d) Hematoma
(e) Laceration

78. _____ is the medical term for a break or cut in the skin.

(a) Abrasion
(b) Avulsion
(c) Contusion
(d) Hematoma
(e) Laceration

79. _____ is the medical term for a scraping injury.

(a) Abrasion
(b) Avulsion
(c) Contusion
(d) Hematoma
(e) Laceration

80. _____ is the medical term for when a flap of skin or tissue is torn loose.

(a) Abrasion
(b) Avulsion
(c) Contusion
(d) Hematoma
(e) Laceration

81. _____ is the medical term for when a flap of skin or tissue is torn completely off.

   (a) Abrasion
   (b) Avulsion
   (c) Contusion
   (d) Hematoma
   (e) Laceration

82. All of the following emergency care measures should be employed for open chest injuries, except

   (a) high-flow oxygen administration.
   (b) placing the patient in a position of comfort (if no spinal injury is suspected).
   (c) application of sterile gauze dressings, moistened with sterile water or saline.
   (d) sealing the chest dressing on three or four edges (depending on local protocol).
   (e) considering all open chest injuries to be life-threatening.

83. All of the following emergency care measures should be employed for open abdominal injuries, except

   (a) high-flow oxygen administration.
   (b) keeping the patient supine and flat even when spinal injury is not suspected (do not allow the patient to raise her/his knees, flexing the hips, because this will increase any hidden abdominal bleeding).
   (c) application of sterile dressings, moistened with sterile water or saline.
   (d) requesting an order for application of the pneumatic anti-shock garment (PASG) if your protocol allows it.
   (e) considering all open abdominal injuries to be life-threatening.

84. A dressing that does not allow air to escape from or enter a wounded area is called

   (a) an abusive dressing.
   (b) a hard dressing.
   (c) a closed dressing.
   (d) an occlusive dressing.
   (e) a soft dressing.

85. When intestines (or other organs) are protruding from an open abdominal wound, the injury is called

   (a) a third degree open abdominal injury.
   (b) an evisceration.

(c) an abdominal hematoma.
(d) a bowel injury.
(e) an intestinal-protrusion injury.

86. Which of the following statements regarding emergency care for an open abdominal injury with protruding intestines is false?

    (a) Gently push the protruding organs back within the abdominal cavity before herniation (intestinal strangulation) or exposure results in the death of an intestinal segment.
    (b) Cover the wound and any exposed organs with a sterile dressing, moisten it with sterile water or saline, and secure it in place.
    (c) Cover the initial, moist dressing with an additional dressing that prevents air or fluid from escaping and helps preserve heat.
    (d) Apply a clean towel or blanket on top of the dressings to preserve body heat.
    (e) If there is no suspicion of spinal injury, and the patient's hips and legs are uninjured, flex the patient's hips and knees to reduce abdominal pain.

87. Which of the following statements regarding emergency medical care of impaled objects is true?

    (a) Do not remove any impaled object that remains embedded in any part of the body.
    (b) Remove all impaled objects before dressing the wound and transporting the patient. Contact the medical director for specific removal instructions.
    (c) An object impaled in the cheek may threaten the patient's airway. Thus, if the object can be removed without twisting or increasing the injury size, remove it.
    (d) All of the above are true.
    (e) None of the above are true.

88. Which of the following statements regarding emergency medical care of avulsions is true?

    (a) Clean the wound surface by rinsing with sterile saline.
    (b) Fold the avulsed tissue back into its normal position.
    (c) Control the bleeding and dress the wound with bulky pressure dressings.
    (d) Both answers (a) and (c) are true.
    (e) All of the above are true.

89. Which of the following statements regarding emergency medical care of full avulsions or amputations is false?

(a) It may be possible to re-attach the amputated or fully avulsed part. Place the part in a clean (if not sterile) container and float it in sterile saline solution for transportation with the patient. Ice should be added to the saline solution if transport time will be longer than 15 minutes.
(b) Place a pressure dressing over the amputation wound (the stump).
(c) Do not use a tourniquet unless all other methods of bleeding control have failed.
(d) All of the above are false.
(e) None of the above are false.

90. Which of the following statements regarding emergency medical care of large, open neck wounds is true?

(a) The blood vessels in the neck are large and may result in life-threatening blood loss.
(b) An air embolism may enter an open neck vein and cause the patient's death. Thus, any open neck wounds should be sealed with a substance that does not allow air to pass through the dressing.
(c) Do not apply pressure to both sides of the patient's neck, simultaneously compressing both carotid arteries.
(d) All of the above are true.
(e) None of the above are true.

91. A first-degree burn is also known as a

(a) superficial burn.
(b) partial thickness burn.
(c) full thickness burn.
(d) Either answer (a) or (b).
(e) Either answer (b) or (c).

92. A third-degree burn is also known as a

(a) superficial burn.
(b) partial thickness burn.
(c) full thickness burn.
(d) Either answer (a) or (b).
(e) Either answer (b) or (c).

93. A reddened skin color will be present only in the area of a

(a) superficial burn.
(b) partial thickness burn.
(c) full thickness burn.
(d) Either answer (a) or (b).
(e) Either answer (b) or (c).

94. The presence of blisters indicates an area of

  (a) superficial burn.
  (b) partial thickness burn.
  (c) full thickness burn.
  (d) Either answer (a) or (b).
  (e) Either answer (b) or (c).

95. Severe pain indicates an area of

  (a) superficial burn.
  (b) partial thickness burn.
  (c) full thickness burn.
  (d) Either answer (a) or (b).
  (e) Either answer (b) or (c).

96. The loss of sensation (little to no pain) indicates an area of

  (a) superficial burn.
  (b) partial thickness burn.
  (c) full thickness burn.
  (d) Either answer (a) or (b).
  (e) Either answer (b) or (c).

97. Determining the percentage of body surface area burned may be accomplished by using the Palmar Surface Area (or Rule of Palm) method. This method consists of using the size of _____ and comparing that palm-percentage measurement to the size of the burn.

  (a) the patient's palm to represent 9 percent of the patient's body surface area
  (b) your palm to represent 9 percent of the patient's body surface area
  (c) the patient's palm to represent 5 percent of the patient's body surface area
  (d) your palm to represent 1 percent of the patient's body surface area
  (e) the patient's palm to represent 1 percent of the patient's body surface area

98. Determining the percentage of body surface area (BSA) burned may be accomplished by using the Rule of Nines method. Using this method, what is the percentage of BSA burned if an adult patient has burned the front of her right arm, the right half of her anterior abdomen, and the front of her right leg?

  (a) 9 percent.
  (b) 13.5 percent.
  (c) 18 percent.
  (d) 22.5 percent.
  (e) 27 percent.

99. Using the Rule of Nines, what is the percentage of BSA burned if an adult patient has burned his anterior chest, anterior abdomen, genital area, and anterior left leg?

    (a) 23.5 percent.
    (b) 36 percent.
    (c) 27 percent.
    (d) 19 percent.
    (e) 28 percent.

100. Using the Rule of Nines, what is the percentage of BSA burned if an 8-year-old patient has burned the front of her right arm, the right half of her anterior chest and abdomen, and the front of her right leg?

    (a) 26 percent.
    (b) 20.5 percent.
    (c) 23 percent.
    (d) 13.5 percent.
    (e) 29.5 percent.

101. Using the Rule of Nines, what is the percentage of BSA burned if an 8-year-old patient has burned his anterior chest, anterior abdomen, genital area, and anterior left leg?

    (a) 26 percent.
    (b) 20.5 percent.
    (c) 23 percent.
    (d) 13.5 percent.
    (e) 29.5 percent.

102. Of the following burns, which one can be considered the least critical?

    (a) Burns that encompass an adult's arm, chest, or leg.
    (b) Burns accompanied by a painful, swollen, or deformed extremity.
    (c) Burns associated with respiratory injury.
    (d) Partial thickness burns of 10 percent of the adult's BSA (not involving the hands, feet, face, or genitalia).
    (e) Moderate burns in young children or elderly patients.

103. Of the following burns, which one can be considered the most critical?

    (a) Partial thickness burns involving the hands, feet, face, or genitalia.
    (b) Partial thickness burns of 15 to 30 percent of the adult's BSA (not involving the hands, feet, face, or genitalia).
    (c) Full thickness burns of 2 to 10 percent of the adult's BSA (not involving the hands, feet, face, or genitalia).

(d) All of the above are equally critical burns.
(e) None of the above are considered critical burns.

104. A burn that encircles a body part (such as an arm, the chest, or a leg) is called

(a) a circumoral burn.
(b) a full thickness burn.
(c) a full surface burn.
(d) a circumferential burn.
(e) an amputating burn.

105. Place the following emergency care measures for thermal burns in the order of their performance (from first performed to last performed).

1. Assess the airway.
2. Assess the patient's breathing.
3. Assess the patient's circulation.
4. Assure personal safety.
5. Manage any airway problems.
6. Stop the burning process, initially with water or saline.
7. Take body substance isolation precautions.
8. Manage any breathing problems.
9. Treat the patient for shock signs and symptoms.
10. Use the Rule of Nines or Palmar Surface Area method to determine the percentage of body surface area burned, along with assessing for burn depth and severity.

(a) 1, 2, 3, 4, 5, 6, 7, 8, 9, and then 10.
(b) 4, 6, 1, 2, 3, 7, 5, 8, 10, and then 9.
(c) 4, 7, 6, 1, 5, 2, 8, 3, 9, and then 10.
(d) 4, 7, 6, 1, 2, 3, 10, 5, 8, and then 9.
(e) Any of the above orders of performance are acceptable. Different patients require different approaches.

106. Which of the following statements regarding emergency care measures for thermal burns is false?

(a) Do not break any blisters.
(b) Request orders from the medical director to apply a topical burn antiseptic (available in ointment or lotion form).
(c) Remove any smoldering clothing (even after the flames are extinguished).
(d) Remove all jewelry from burned extremities as soon as possible.
(e) Do not bandage burned hands and feet until you have separated burned digits with sterile gauze pads.

107. Which of the following statements regarding emergency care measures for chemical burns is false?

(a) Dry powders should be brushed off before any flushing is done.
(b) Flushing of the chemical burn area should be done for at least 20 minutes and can be done while en route to the receiving emergency department.
(c) Do not contaminate unexposed areas when flushing.
(d) Remove all clothing, shoes, socks, and jewelry before flushing.
(e) Treat the patient for shock.

108. Which of the following statements regarding emergency care measures for electrical burns is false?

(a) A doubled pair of latex gloves, or a large, dry tree branch, will protect the EMT from electrical shock while removing a patient from an electrical source.
(b) Monitor the patient closely for respiratory arrest.
(c) Monitor the patient closely for cardiac arrest (consider the need for AED).
(d) Electrical burns usually are more severe than their outward appearance.
(e) Look for both an entrance and an exit wound.

109. _____ may be defined as any material placed on a wound to control bleeding and to prevent further contamination and infection.

(a) Bandages
(b) Dressings
(c) Splints
(d) Either answer (a) or (c).
(e) Either answer (b) or (c).

110. _____ may be defined as any material used to secure other material to a wound to control bleeding and to prevent further contamination and infection.

(a) Bandages
(b) Dressings
(c) Splints
(d) Either answer (a) or (c).
(e) Either answer (b) or (c).

111. Which of the following statements regarding open wound care is false?

   (a) Expose the entire wound so that it can be completely covered by sterile material.
   (b) Separate injured digits with gauze pads and leave the tips of fingers and toes exposed.
   (c) If blood soaks through part of the dressing, remove the soiled material and replace it with fresh material.
   (d) Do not apply bandages too tightly. The patient's distal pulse should remain present (unless it was absent before wound care).
   (e) None of the above are false.

112. Which of the following statements regarding the mechanism of injury required to damage bones is false?

   (a) A mechanism of injury involving direct force (a direct impact to the injured part) may damage bones.
   (b) A mechanism of injury involving twisting forces (a twisting of the injured part) may damage bones.
   (c) A mechanism of injury involving indirect force (an impact with a body area other than the part) will not damage bones.
   (d) A damaged bone may be associated with either a closed or an open soft-tissue wound.
   (e) None of the above are false.

113. Which of the following statements regarding bone injuries is false?

   (a) A fracture is best defined as when there is any sort of break in the bone (even just a crack).
   (b) A dislocation is best defined as when there is an alteration of the normal alignment or placement of bones, without an actual break in the bones.
   (c) As an EMT, it is vitally important to emergency care that you be able to differentiate between fractures and dislocations.
   (d) Any painful, swollen, and/or deformed extremity should be treated as though it were a fracture until proven otherwise.
   (e) None of the above are false.

114. Using the following emergency care steps, select the care measures appropriate for treatment of bone or joint injuries, and place them in the order of their correct performance (from first performed to last performed). Some measures may be repeated (performed more than once).

1. Apply cold packs to painful, swollen, or deformed extremity areas.
2. Assess the pulse, range of motion, and sensation in the areas distal to the injury.
3. Control any bleeding.
4. Dress any open wounds with a sterile dressing.
5. In preparation for transport, elevate the injured extremity.
6. In preparation for transport, keep the injured part at or below the level of the patient's heart.
7. Manage any life-threatening injuries.
8. Perform an initial assessment.
9. Splint injuries to minimize additional injury.

   (a) 8, 7, 3, 4, 2, 9, 2, 1, and 6.
   (b) 8, 7, 3, 4, 2, 9, 2, 1, and 5.
   (c) 1, 2, 3, 4, 6, 7, 8, and 9.
   (d) 8, 7, 3, 4, 6, 8, 9, 2, and 1.
   (e) 3, 8, 7, 4, 6, 8, 9, 2, and 1.

115. Which of the following statements regarding general rules of splinting is false?

   (a) Never intentionally replace protruding bone ends.
   (b) An injured extremity always should be immobilized from the joint above the injury to the joint below the injury (proximal and distal joint immobilization).
   (c) Never attempt to realign a deformed extremity. Always "splint it as it lies."
   (d) If no immediate danger or life-threats are found, splint the patient before moving the patient.
   (e) If a patient appears to be in life-threat from other injuries or conditions, disregard specific extremity immobilization. Instead, treat the life-threatening injuries or conditions while immobilizing the patient on a long backboard.

116. Improper splinting may result in

   (a) splint compression of (and/or damage to) nerves, blood vessels, or body tissues.
   (b) death of the patient whose transport was delayed to accomplish splinting.

(c) reduction of circulation distal to the splinted part.
(d) aggravation of the bone or joint injury that is being (or has been) splinted.
(e) Any of the above.

117. A traction splint may be applied to which of the following injuries?

(a) An isolated, painful, swollen, and deformed mid-thigh injury.
(b) A painful, swollen, and deformed knee injury.
(c) A painful, swollen, and deformed lower leg injury.
(d) Answers (a) and/or (b) only.
(e) Answers (a) and/or (c) only.

118. The use of a traction splint is contraindicated in

(a) a hip injury.
(b) a pelvic injury.
(c) a partial mid-thigh amputation or a mid-thigh avulsion with possible bone separation (where the distal limb is connected only by tissue).
(d) Any of the above.
(e) None of the above.

119. Mechanisms of injury that may indicate an associated spinal injury include all of the following, except

(a) isolated, blunt trauma to the mid-thigh (such as a blow from a large bat).
(b) falls or diving accidents where the patient lands feet first.
(c) any unconscious trauma victim.
(d) soft rope hangings.
(e) isolated, blunt trauma to the head.

120. Of the following mechanisms of injury, which is the least likely to cause spinal injury?

(a) Penetrating trauma to the head, neck, or torso (such as a gunshot wound).
(b) A pedestrian-versus-vehicle accident.
(c) A lateral fall to soft dirt from standing.
(d) A restrained patient involved in a moderate- to high-speed motor vehicle accident.
(e) An unrestrained patient involved in a moderate- to high-speed motor vehicle accident.

121. Which of the following statements regarding assessment of spinal injury mechanisms, signs, and symptoms is true?

    (a) The possibility of spinal injury is ruled out if the patient already is walking, moving all extremities, and denies neurological or spinal pain complaints.

    (b) When the mechanism of injury suggests the potential for spinal injury, but the patient denies any spinal complaints, the patient should be directed to perform range of motion tests to determine if a hidden spine injury may be present.

    (c) If a victim of isolated head trauma, that did not involve a direct blow to the spine, denies neurological or spinal pain complaints, the patient does not need to be treated for a spinal injury.

    (d) All of the above are true.

    (e) None of the above are true.

122. Which of the following statements regarding head (scalp, skull, and brain) injuries is false?

    (a) Profuse bleeding from the scalp is always a life-threatening situation. (The scalp itself is too thin to bleed very much. Impressive bleeding from a simple scalp wound indicates serious brain injury.)

    (b) Nontraumatic brain injuries may occur due to clots or hemorrhaging within the brain.

    (c) Nontraumatic brain injuries can be a cause of altered mental status.

    (d) Nontraumatic brain injuries can produce the same signs and symptoms as traumatic brain injuries.

    (e) None of the above are false.

*The following 20 questions (123 through 142) are an **elective** group of questions about traumatic conditions, emergencies, and/or medical terminology. Most of these questions represent information that is **not** DOT-required knowledge for the EMT-Basic but may be included in local or state examinations. Page numbers keyed to Brady's* **Emergency Care,** *7th ed., are provided for these questions in the answer key.*

123. Functions of blood include all of the following, except

    (a) transportation of nutrients to the cells of the body and transportation of waste products away from the cells of the body.

    (b) determining the normal color of a person's skin (as in the skin color of White, Black, Indian, and Asian persons).

(c) regulation of body functions, via transportation of hormones and electrolytes (chemicals important to body functions) to target organs.
(d) defense against disease organisms.
(e) assisting with body temperature regulation.

124. _____ is the specific medical name for shock from failure of the heart to adequately pump blood to the body's vital tissues.

(a) Heart failure shock
(b) Cardiac failure shock
(c) Cardiogenic shock
(d) Cardiopulmonary shock
(e) Heterogenic shock

125. _____ is the specific medical name for shock caused by severe, systemic infection (infection involving all body systems).

(a) Infectious shock
(b) Septic shock
(c) Vessel shock
(d) Total body shock (TBS)
(e) Heterogenic shock

126. Shock may be produced by a systemic infection because

(a) systemic infections release toxins that dilate the body's blood vessels, enlarging the body's blood container, causing a "relative" hypovolemia.
(b) systemic infections release toxins that constrict the body's blood vessels, enlarging the body's blood container, causing a "relative" hypovolemia.
(c) systemic infections release toxins that dilate the body's blood vessels, diminishing the body's blood container, causing a "relative" hypovolemia.
(d) systemic infections release toxins that constrict the body's blood vessels, diminishing the body's blood container, causing a "relative" hypovolemia.
(e) None of the above. Infections may make someone feel terribly ill, but they do not produce any form of "shock."

127. _____ is the specific medical name for shock caused by a systemic body reaction to an allergen.

(a) Anaphylactic shock
(b) Septic shock
(c) Allergy defense shock
(d) Systemic shock
(e) Total body shock (TBS)

128. _____ is the specific medical name for shock caused by spinal cord injury.

   (a) Cord shock
   (b) Spinal tap shock
   (c) Cervical shock
   (d) Neurogenic shock
   (e) CNS shock

129. Shock may be produced by spinal cord injury because

   (a) all feeling in the body becomes absent and all body functions shut down.
   (b) the heart no longer receives electrical impulses to pump the blood, so spinal cord injury causes heart failure.
   (c) the diameter of the body's blood vessels (below the level of injury) becomes constricted, and blood is no longer allowed to flow through them.
   (d) the diameter of the body's blood vessels (below the level of injury) becomes dilated, and there is no longer enough blood to fill them.
   (e) spinal cord injury always involves internal bleeding and immediately leads to shock from actual blood loss.

130. Shock usually occurs in stages. The stage called _____ is when shock is developing, but the patient's body still is able to maintain perfusion to vital organs.

   (a) decompensated shock
   (b) compensated shock
   (c) partial shock
   (d) incomplete shock
   (e) complete shock

131. The stage called _____ is when shock has fully developed, and the patient's body no longer is able to maintain perfusion to vital organs.

   (a) decompensated shock
   (b) compensated shock
   (c) partial shock
   (d) incomplete shock
   (e) complete shock

132. When air accumulates in the pleural space (the space between the lining of the interior chest wall and the lining of the lung), a serious condition occurs. Which of the following statements regarding this condition is true?

   (a) Air may enter a pleural space via an external wound.
   (b) Air may enter a pleural space via an internal lung rupture.

(c) Accumulation of air in a pleural space will diminish that lung's ability to expand and adequately provide for gas exchange.
(d) Only answers (a) and (c) are true.
(e) Answers (a), (b), and (c) are true.

133. The phrase **sucking chest wound** refers to
   (a) an external wound allowing air into that lung's pleural space.
   (b) an internal wound leaking air into that lung's pleural space.
   (c) an incident involving oral trauma that causes air to be "sucked" into the pleural space via an opening in the oropharnyx.
   (d) Either answer (a) or (c).
   (e) Either answer (b) or (c).

134. When local protocol calls for an occlusive dressing to be applied to an open chest wound and sealed on all four sides, the fourth side should be sealed immediately after the patient has
   (a) been spinally immobilized.
   (b) forcefully inhaled.
   (c) forcefully exhaled.
   (d) been placed on supplemental oxygen.
   (e) been moved to the ambulance (and not before).

135. When local protocol calls for an occlusive dressing to be applied to an open chest wound and sealed on only three sides, the fourth (open) side serves as a
   (a) suction route.
   (b) one-way valve, allowing trapped air to escape, but preventing external air from being drawn into the wound.
   (c) two-way valve, allowing trapped air to escape and oxygen to be drawn in.
   (d) Both answers (a) and (b).
   (e) Both answers (a) and (c).

136. The condition of having air trapped in the pleural space (moderately interfering with lung function on that side) is called
   (a) an aerothorax.
   (b) a pneumothorax.
   (c) a tension pneumothorax.
   (d) a hemothorax.
   (e) a hemopneumothorax.

137. The condition of having blood trapped in the pleural space (moderately interfering with lung function on that side) is called

   (a) an aerothorax.
   (b) a pneumothorax.
   (c) a tension pneumothorax.
   (d) a hemothorax.
   (e) a hemopneumothorax.

138. The condition of having a large amount of air trapped in the pleural space (severely interfering with lung function on the affected side and possibly interfering with heart and opposite lung function) is called

   (a) an aerothorax.
   (b) a pneumothorax.
   (c) a tension pneumothorax.
   (d) a hemothorax.
   (e) a hemopneumothorax.

139. The condition of having blood and air trapped in the pleural space (moderately to severely interfering with lung function on that side) is called

   (a) an aerothorax.
   (b) a pneumothorax.
   (c) a tension pneumothorax.
   (d) a hemothorax.
   (e) a hemopneumothorax.

140. All of the following are signs and symptoms of traumatic asphyxia, except

   (a) a patient who may be wildly and frantically staggering about the scene, loudly screaming, and complaining of severe chest pain and difficulty breathing.
   (b) obvious distention of the patient's jugular veins, with noticeably bloodshot and bulging eyes.
   (c) a swollen and/or protruding appearance of the patient's lips and/or tongue.
   (d) noticeable cyanosis of the patient's shoulders, neck, face, and head.
   (e) possible deformity of the chest.

141. An external or internal wound to the area surrounding the heart may allow blood to accumulate between the heart and the sac that encloses it. The accumulation of blood in this area will begin to interfere with the heart's ability to expand and fully fill with blood, thus decreasing the heart's ability to pump a normal amount of blood out to the body. This condition is called

    (a) cardiac bypass.
    (b) cardiac tamponade.
    (c) cardiopneumo thorax.
    (d) cardiothorax.
    (e) the "bends."

142. Signs and symptoms of a heart being squeezed by the accumulation of blood in its surrounding sac include all of the following, except

    (a) distended jugular veins.
    (b) a weakening pulse.
    (c) a falling systolic blood pressure with a rising or unchanging diastolic blood pressure.
    (d) a rising systolic blood pressure with a falling or unchanging diastolic blood pressure.
    (e) a mechanism of injury that suggests blunt or penetrating chest trauma.

The answer key for Test Section Five is on pages 369 through 372.

Test Section Six

This test section covers the following subjects:

* Age Group Definitions for Infants and Children
* Developmental Differences Between Age Groups
* Pediatric Airway Differences
* General Special Assessment Considerations for Infants and Children
* General Special Emergency Care Considerations for Infants and Children
* Pediatric Seizures, Poisonings, Fevers, and Drownings
* Sudden Infant Death Syndrome
* Pediatric Trauma, Child Abuse, and Child Neglect

1994 Revised EMT-Basic National Standards Review Self-Test

1. An infant is best defined as a child from the age of birth to

    (a) 4 months.
    (b) 6 months.
    (c) 12 months.
    (d) 18 months.
    (e) 24 months.

2. A toddler is best defined as a child from the age of

    (a) 6 months to 2 years.
    (b) 1 year to 3 years.
    (c) 18 months to 3 years.
    (d) 24 months to 2 years.
    (e) 2 years to 5 years.

3. A preschooler is best defined as a child from the age of

    (a) 3 years to 6 years.
    (b) 2 years to 8 years.
    (c) 5 years to 9 years.
    (d) birth to 5 years (or 4 years, if born in the fall months).
    (e) 2 years to 5 years.

4. A school-age child is best defined as a child from the age of

    (a) 6 years to 18 years.
    (b) 8 years to 18 years.
    (c) 9 years to 12 years.
    (d) 4 years or 5 years to 18 years.
    (e) 6 years to 12 years.

5. An adolescent is best defined as a child from the age of

    (a) 6 years to 18 years.
    (b) 8 years to 18 years.
    (c) 13 years to 15 years.
    (d) 12 years to 18 years.
    (e) 13 years to 20 years.

TEST SECTION SIX

Some common pediatric characteristics or concerns can be anticipated, depending on the child's age and stage of development. Use the following list of characteristics to answer the next four questions (questions 6 through 9).

1. A fear of needles
2. Being uncomfortable with their changing bodies
3. Easily losing body heat—they need to be kept warm
4. A high degree of modesty
5. Considering illness or injury as "punishment" for having done something "bad"
6. A dislike of having their clothing removed
7. A dislike of being separated from their parents
8. A dislike of being touched (by strangers)
9. Experiencing fear of suffocation when an oxygen mask is placed on their face
10. Fearing that they may be permanently disfigured
11. Fearing that they may be permanently injured
12. Having minimal stranger anxiety

6. Common concern characteristics of newborns and infants usually include

(a) 1, 2, 7, and 8.
(b) 1, 3, 7, and 12.
(c) 3, 4, 8, and 12
(d) 3, 7, 9, and 12.
(e) 1, 2, 3, 7, and 12.

7. Common concern characteristics of toddlers usually include

(a) 1, 5, 6, 7, 8, and 9.
(b) 2, 3, 4, 5, and 12.
(c) 2, 7, 8, 10, and 11.
(d) 1, 2, 3, 4, 5, 6, 7, 8, 9, 10, 11, and 12.
(e) None of the above (toddlers are unusually trusting and eager for emergency care).

8. Common concern characteristics of preschoolers and school-age children usually include

(a) 2, 3, 5, 9, and 12.
(b) 2, 3, 4, 5, 6, 11, and 12.
(c) 1, 4, 6, 7, 8, 9, 10, and 11.
(d) 1, 2, 3, 4, 5, 6, 7, 8, 9, 10, 11, and 12.
(e) None of the above (preschoolers and school-age children are unusually trusting and eager for emergency care).

9. Common concern characteristics of adolescents usually include
    (a) 1, 2, 3, 9, 10, 11, and 12.
    (b) 2, 4, 10, and 11.
    (c) 1, 3, 4, 7, 8, 9, 10, and 11.
    (d) 1, 2, 3, 4, 5, 6, 7, 8, 9, 10, 11, and 12.
    (e) None of the above (teenagers are unusually trusting and eager for emergency care).

10. Which of the following statements regarding anatomical and physiological pediatric airway considerations is false?
    (a) Throughout their respiratory system, infants and children have smaller airway structures than adults. Thus, it takes less swelling or secretions to block pediatric airways.
    (b) The tongues of infants and children take up more space in the mouth than the tongues of adults. Thus, it is easier for the pediatric airway to become obstructed by the tongue.
    (c) Infants breathe only with their mouth. Thus, it rarely is necessary to suction the infant's nostrils.
    (d) The trachea is softer and narrower in infants and children. Thus, positioning for an open pediatric airway is different than positioning for an open adult airway.
    (e) None of the above are false.

11. Open airway positioning for infants and children may be assisted by placing a folded towel under the patient's
    (a) head to aid in hyperextension (in the absence of spinal trauma).
    (b) neck to maintain neutral positioning of the airway.
    (c) shoulders to maintain neutral positioning of the airway.
    (d) Both answers (a) and (b).
    (e) Both answers (a) and (c).

12. When clearing a complete airway obstruction in children _____, use back blows and chest thrusts.
    (a) less than 1 year old
    (b) from 1 year to 8 years old
    (c) over 8 years old
    (d) from birth to 8 years old
    (e) None of the above (this technique is no longer used).

13. When clearing a complete airway obstruction in children _____, use abdominal thrusts (the Heimlich maneuver).
    (a) less than 1 year old
    (b) from 1 year to 8 years old (only)
    (c) over 1 year old
    (d) from birth to 8 years old
    (e) of all ages

14. When clearing a complete airway obstruction in children _____, use blind finger sweeps to clear the oropharnyx of secretions or obstructive material.

(a) less than 1 year old
(b) from 1 year to 8 years old
(c) over 8 years old (only)
(d) from birth to 8 years old
(e) of all ages

15. When clearing a complete airway obstruction in children _____, manually remove any visible foreign material from the airway.

(a) less than 1 year old
(b) from 1 year to 8 years old
(c) over 8 years old
(d) from birth to 8 years old
(e) of all ages

16. Oral airway insertion for an infant or child consists of using

(a) an entirely different method of airway adjunct sizing than that used for an adult.
(b) a tongue depressor to push and lift the tongue out of the way, then inserting the adjunct into the airway without rotation.
(c) the same method of airway adjunct sizing as that used for an adult.
(d) Both answers (a) and (b).
(e) Both answers (b) and (c).

17. Which of the following statements regarding oxygenation of infants and children is false?

(a) Nonrebreather-administrated oxygen is the preferred method of oxygenation.
(b) Blow-by oxygenation may be accomplished by holding a pediatric nonrebreather mask or oxygen tubing approximately 2 inches away from the pediatric patient's face.
(c) Blow-by oxygenation may be accomplished by inserting oxygen tubing into the bottom of a paper cup directed at the pediatric patient's face.
(d) Blow-by oxygenation may be accomplished by inserting oxygen tubing into the bottom of a Styrofoam cup directed at the pediatric patient's face.
(e) None of the above are false.

18. Artificial ventilations should be delivered to an infant or child at a rate of

    (a) 12 per minute (1 ventilation every 5 seconds).
    (b) 60 per minute (1 ventilation every second).
    (c) 15 per minute (1 ventilation every 4 seconds).
    (d) 30 per minute (1 ventilation every 2 seconds).
    (e) 20 per minute (1 ventilation every 3 seconds).

19. Respiratory assessment of an infant or child includes

    (a) noting chest expansion, symmetry, and effort of breathing.
    (b) observing for nasal flaring, stridor, crowing, or retractions.
    (c) listening for any noisy breathing, especially grunting.
    (d) Answers (a) and (b) only.
    (e) Answers (a), (b), and (c).

20. The normal (resting) pulse rate range for an infant is

    (a) 110 to 210 beats per minute.
    (b) 100 to 200 beats per minute.
    (c) 80 to 140 beats per minute.
    (d) 60 to 100 beats per minute.
    (e) 60 to 90 beats per minute.

21. The normal (resting) pulse rate range for a preschooler is

    (a) 100 to 200 beats per minute.
    (b) 80 to 120 beats per minute.
    (c) 60 to 100 beats per minute.
    (d) 60 to 90 beats per minute.
    (e) 50 to 80 beats per minute.

22. The normal (resting) respiratory rate for a toddler is

    (a) 30 to 50 breaths per minute.
    (b) 20 to 30 breaths per minute.
    (c) 12 to 20 breaths per minute.
    (d) 8 to 15 breaths per minute.
    (e) 8 to 12 breaths per minute.

23. Infants and children normally have different pulse rate ranges than adult patients. Which of the following general statements regarding infant and child pulse rates is false?

    (a) A maintained pulse rate of greater than 100 in an infant or child is a cause for serious illness or injury concern.
    (b) A maintained pulse rate of lower than 60 in an infant or child is not a cause for serious illness or injury concern.

(c) In infants and children, maintenance of a faster pulse rate (100 to 120) is a much greater concern than maintenance of a slower pulse rate (40 to 60).
(d) Only answers (a) and (b) are false.
(e) All of the above are false.

24. Use the appropriate size blood pressure cuff to assess the blood pressure of children

    (a) over 12 years old, only.
    (b) over 8 years old, only.
    (c) over 3 years old, only.
    (d) over 1 year old, only.
    (e) of all ages (including infants).

25. The Detailed Physical Exam for infants and children

    (a) is exactly the same as for adults.
    (b) should be done in a head-to-toe manner of order.
    (c) should be done in a trunk-to-head manner of order.
    (d) Both answers (a) and (b).
    (e) Both answers (a) and (c).

26. Which of the following statements regarding emergency care for an alert pediatric patient with a partial airway obstruction is true?

    (a) Offer oxygen to the child, but do not agitate the child.
    (b) Do not allow the parent to sit the child on a lap (parents tend to "bounce" children and may cause the obstruction to become worse).
    (c) Allow the child to sit in a position of comfort; do not force the child to lay flat.
    (d) Both answers (a) and (b) are true.
    (e) Both answers (a) and (c) are true.

27. There are special considerations to remember when assessing and treating the pediatric patient in respiratory distress. Which of the following special considerations is false?

    (a) For the pediatric patient in respiratory distress, a slow pulse indicates a serious emergency.
    (b) The observation of cyanosis is a late finding in children, indicating a seriously ill, very critical patient.
    (c) Pediatric patients rarely require the strong medications contained in respiratory inhalers. Thus, EMT-Basics are not allowed to assist with pediatric inhaler use.
    (d) EMT-assisted usage of handheld inhalers is the same for the child as for the adult, as long as the same indications and contraindications have been considered.
    (e) None of the above are false.

28. When exhaling into the pocket face mask to ventilate the pediatric patient, each exhalation (ventilation) should last

　　(a) ½ to 1 second.
　　(b) 1 to 1½ seconds.
　　(c) 1½ to 2 seconds.
　　(d) 2 to 2½ seconds.
　　(e) 2½ to 3 seconds.

29. When using a flow-restricted, oxygen-powered ventilation device to deliver ventilations to a pediatric patient, ventilate the patient every ___ seconds.

　　(a) 8
　　(b) 5
　　(c) 3
　　(d) Either answer (a) or (b).
　　(e) None of the above; these devices are not to be used on children.

30. The dosage protocol for EMT-B-assisted infant or child epinephrine auto-injector use is

　　(a) assist with only one infant/child auto-injector use (0.15 mg of medication).
　　(b) if the patient has **both** respiratory distress and signs and symptoms of shock, assist with two simultaneous infant/child auto-injector uses (0.3 mg of medication, total).
　　(c) assist with one infant/child auto-injector use (0.15 mg of medication), followed by another assisted injection (if ordered) every 5 minutes until the patient's injectors are all used or you arrive at the emergency department.
　　(d) if the patient has **both** respiratory distress and signs and symptoms of shock, assist with two simultaneous infant/child auto-injector uses (0.6 mg of medication) every 5 minutes until the patient's injectors are all used or you arrive at the emergency department.
　　(e) None of the above. Infants and children are not prescribed epinephrine auto-injectors.

31. Which of the following statements regarding pediatric seizures is false?

　　(a) Seizures in children who have chronic seizure disorders rarely are life-threatening.
　　(b) In the prehospital setting, all pediatric seizures, including febrile (fever) seizures, should be considered life-threatening.
　　(c) Seizures may be caused by trauma, or trauma may occur during the seizure.
　　(d) None of the above are false.
　　(e) Both answers (a) and (b) are false.

TEST SECTION SIX

32. Which of the following statements regarding treatment of the conscious pediatric poisoning patient is true?

(a) Administer oxygen and monitor vital signs closely.
(b) Contact the medical director to report the poisoning substance.
(c) Depending on the poisoning substance, request orders to administer activated charcoal.
(d) Both answers (a) and (b) are true.
(e) Answers (a), (b), and (c) are true.

33. Which of the following statements regarding treatment of the unconscious pediatric poisoning patient is true?

(a) Administer oxygen and artificial ventilations, and monitor vital signs closely.
(b) Contact the medical director to report the poisoning substance.
(c) Depending on the poisoning substance, request orders to administer activated charcoal.
(d) Both answers (a) and (b) are true.
(e) Answers (a), (b), and (c) are true.

34. Which of the following statements regarding pediatric fevers is false?

(a) Fevers often accompany simple (non-life-threatening) childhood diseases such as measles or chicken pox.
(b) Never consider a child's fever as an unimportant sign of simple illness.
(c) A fever accompanied by a rash may indicate a serious illness.
(d) Both answers (a) and (c) are false.
(e) None of the above are false.

35. Which of the following statements regarding pediatric patients in shock is false?

(a) Pediatric shock most often occurs because of cardiac failure (children will compensate for all other causes until their heart "gives out").
(b) It takes very little blood or fluid loss to produce shock in the pediatric patient.
(c) Vomiting and/or diarrhea may quickly dehydrate the pediatric patient and result in shock.
(d) Children have strong, resilient bodies that can compensate for shock longer than an adult. Thus, they may appear fine but be in the initial stage of shock.
(e) Once children are no longer able to compensate for shock, they deteriorate much more rapidly than adults.

36. All near-drowning victims must be transported to the hospital, even if they seem to fully recover at the scene. This is because

   (a) pediatric drowning is most often the result of child abuse, and the parents must be investigated before the child is allowed to return home with them.
   (b) adolescent drowning is most often the result of illegal alcohol ingestion, and the police may want to investigate how the patient obtained the alcohol.
   (c) "secondary drowning syndrome" may occur within minutes to hours after the patient resumes normal breathing.
   (d) artificial ventilation always causes lung damage when performed for more than one minute.
   (e) protocol demands that all patients be transported by ambulance.

37. Sudden infant death syndrome (SIDS) is caused by

   (a) child abuse (often without external signs of abuse).
   (b) external suffocation, either purposefully (by parents) or accidentally (by bed covers).
   (c) aspiration of vomitus and subsequent suffocation.
   (d) Either answer (b) or (c).
   (e) None of the above.

38. Emergency care for the SIDS patient includes

   (a) performing resuscitation methods for all SIDS babies, unless the child has rigor mortis (a stiff, cold body in a warm environment).
   (b) avoiding any comments that might suggest blame to the parents.
   (c) reassuring the parents that SIDS occurs in apparently healthy babies, without any warning.
   (d) ensuring that the parents receive emotional support and counseling.
   (e) All of the above.

39. Which of the following statements regarding pediatric trauma is false?

   (a) Trauma is the second leading cause of death in infants and children (second only to cardiac failure).
   (b) Blunt trauma is the most common pediatric trauma mechanism.

(c) Pediatric respiratory arrest is common secondary to head injuries and may occur during transport.
(d) The most common cause of hypoxia in the unconscious pediatric head injury patient is obstruction of the airway by the tongue.
(e) Sand bags should never be used to stabilize the pediatric patient's head.

40. Which of the following statements regarding pediatric trauma is false?

     (a) Children have very soft, pliable ribs. They may have significant internal chest injuries without any external signs.
     (b) The abdomen is a more common site of injury in children than in adults.
     (c) Always consider hidden abdominal injury in the pediatric multiple trauma patient who is deteriorating without external signs of serious injury.
     (d) Children have very flexible bones and often are frightened by splinting techniques. Therefore, only apply splints to extremities with obvious deformities (simple pain and swelling is not an indication for splinting in the pediatric patient).
     (e) Pneumatic antishock garments (PASGs) should be used only if they fit the patient. Never place both of a child's legs inside an adult PASG leg section.

41. Signs and symptoms of possible child abuse include all of the following, except

     (a) multiple bruises in various stages of healing.
     (b) an injury that doesn't seem to fit the mechanism described by the caregiver present.
     (c) repeated calls to the same address.
     (d) a parent who seems unusually concerned about a seemingly innocent injury.
     (e) a parent who appears angry that the child is "always falling down or getting hurt."

42. Signs and symptoms of possible child neglect include

     (a) the absence of adult supervision.
     (b) a child who appears malnourished.
     (c) a living environment that appears unsafe.
     (d) Answers (b) and (c) only.
     (e) Answers (a), (b), and (c).

43. Which of the following statements regarding EMT actions, when suspicious of child abuse or neglect, is false?

(a) Report your suspicions that abuse or neglect is involved to the emergency department staff.

(b) Clearly document your conclusion that the child was abused and/or neglected on the patient trip report. In this way, more attention will be paid to your assessment of the child's situation, and you will not be accused of "missing" the signs of abuse or neglect.

(c) Avoid accusing or confronting the parties suspected of abuse or neglect.

(d) Document only your objective findings (what you saw, heard, and so on), not your suspicion of child abuse or neglect.

(e) If you have any suspicion of abuse or neglect, transport the child to the emergency department (even when the injuries do not warrant ambulance transport).

The answer key for Test Section Six is on pages 373 through 374.

Test Section Seven

This test section covers the following subjects:

* Ambulance Operations
* Gaining Access
* Hazardous Materials Incident Management
* Multiple-casualty Incident Management

1994 Revised EMT-Basic National Standards Review Self-Test

1. When operating an emergency vehicle with lights and sirens engaged,
   (a) the emergency vehicle driver is just as liable as any other motorist for the occurrence of accidents due to negligent driving practices.
   (b) other motorists must yield the right-of-way to the emergency vehicle. If they do not, they will be found at fault for any type of accident that occurs.
   (c) stop signs may be ignored.
   (d) flashing red signals may be ignored.
   (e) red stop signals may be ignored.

2. When operating with lights and sirens engaged, the emergency vehicle
   (a) may exceed the posted speed limit without any liability.
   (b) does not need to signal turns.
   (c) may pass other vehicles without signaling or "clearing" the passing lane.
   (d) may pass an off-loading school bus even when its red warning lights are blinking.
   (e) may disregard regulations governing direction of travel (may drive eastbound in a westbound lane of traffic), but only if using proper caution and a regard for the safety of others.

3. When operating without lights and sirens engaged, the emergency vehicle
   (a) may exceed the posted speed limit without any liability.
   (b) does not need to signal turns.
   (c) may park anywhere, including in a lane of traffic, as long as personal property or lives are not threatened.
   (d) must follow every traffic rule and regulation that any other vehicle is subject to.
   (e) must follow only the traffic rules and regulations that apply to vehicles using lights and sirens.

4. Which of the following statements regarding the use of sirens is false?
   (a) Some states require the use of sirens anytime an emergency vehicle is traveling with its emergency lights engaged.
   (b) Studies have shown that, the longer a siren is sounded (especially in one sound pattern), the more likely it is that motorists will hear it and yield the right-of-way.

(c) An ill or injured patient may experience increased anxiety and discomfort when transported with lights and sirens in continuous use.
   (d) Use of sirens may cause hearing loss for the unprotected emergency vehicle operator.
   (e) None of the above are false.

5. Which of the following statements regarding the use of lights and sirens is false?
   (a) Some states require that an emergency vehicle, using lights and sirens, must come to a complete stop at a red stoplight or stop sign, before proceeding through the intersection.
   (b) Some states require that an emergency vehicle, using lights and sirens, must slow down at a red stoplight or stop sign, proceeding through the intersection only after determining that other motorists are yielding the right-of-way.
   (c) Most states require that lights and sirens be used only for situations that threaten life and/or limb, and then only with due regard for the safety of the public.
   (d) In any state, if an emergency vehicle operator does not drive with due regard for the safety of others, the operator may be ticketed, sued, or even incarcerated.
   (e) None of the above are false.

6. Which of the following statements regarding the use of sirens is false?
   (a) Modern-day sirens are designed specifically to penetrate buildings, dense shrubbery, and/or civilian vehicle sound-proofing.
   (b) Even when they can hear them, motorists may ignore emergency vehicle sirens.
   (c) Motorists listening to loud radios or car stereos may not hear a siren.
   (d) Motorists sometimes panic when they hear a siren.
   (e) None of the above are false.

7. The faster an emergency vehicle travels,
   (a) the more likely it is to be involved in a collision.
   (b) the greater the distance required to stop.
   (c) the more lives will be saved.
   (d) Both answers (a) and (b).
   (e) Answers (a), (b), and (c).

8. Which of the following statements regarding an escorted emergency vehicle (with both vehicles using lights and sirens) is true?
    (a) The escort vehicle should be followed as closely as possible so that motorists will not have room to pull in between you and the escort.
    (b) The use of an escort vehicle is extremely hazardous and should be used only when the escorted operator absolutely requires guidance.
    (c) The use of an escort vehicle increases the safety of both vehicles' operators and passengers.
    (d) Both answers (a) and (b) are true.
    (e) Both answers (a) and (c) are true.

9. The most common site of emergency vehicle accidents is
    (a) within 5 blocks of the emergency facilities.
    (b) in a parking lot.
    (c) at an intersection.
    (d) along a busy, grid-locked city street.
    (e) along a busy, grid-locked interstate highway.

10. Duties of the EMT-Basic who is not trained in rescue and/or extrication techniques include all of the following, except
    (a) assessment and administration of necessary care to the patient before extrication.
    (b) assuring that the patient is removed in a manner that will not cause further injury.
    (c) directing the efforts of all rescue and/or extrication personnel.
    (d) cooperation with the activities of rescue and/or extrication personnel.
    (e) assuring that the activities of rescue and/or extrication personnel do not interfere with patient safety and care.

11. Duties of the EMT-Basic who is also trained in rescue and/or extrication techniques include
    (a) first assuring that at least one EMS/rescue provider will be focusing on the patient's needs prior to beginning rescue and/or extrication (establishing assigned duties).
    (b) assuring that patient care precedes extrication unless delayed movement would endanger the life of the patient or other rescuers.
    (c) assuring that the activities of rescue and/or extrication personnel do not interfere with patient safety and care.
    (d) Answers (a) and (b) only.
    (e) Answers (a), (b), and (c).

12. The number one priority for all EMS, rescue, and/or extrication personnel is

    (a) patient safety and appropriate care.
    (b) personal protection and safety of other team members.
    (c) cervical-spine precautions for the patient.
    (d) gaining access at any cost.
    (e) representing the service well when filmed by news crews.

13. The number two priority for all EMS, rescue, and/or extrication personnel is

    (a) patient safety and appropriate care.
    (b) personal protection and safety of other team members.
    (c) cervical-spine precautions for the patient.
    (d) gaining access at any cost.
    (e) representing the service well when filmed by news crews.

14. The EMT who is untrained in rescue and/or extrication operation may

    (a) engage in simple access rescue techniques without special training or equipment.
    (b) engage in complex access rescue techniques without training or special equipment.
    (c) direct the activities of all other rescue/extrication personnel (as "medical officer," the EMT is in command of any scene that involves patients).
    (d) Both answers (a) and (b).
    (e) Both answers (a) and (c).

The following 4 questions (questions 15 through 18) pertain to the same scenario.

15. You and your crew are responding southbound on a north/south highway. The wind is blowing from the north. As you near the scene of the accident, you notice that some kind of a tanker truck is on its side, about 25 feet east of the highway. There is a dust cloud (or odd-looking smoke) seeping from a break in the tank. You park your vehicle

    (a) on the east side of the highway, at least 100 feet before reaching the truck accident site.
    (b) on the west side of the highway, at least 100 feet before reaching the truck accident site.
    (c) on the east side of the highway, at least 100 feet past the truck accident site.
    (d) on the west side of the highway, at least 100 feet past the truck accident site.
    (e) immediately between the truck site and the highway (to provide quick site access).

16. You and your crew are not trained in (or equipped for) hazardous materials handling. Your first tasks after parking your vehicle include all of the following, except

(a) establishing a "safe zone" and a "danger zone," and verbally directing anyone standing in the danger zone to leave it.
(b) removing patients from the danger zone.
(c) attempting to identify the tanker contents from a safe distance.
(d) directing unnecessary people away from the site (politely asking them to leave the area if not involved in the accident).
(e) staying in the safe zone and radioing for appropriate support resources.

17. To identify the contents of the tanker truck, you should

(a) use binoculars to search for and read any hazardous material placard that is posted on the tank.
(b) interview the conscious driver in the safe zone (while another EMT is assessing and caring for her/him).
(c) search the overturned cab for the bill of lading or shipping papers.
(d) Answers (a) and (b) only.
(e) Answers (a), (b), and (c).

18. Although some studies show that vehicles are correctly placarded only 50 to 75 percent of the time, if you see a hazardous material placard, you may identify the indicated material by

(a) looking up the placard's numbers, shape, and/or colors in **Hazardous Materials, The Emergency Response Handbook**, if it is carried in your vehicle.
(b) having your dispatcher look up the placard's numbers, shape, and/or colors in **Hazardous Materials, The Emergency Response Handbook**, if the book is kept at dispatch.
(c) having your dispatcher call CHEMTREC, a 24-hour hotline number (800-424-9300), to report the placard's numbers, shape, and/or colors.
(d) Answers (a) and (b) only.
(e) Answers (a), (b), and (c).

19. A multiple-casualty incident (MCI), sometimes called a multiple-casualty situation (MCS), is best defined as

(a) any incident or situation involving 3 or more patients.
(b) any incident or situation involving more patients than rescuers.

(c) any incident or situation involving 25 or more patients.
(d) any event that places a great demand on EMS equipment or personnel resources.
(e) any incident or situation involving 50 or more patients.

20. An incident management system is a system developed by local jurisdictions for planned and coordinated response to MCIs. This system should provide for

    (a) an orderly means of communication between other agencies and resources.
    (b) a central means of coordinating multiple agencies and resources.
    (c) an easier and smoother interaction between different agencies and resources.
    (d) Answers (a) and (b) only.
    (e) Answers (a), (b), and (c).

21. The first EMT to arrive on the scene of an obvious MCI should immediately

    (a) begin counting the number of patients, so that a "false alarm" will not be sounded.
    (b) initiate the incident management system for MCI response.
    (c) begin clearing uninjured and/or uninvolved persons away from the scene so that an accurate count can be made.
    (d) begin treating patients.
    (e) establish a danger zone and a safe zone.

22. The process called *triage* comes from the French word that means

    (a) "to select."
    (b) "determine the first."
    (c) "to sort."
    (d) "determine the worst."
    (e) "determine the best."

23. During an MCI, the goal of initial triage is to

    (a) save the greatest number of lives possible, given the available resources.
    (b) decide which patients require rapid treatment and transportation and which patients can wait.
    (c) obtain the name, age, and address of each patient before confusion (and/or unconsciousness) prohibits patient identification.
    (d) Answers (a) and (b) only.
    (e) Answers (a), (b), and (c).

During initial triage, patients are sorted into four different categories. Use the following list of patient conditions and injuries to answer the last four questions in this test section (questions 24 through 27). Each number should be used only once.

1. Airway and breathing difficulties
2. Back injuries with obvious spinal cord damage
3. Back injuries without obvious spinal cord damage
4. Burns of 100 percent body surface area (incineration)
5. Burns without airway problems
6. Cardiac arrest
7. Crushing head injury with exposed brain matter
8. Decapitation
9. Decreased mental status
10. Major or multiple bone or joint injuries
11. Minor, but painful, extremity injuries
12. Minor soft-tissue injuries
13. Minor swelling and deformity of an extremity
14. Patients with severe medical problems
15. Severe burns
16. Shock (hypoperfusion)
17. Uncontrolled or severe bleeding

24. Highest-priority patients, those who should receive the most rapid treatment and transportation when resources are limited, are called "Priority 1" patients. From the previous list, select six patients to be Priority 1 patients.

(a) 1, 2, 6, 14, 15, and 17.
(b) 2, 6, 10, 14, 15, and 17.
(c) 1, 9, 14, 15, 16, and 17.
(d) 2, 4, 6, 14, 15, and 16.
(e) 1, 6, 10, 14, 15, and 16.

25. When resources are limited, second-priority patients are those who should receive rapid treatment and transportation after Priority 1 patients have been managed. These patients are called "Priority 2" patients. From the previous list, select four patients to be Priority 2 patients.

(a) 2, 3, 5, and 10.
(b) 1, 3, 5, and 9.
(c) 3, 5, 9, and 14.
(d) 3, 5, 9, and 17.
(e) 3, 5, 11, and 16.

26. Priority 3 patients are sometimes called "the walking wounded." These are patients who may wait the longest before their treatment and transportation is arranged. From the previous list, select three patients to be Priority 3 patients.

    (a) 9, 12, and 13.
    (b) 11, 12, and 13.
    (c) 12, 13, and 14.
    (d) 12, 13, and 16.
    (e) 3, 5, and 12.

27. The final triage category is called either "Priority 4" or "Priority 0." These are victims who will not receive treatment and transportation. Of the patients previously listed, when resources are limited, which would be Priority 4 patients?

    (a) 4, 7, and 8.
    (b) 4 and 8.
    (c) 7 and 8.
    (d) 4, 6, 7, and 8.
    (e) 1, 4, 6, 7, and 8.

The answer key for Test Section Seven is on page 375.

Test Section Eight

8

This test section covers the following subjects:

* Airway Anatomy Review (repeated per DOT emphasis)
* Adult Orotracheal Intubation
* Pediatric Orotracheal Intubation
* Nasogastric Tube Insertion
* Endotracheal Tube Suctioning

1994 Revised EMT-Basic National Standards Review Self-Test

1. When breathing through the mouth, air first enters the
   - (a) pharynx.
   - (b) nasopharynx.
   - (c) larynx.
   - (d) hypopharynx.
   - (e) oropharynx.

2. When breathing through the nose, air first enters the
   - (a) pharynx.
   - (b) nasopharynx.
   - (c) larynx.
   - (d) hypopharynx.
   - (e) oropharynx.

3. The area that lies directly above the openings of the windpipe and the tube leading to the stomach is called the
   - (a) pharynx.
   - (b) nasopharynx.
   - (c) larynx.
   - (d) hypopharynx.
   - (e) oropharynx.

4. A leaf-shaped valve that prevents food and liquid from entering the windpipe is called the
   - (a) cricoid cartilage.
   - (b) larynx.
   - (c) valecula.
   - (d) epiglottis.
   - (e) trachea.

5. A groove-like space (sometimes considered a structure) that is immediately anterior to the leaf-shaped valve that prevents food and liquid from entering the windpipe is called the
   - (a) cricoid cartilage.
   - (b) larynx.
   - (c) valecula.
   - (d) epiglottis.
   - (e) trachea.

6. The medical term for the windpipe is the

   (a) cricoid cartilage.
   (b) larynx.
   (c) valecula.
   (d) epiglottis.
   (e) trachea.

7. The firm ring that forms the lower portion of the voice box is the

   (a) cricoid cartilage.
   (b) larynx.
   (c) valecula.
   (d) epiglottis.
   (e) trachea.

8. The medical term for the voice box is the

   (a) cricoid cartilage.
   (b) larynx.
   (c) valecula.
   (d) epiglottis.
   (e) trachea.

9. The windpipe divides into two large air tubes at a junction called the **carina**. The medical term for these air tubes is the

   (a) right or left rhonchi.
   (b) right or left bronchi.
   (c) right or left alveoli.
   (d) anterior or posterior rhonchi.
   (e) anterior or posterior bronchi.

10. At the end of the respiratory "tree" are groups of tiny sacs. These sacs are called the

   (a) rhonchi.
   (b) bronchi.
   (c) alveoli.
   (d) petechia.
   (e) cilia.

11. The narrowest area of an infant's or child's airway is at the level of the

   (a) cricoid cartilage.
   (b) larynx.
   (c) valecula.
   (d) epiglottis.
   (e) trachea.

12. An endotracheal tube is designed to be inserted through the _____ and into the _____.

    (a) cricoid cartilage/larynx
    (b) larynx/trachea
    (c) valecula/larynx
    (d) epiglottis/valecula
    (e) trachea/larynx

13. The medical term **intubation** is best defined as

    (a) an airway maneuver that is too advanced for EMT-Basics.
    (b) the insertion of a tube into the mouth.
    (c) the insertion of a tube.
    (d) the insertion of a tube into the esophagus.
    (e) the insertion of a tube through the nose.

14. The medical phrase **orotracheal intubation** is best defined as

    (a) the insertion of a tube into the trachea via the nose.
    (b) the insertion of a tube into the trachea via the mouth.
    (c) the insertion of a tube into the esophagus via the mouth.
    (d) the insertion of a tube into the esophagus via the nose.
    (e) the insertion of any tube through the nose or mouth.

15. A **laryngoscope** is best defined as an illuminating tool that is inserted into the pharynx and used to visualize the pharynx and

    (a) larynx (vocal cords).
    (b) cricoid cartilage (vocal cords).
    (c) vocal cords (cricoid cartilage).
    (d) trachea (cricoid cartilage).
    (e) nasopharynx.

16. All of the following advantages accompany the performance of orotracheal intubation, except that it

    (a) provides for complete control of the patient's airway.
    (b) minimizes the risk of aspiration.
    (c) allows for better suctioning of the esophagus.
    (d) allows for better oxygen delivery to the lungs.
    (e) allows for deeper suctioning of the airways.

17. Complications of orotracheal intubation include all of the following, except

    (a) physical stimulation of the airway producing a dangerously rapid heart rate.
    (b) trauma to lips, teeth, tongue, gums, and/or airway structures.

(c) inadequate oxygenation due to prolonged intubation attempts.
(d) right main-stem intubation.
(e) esophageal intubation.

18. Complications of orotracheal intubation include all of the following, except
    (a) stimulation of vomiting.
    (b) self-extubation by the patient who regains consciousness.
    (c) physical stimulation of the airway, producing a dangerously slow heart rate.
    (d) unrecognized accidental extubation during moving or transporting the patient.
    (e) self-extubation by the unconscious patient.

19. The most serious complication of orotracheal intubation is
    (a) airway stimulation that produces a rapid heart rate.
    (b) right main-stem intubation.
    (c) esophageal intubation.
    (d) stimulation of vomiting.
    (e) self-extubation by the patient who regains consciousness.

20. Laryngoscope blades come in two general types, curved and straight. Each type of blade comes in a variety of sizes, from the smallest size (_____) to the largest size (_____).
    (a) 6/0
    (b) 3/0
    (c) 0/6
    (d) 0/4
    (e) 4/1

21. The straight laryngoscope blade (also called a "Miller" or "Wisconsin" blade) is designed to be inserted so that the tip of the blade
    (a) enters the valecula and lifts it, indirectly lifting the epiglottis, so that the lower airway opening can be visualized.
    (b) is placed under the epiglottis, directly lifting it, to visualize the lower airway opening.
    (c) enters the epiglottis, just above the cricoid cartilage, to indirectly lift the valecula, so that the lower airway opening can be visualized.
    (d) is placed into the valecula, sliding it to the right side, to visualize the cricoid cartilage opening to the airway.
    (e) enters the cricoid cartilage, just above the valecula, to indirectly lift the cricoid cartilage and visualize the lower airway opening.

22. The curved laryngoscope blade (also called a "MacIntosh" blade) is designed to be inserted so that the tip of the blade

   (a) enters the valecula and lifts it, indirectly lifting the epiglottis, so that the lower airway opening can be visualized.
   (b) is placed under the epiglottis, directly lifting it, to visualize the lower airway opening.
   (c) enters the epiglottis, just above the cricoid cartilage, to indirectly lift the valecula, so that the lower airway opening can be visualized.
   (d) is placed into the valecula, sliding it to the right side, to visualize the cricoid cartilage opening to the airway.
   (e) enters the cricoid cartilage, just above the valecula, to indirectly lift the cricoid cartilage and visualize the lower airway opening.

23. The average size of an endotracheal tube required by an adult male is

   (a) 9.5 to 10.0 millimeters in diameter.
   (b) 8.5 to 9.5 millimeters in diameter.
   (c) 8.0 to 8.5 millimeters in diameter.
   (d) 7.5 to 8.5 millimeters in diameter.
   (e) 7.0 to 8.0 millimeters in diameter.

24. The average size of an endotracheal tube required by an adult female is

   (a) 9.5 to 10.0 millimeters in diameter.
   (b) 8.5 to 9.5 millimeters in diameter.
   (c) 8.0 to 8.5 millimeters in diameter.
   (d) 7.5 to 8.5 millimeters in diameter.
   (e) 7.0 to 8.0 millimeters in diameter.

25. In an emergency, an endotracheal tube that is _____ millimeters in diameter may be used for any adult.

   (a) 9.5
   (b) 8.5
   (c) 7.5
   (d) 6.0
   (e) 5.0

26. At the top of the endotracheal tube is an adapter that is designed to connect the tube with a bag-valve for ventilation. Because there are many manufacturers of both bag-valve-mask devices and endotracheal tubes, this adapter (and the port of the bag-valve) must be a standard size on all brands. The standard size of the adapter at the top end of an endotracheal tube is

(a) 5 millimeters.
(b) 10 millimeters.
(c) 15 millimeters.
(d) 20 millimeters.
(e) 25 millimeters.

27. Many endotracheal tubes have a small hole opposite to the beveled, bottom end of the endotracheal tube. This hole is called "Murphy's eye" and is designed to

(a) be a port through which an endotracheal suctioning device is passed.
(b) decrease the chance of endotracheal tube obstruction.
(c) allow for extra ventilation, in case the selected endotracheal tube is too small for the patient.
(d) Answers (a) and (b) only.
(e) Answers (a), (b), and (c).

28. At the far end of adult endotracheal tubes is an inflatable cuff. The purpose of this cuff is to

(a) anchor the tube in place (the inflated cuff is larger than the cricoid cartilage). Thus, if tape or tube-tying materials are not immediately available, they are unnecessary.
(b) keep vomitus from entering the endotracheal tube.
(c) keep air from leaking around the tube (escaping, rather than ventilating the patient).
(d) Answers (a) and (b) only.
(e) Answers (b) and (c) only.

29. The endotracheal tube's inflatable cuff holds _____ of air.

(a) 5 cc
(b) 10 cc
(c) 15 cc
(d) 20 cc
(e) 30 cc

30. The endotracheal tube's cuff is inflated by injecting air into the inflation valve at the top of the endotracheal tube. Just beyond the inflation valve is a pilot balloon. The pilot balloon is designed to

   (a) verify that the inflated cuff retains its air.
   (b) hold air in the cuff.
   (c) provide an injection site for medications that are administered through the endotracheal tube.
   (d) Both answers (a) and (b).
   (e) Both answers (a) and (c).

31. The length of a standard adult endotracheal tube is

   (a) 15 centimeters.
   (b) 20 centimeters.
   (c) 25 centimeters.
   (d) 33 centimeters.
   (e) 47 centimeters.

32. In the average adult, the distance between the teeth and the carina is

   (a) 15 centimeters.
   (b) 20 centimeters.
   (c) 25 centimeters.
   (d) 33 centimeters.
   (e) 47 centimeters.

33. In the average adult, the distance between the teeth and the suprasternal notch is

   (a) 15 centimeters.
   (b) 20 centimeters.
   (c) 25 centimeters.
   (d) 33 centimeters.
   (e) 47 centimeters.

34. In the average adult, the distance between the teeth and the vocal cords is

   (a) 15 centimeters.
   (b) 20 centimeters.
   (c) 25 centimeters.
   (d) 33 centimeters.
   (e) 47 centimeters.

35. A malleable metal stylet is often used to provide extra stiffness and shape to the endotracheal tube during intubation. Prior to intubation, this stylet should be inserted until the tip of the stylet is

  (a) visible just beyond the endotracheal tube's distal opening.
  (b) between the Murphy's eye and the endotracheal tube's distal opening.
  (c) protruding from Murphy's eye.
  (d) at the distal end of the inflatable cuff, approximately ¼ inch before reaching Murphy's eye.
  (e) Any of the above are acceptable.

36. Which of the following statements regarding lubricants used for intubation is false?

  (a) Only water-soluble lubricants should be used.
  (b) The stylet may be lubricated to allow for easy removal after intubation.
  (c) A lubricant should be applied to the endotracheal tube prior to intubation.
  (d) If a water-soluble lubricant is not available, Vaseline jelly (or the like) may be used.
  (e) None of the above are false.

37. Indications for performance of orotracheal intubation include all of the following, except

  (a) inability to ventilate the apneic patient.
  (b) to protect the airway of a patient who is unresponsive to any painful stimuli.
  (c) to protect the airway of a patient who has no gag reflex.
  (d) cardiac arrest.
  (e) to secure the airway of an unconscious patient who coughs when attempts to insert an oral airway are made.

38. Prior to any intubation attempt, the patient should be _____ with 100 percent oxygen, using the bag-valve-mask and an oral airway, at a rate of _____ ventilations per minute.

  (a) normally ventilated / 12
  (b) normally ventilated / 10
  (c) hyperventilated / 24
  (d) hyperventilated / 60
  (e) slowly, but fully, ventilated / 12

39. Which of the following statements regarding assembling and preparing the equipment needed for orotracheal intubation is false?

    (a) A suction unit with a rigid tip suction catheter must be functional and within easy reach.
    (b) The cuff of the selected endotracheal tube should be inflated and tested for leaks.
    (c) A syringe for injection of air should be attached to the endotracheal tube cuff inflation valve and remain attached during intubation.
    (d) A securing device must be within easy reach.
    (e) None of the above are false.

40. Correct positioning of the patient's head (to achieve correct airway alignment) is vitally important to successful orotracheal intubation. When trauma is not suspected, the patient should be positioned with her/his

    (a) head and neck in a neutral position, using manual, in-line stabilization.
    (b) neck flexed and chin lifted.
    (c) head tilted back and chin lifted.
    (d) Either answer (a) or (b).
    (e) Either answer (b) or (c).

41. When orotracheal intubation is required for a trauma patient, the patient should be positioned with her/his

    (a) head and neck in a neutral position, using manual, in-line stabilization.
    (b) neck flexed and chin lifted.
    (c) head tilted back and chin lifted.
    (d) Either answer (a) or (b).
    (e) Either answer (b) or (c).

42. When beginning orotracheal intubation, the _____ should be held in the left hand, and the _____ should be held in the right hand.

    (a) suction catheter/laryngoscope
    (b) endotracheal tube/laryngoscope
    (c) laryngoscope/endotracheal tube
    (d) suction catheter/endotracheal tube
    (e) Any of the above (right-handed and left-handed providers will use the technique most comfortable for them).

43. When using the laryngoscope to visualize the glottic opening, the EMT should

  (a) lift the patient's mandible up and away from the patient.
  (b) use a sweeping motion to lift the tongue up and to the left.
  (c) gently use the teeth as a fulcrum for the laryngoscope handle to achieve the best visualization possible.
  (d) Both answers (a) and (b).
  (e) Either answer (a) or (c), and answer (b).

44. Application of **Sellick's maneuver** during attempts at orotracheal intubation may be helpful. Which of the following statements regarding Sellick's maneuver is false?

  (a) Sellick's maneuver consists of another rescuer using her/his thumb and index finger to apply direct pressure to the patient's anterior neck, at the cricoid cartilage level.
  (b) Sellick's maneuver consists of the intubating rescuer using the laryngoscope to apply direct pressure to the patient's cricoid cartilage.
  (c) Sellick's maneuver will help to compress the esophagus, thus reducing the risk of vomiting during intubation.
  (d) Sellick's maneuver may help to bring the glottic opening into better view.
  (e) None of the above are false.

45. Visualization of the glottic opening

  (a) must be maintained until the endotracheal tube has entered the opening.
  (b) is important before inserting the endotracheal tube. After visualization, keep the patient and laryngoscope steady as you pass the tube into the opening (that you can no longer see).
  (c) is preferred. However, if no opening can be visualized, do not delay intubation. Make several attempts to pass the endotracheal tube without visualization (this is often called "blind intubation").
  (d) Both answers (b) and (c).
  (e) None of the above.

46. Gently insert the endotracheal tube through the glottic opening until

  (a) the cuff just passes the vocal cords.
  (b) the cuff is halfway through the vocal cords.
  (c) the cuff has passed the vocal cords by at least 10 centimeters.
  (d) the tube is advanced so that the bag-valve adapter is even with the patient's teeth.
  (e) the tube cannot be advanced any farther.

47. After the tube has been placed, the EMT should

    (a) remove the stylet (if one was used).
    (b) inflate the endotracheal tube's cuff.
    (c) have the bag-valve device attached to the endotracheal tube.
    (d) Answers (a) and (c) only.
    (e) Answers (a), (b), and (c).

48. The most accurate way to confirm the correct placement of the endotracheal tube is to

    (a) auscultate for breath sounds over the epigastrium.
    (b) auscultate for breath sounds over the apex of the left lung.
    (c) auscultate for breath sounds over the apex of the right lung.
    (d) visualize the endotracheal tube passing through the vocal cords of the glottic opening.
    (e) Any of the above (all are equally accurate methods of tube placement confirmation).

49. When verifying correct placement of the endotracheal tube with a stethoscope, the first place the EMT should listen is over the

    (a) epigastrium.
    (b) apex of the left lung.
    (c) apex of the right lung.
    (d) base of the left lung.
    (e) base of the right lung.

50. If breath sounds are present and clear on the right, but diminished or absent on the left, the EMT should

    (a) immediately secure the endotracheal tube and hyperventilate the patient (the patient has an absent or collapsed left lung and requires excessive ventilation as soon as possible).
    (b) remove the endotracheal tube and immediately re-attempt orotracheal intubation with a fresh tube.
    (c) deflate the endotracheal tube cuff and (without completely removing the tube) slowly withdraw the tube, while auscultating for improved breath sounds on the left.
    (d) remove the endotracheal tube and immediately re-attempt orotracheal intubation with the same tube.
    (e) remove the endotracheal tube and immediately discontinue any further attempts at orotracheal intubation.

51. If breath sounds are present only in the epigastrium, the EMT should

(a) immediately secure the endotracheal tube and hyperventilate the patient (both the patient's lungs have collapsed and excessive ventilation is needed as soon as possible).
(b) recognize that an esophageal intubation can be fatal for the patient, immediately deflate the endotracheal tube cuff, and completely remove the tube.
(c) deflate the endotracheal tube cuff and (without completely removing the tube) slowly withdraw the tube, while auscultating for improved breath sounds in the lungs.
(d) remove the endotracheal tube and immediately re-attempt orotracheal intubation with the same tube.
(e) remove the endotracheal tube and immediately discontinue any further attempts at orotracheal intubation.

52. When breath sounds are heard over both the right and left lungs, and no sounds are heard in the epigastrium, the EMT should have the tube held in place while the patient is appropriately ventilated and

(a) make sure that the endotracheal tube cuff is inflated.
(b) secure the tube in place, noting the distance that the tube has been inserted.
(c) insert an oral airway into the patient's mouth to serve as a bite block.
(d) Answers (a) and (b) only.
(e) Answers (a), (b), and (c).

53. Following successful orotracheal intubation, the EMT should continue with patient care and transportation, remembering that

(a) breath sounds do not need to be reassessed after the endotracheal tube is secured.
(b) the external endotracheal tube depth measurement should be checked frequently, to be sure it shows no tube movement.
(c) breath sounds must be frequently reassessed, especially following every major movement of the patient.
(d) Answers (a) and (b) only.
(e) Answers (b) and (c) only.

54. Indications for orotracheal intubation of pediatric patients include all of the following, except

    (a) when prolonged artificial ventilation will be required.
    (b) when adequate artificial ventilation cannot be achieved by other means.
    (c) the pediatric cardiac arrest patient.
    (d) the pediatric respiratory arrest patient.
    (e) when attempts to insert an oral airway cause the pediatric patient to cough and sputter.

55. The average size of pediatric endotracheal tubes required by the premature infant is

    (a) 1.0 millimeter in diameter.
    (b) 2.0 millimeters in diameter.
    (c) 3.0 to 3.5 millimeters in diameter.
    (d) 4.0 millimeters in diameter.
    (e) 5.0 to 6.0 millimeters in diameter.

56. The average size of pediatric endotracheal tubes required by (full-term) newborns and small infants is

    (a) 1.0 millimeter in diameter.
    (b) 2.0 millimeters in diameter.
    (c) 3.0 to 3.5 millimeters in diameter.
    (d) 4.0 millimeters in diameter.
    (e) 5.0 to 6.0 millimeters in diameter.

57. The average size of pediatric endotracheal tubes required by large infants (up to 1 year of age) is

    (a) 1.0 millimeter in diameter.
    (b) 2.0 millimeters in diameter.
    (c) 3.0 to 3.5 millimeters in diameter.
    (d) 4.0 millimeters in diameter.
    (e) 5.0 to 6.0 millimeters in diameter.

58. A generic, mathematical formula for selecting the best endotracheal tube size for the pediatric patient is: the patient's _____ plus 16, divided by 4, equals the tube size.

    (a) age
    (b) weight
    (c) height
    (d) Either answer (a) or (b).
    (e) Either answer (b) or (c).

59. Another means of selecting the best endotracheal tube size for the pediatric patient is to select a tube with a diameter that is the same size as the patient's

(a) thumb.
(b) small finger.
(c) nostril opening.
(d) Either answer (a) or (c).
(e) Either answer (b) or (c).

60. Which of the following statements regarding intubation of pediatric patients and the use of endotracheal tubes without inflatable cuffs is true?

(a) Children from birth to the age of 8 years should not be intubated with a cuffed endotracheal tube.
(b) Uncuffed endotracheal tubes are only for infants.
(c) Children between the ages of 3 and 8 years should not be intubated with a cuffed endotracheal tube. For infants and children over age 8, cuffed endotracheal tubes should be used.
(d) For small children (including infants), uncuffed endotracheal tubes should be used. For large children (even as young as 5 or 6 years old), cuffed endotracheal tubes should be used.
(e) None of the above are true.

61. Which of the following statements regarding laryngoscope blades and orotracheal intubation of pediatric patients is false?

(a) The EMT should have both curved and straight blades in pediatric sizes.
(b) The straight blade is preferred for intubation of infants and very small children.
(c) Only the curved blade should be used for intubation of older (larger) children.
(d) None of the above are false.
(e) Both answers (b) and (c) are false (the correct answers are the opposite).

62. Which of the following statements regarding orotracheal intubation procedures for pediatric patients is false?

   (a) The procedure for orotracheal intubation of children is generally the same as for adult orotracheal intubation.
   (b) The rate of ventilation before and after intubation is faster for children than for adults.
   (c) Orotracheal intubation may stimulate slow heart rates in pediatric patients. However, this heart rate stimulation is not a concern for pediatric patients (as it is for adults). Do not be preoccupied with, or distracted by, heart rate monitoring during intubation of infants and children.
   (d) Just as in adults, if trauma is suspected, the pediatric patient's head and neck must be manually stabilized in a neutral, in-line position during intubation.
   (e) None of the above are false.

63. Correct positioning of the pediatric patient's head (to achieve correct airway alignment) is vitally important to successful orotracheal intubation. When trauma is not suspected, the patient should be positioned with her/his

   (a) head and neck hyperextended as far as possible.
   (b) neck flexed forward and chin lifted.
   (c) head extended only slightly and chin lifted (the "sniffing" position).
   (d) Either answer (a) or (b).
   (e) Either answer (b) or (c).

64. If good visualization of the pediatric glottic opening is not well achieved by the previously mentioned head positioning, the EMT should

   (a) flex the head and neck forward more.
   (b) flex the head and neck backward more
   (c) turn the head slightly to the left side.
   (d) turn the head slightly to the right side.
   (e) use folded towels (or the like) to raise the patient's shoulders one or more inches.

65. In infants and small children, the best indications of a correctly placed tube and adequately delivered ventilations include an improvement in skin color and when

   (a) breath sounds are heard on the left side of the patient's chest.
   (b) breath sounds are heard on the right side of the patient's chest.

(c) epigastric sounds are heard (children are "belly" breathers).
(d) the chest gently rises and falls with each ventilation.
(e) the abdomen rises with each ventilation (children are "belly" breathers).

66. If the endotracheal tube is properly placed (you saw it go through the glottic opening and there are no gastric sounds on ventilation), but the child's chest does not expand adequately with ventilation, the problem probably is an endotracheal tube that is

(a) blocked by secretions. The tube should be suctioned. If suctioning fails, the tube should be removed and replaced with a fresh tube, after hyperventilation.
(b) too small for the patient, and air is escaping around the tube at the glottic opening. The tube should be removed and replaced with a larger tube, after hyperventilation.
(c) too large for the patient. The cricoid cartilage is pinching off the tube, and air is not reaching the lungs. The tube should be removed and replaced with a smaller tube, after hyperventilation.
(d) Either answer (a) or (b).
(e) Any of the above.

67. The purpose of prehospital insertion of a nasogastric tube (NG tube) is to

(a) confirm the placement of the endotracheal tube.
(b) administer glucose to an unresponsive diabetic patient before transportation to the emergency department.
(c) reduce gastric distention caused by air in the stomach and proximal bowel.
(d) Answers (a) and (b) only.
(e) Answers (a), (b), and (c).

68. Which of the following is an indication for prehospital insertion of a nasogastric tube in the pediatric patient?

(a) Inability to ventilate the infant or child due to gastric distention (which often occurs in infants and children from bag-valve-mask ventilations prior to orotracheal intubation).
(b) An unconscious infant or child with gastric distention.
(c) An infant or child with an altered level of consciousness from head trauma (head injuries are often accompanied by profuse vomiting).
(d) Answers (a) and (b) only.
(e) Answers (a), (b), and (c).

69. Which of the following statements regarding complications of nasogastric tube insertion is false?

  (a) The NG tube may accidentally enter the trachea, especially if the patient has not been intubated with an endotracheal tube.
  (b) Passing of the NG tube may cause nasal trauma, with severe bleeding, or may stimulate vomiting.
  (c) Although it is a rare occurrence, if the patient has major facial or head trauma, the NG tube may pass into the cranium through a basilar skull fracture. (This is why insertion of a nasogastric tube is **contraindicated** in patients with major facial or head trauma. Consider insertion of an **oro**gastric tube, instead.)
  (d) None of the above are false.
  (e) All of the above are false. Nasogastric tube insertion is not accompanied by complications when the procedure is performed correctly.

70. Which of the following are steps for NG tube insertion?

  1. Be sure that the patient is being oxygenated before and during the procedure.
  2. Select the correct NG tube:
       8.0 French for newborns and infants
       10.0 French for toddlers and preschoolers
       12 French for school-aged children
       14 to 16 French for adolescents
  3. Measure the NG tube from the tip of the patient's nose, around the ear, to below the xyphoid process.
  4. Measure the NG tube from the tip of the patient's nose, down to the xyphoid process.
  5. Lubricate the distal end of the NG tube.
  6. Do not allow lubrication to touch the NG tube (lubricants will degrade the tube's plastic).
  7. Insert the tube into the patient's nose, gently passing the tube downward, along the nasal floor.
  8. Insert the length of tube previously measured as being correct for the patient's size.
  9. Attach a syringe to the exterior end of the tube, and withdraw (aspirate) stomach contents to check for correct tube placement.
  10. Attach a syringe to the exterior end of the tube, and inject 10 to 20 cc of air while auscultating the epigastrium, to check for correct tube placement (a bubbling rush of air will be heard in the stomach if the tube is correctly placed).

11. Remove the syringe and attach the tube to a suction device to aspirate stomach contents.
12. Secure the tube in place by taping it to the sides and/or top of the patient's nose.

   (a) 1, 2, 3, 5, 7, 8, 9, 10, 11, and 12 only.
   (b) 1, 2, 3 or 4, 5, 7, 8, 9, 10, and 12 only.
   (c) 1, 2, 4, 6, 7, 8, 9, 10, 11, and 12 only.
   (d) 1, 4, 6, 7, 8, 9, 10, and 12 only.
   (e) None of the above (every system does it differently).

71. Suctioning of the lower airway via the endotracheal tube is sometimes called "deep suctioning." The medical phrase for this suctioning technique is

   (a) French suctioning (because a French catheter is used).
   (b) orotracheal suctioning.
   (c) intubational suctioning.
   (d) pulmonary suctioning.
   (e) tubal suctioning.

72. Indications for deep suctioning include

   (a) when moist, bubbling noises are heard while ventilating the patient, indicating excess secretions in the lower airway.
   (b) when secretions are visible, bubbling up into the endotracheal tube.
   (c) poor and/or decreasing compliance (chest excursion) noticed while ventilating the patient.
   (d) Answers (a) and (b) only (poor compliance means the tube is in the wrong place and should be removed immediately).
   (e) Answers (a), (b), and (c).

73. Using a sterile technique to perform deep suctioning of the lower airway

   (a) is an unrealistic expectation for prehospital emergency care and may be disregarded.
   (b) is unnecessary, because the suction catheter will be inside the endotracheal tube and will not contact patient tissues.
   (c) is very important. This is an invasive form of suctioning. A contaminated suction catheter would introduce dangerous pathogens to the highly susceptible tissue of the patient's lungs.
   (d) will require too much time and would threaten the patient's life by increasing hypoxia from the continued secretion interference. A "clean" technique is acceptable.
   (e) is only done in school and for testing situations. In "real life," only a fool would bother with sterile techniques.

74. Before inserting the soft ("French") suction catheter, the EMT should
    (a) estimate the length of catheter to be inserted, by measuring from the patient's lips, to her/his ear, to her/his nipple line.
    (b) preoxygenate the patient by hyperventilating with a high concentration of oxygen.
    (c) deflate the endotracheal tube's cuff.
    (d) Answers (a) and (b) only.
    (e) Answers (a), (b), and (c).

75. Suction should be engaged
    (a) while inserting the catheter. This will assist in the passage of the catheter down the endotracheal tube. Discontinue suctioning once the desired level of catheter advancement has been reached. Withdraw the tube without suction.
    (b) once the desired level of catheter advancement has been reached. Suction while remaining at that level. Withdraw the tube without suction.
    (c) only after the desired level of catheter advancement has been reached. Suction while withdrawing the catheter, twisting the catheter back and forth as you withdraw.
    (d) Either answer (a) or (b) only.
    (e) Answers (a), (b), or (c).

76. The suction catheter should be advanced
    (a) until resistance is met or the desired, premeasured length of catheter is inserted (as far as the carina).
    (b) until 33 centimeters of catheter have been inserted (the length of an average adult endotracheal tube). If it were advanced any further, the nonsterile catheter would have contact with patient tissues and contaminate the patient.
    (c) as far as it will continue to insert (well past the carina). In this way, actual intralung suctioning is accomplished (hence the name "deep suctioning").
    (d) only until its tip no longer can be visualized in the exposed endotracheal tube (some systems will advance it an additional 3 centimeters, but no more than that).
    (e) Any of the above lengths (every system is different).

77. The patient may be deep-suctioned for a maximum of _____ at a time. Hyperventilation of the patient must be repeated before suctioning again.
    (a) 5 seconds
    (b) 15 seconds

(c) 20 seconds
(d) 30 seconds
(e) 1 minute

78. Complications of deep suctioning via the endotracheal tube include all of the following, except

(a) oxygen deprivation (hypoxia) and cardiac arrhythmias.
(b) stimulation of the patient's cough reflex (when the carina is reached).
(c) damage to the airway's lining (mucosa).
(d) spasm of the vocal cords.
(e) bronchospasm (if the catheter advances past the carina).

The answer key for Test Section Eight is on pages 376 through 378.

Test Section Nine

This test section covers the following subjects:

* Assisting with Endotracheal Intubation
* Assisting with ECG Application and Use
* Pulse Oximeter Use
* Assisting with IV Therapy
* Infectious Diseases

1994 Revised EMT-Basic National Standards Review Self-Test

AUTHORS' NOTE: *Each group of this section's questions is headed by the group's subject title. In this way, subjects unrelated to an EMT's local requirements may be skipped.*

1. Prior to any intubation attempt, the patient should be _____ with 100 percent oxygen, using the bag-valve-mask and an oral airway, at a rate of _____ ventilations per minute.

    (a) normally ventilated/12
    (b) normally ventilated/10
    (c) hyperventilated/24
    (d) hyperventilated/60
    (e) slowly, but fully, ventilated/12

2. Correct positioning of the patient's head (to achieve correct airway alignment) is vitally important to successful orotracheal intubation. When trauma is not suspected, the patient should be positioned with her/his

    (a) head and neck in a neutral position. The assisting EMT may be required to provide manual, in-line stabilization during intubation.
    (b) neck flexed and chin lifted. The assisting EMT may be required to maintain neck flexion during intubation.
    (c) head tilted back and chin lifted. The assisting EMT usually will not be required to assist with this head positioning.
    (d) Either answer (a) or (b).
    (e) Either answer (b) or (c).

3. When orotracheal intubation is required for a trauma patient, the patient should be positioned with her/his

    (a) head and neck in a neutral position. The assisting EMT may be required to provide manual, in-line stabilization during intubation.
    (b) neck flexed and chin lifted. The assisting EMT may be required to maintain neck flexion during intubation.
    (c) head tilted back and chin lifted. The assisting EMT usually will not be required to assist with this head positioning.
    (d) Either answer (a) or (b).
    (e) Either answer (b) or (c).

4. Application of **Sellick's maneuver** during attempts at orotracheal intubation may be helpful. Which of the following statements regarding Sellick's maneuver is false?
    (a) Sellick's maneuver consists of the assisting EMT using her/his thumb and index finger to apply direct pressure to the patient's anterior neck, at the cricoid cartilage level, while the intubating EMT searches for the glottic opening.
    (b) Sellick's maneuver consists of the intubating EMT using the laryngoscope to apply direct pressure to the patient's cricoid cartilage. An assisting EMT may be asked to maintain neck flexion during this maneuver.
    (c) Sellick's maneuver will help to compress the esophagus, thus reducing the risk of vomiting during intubation.
    (d) Sellick's maneuver may help to bring the glottic opening into better view for the intubating EMT.
    (e) None of the above are false.

5. Ventilating the intubated patient
    (a) is no different from ventilating any other patient with the bag-valve-mask. Once the endotracheal tube is secured, simply maintain the mask seal and compress the bag in the usual manner.
    (b) requires strict attention to avoid dislodging the endotracheal tube, even after the tube has been secured to the patient.
    (c) requires strict observation of the centimeter marks along the side of the endotracheal tube. Note what centimeter number is at the level of the patient's teeth and ensure that the tube stays at that level.
    (d) requires strict attention to avoid dislodging the endotracheal tube while the tube is being secured to the patient. Once secured, the endotracheal tube requires no further special attention.
    (e) Both answers (b) and (c).

6. While ventilating the intubated patient, if the endotracheal tube appears to sink lower into the patient's airway, you should
    (a) pull it back up, and resume ventilation of the patient. Do not interrupt ventilations or the activities of others.
    (b) leave it where it is; there is no need for concern. The endotracheal tube has a cuff at its distal end which will hold the tube's opening in the correct place, even though the exposed section of the tube appears shorter. Do not interrupt ventilations or the activities of others.
    (c) immediately notify the intubating EMT. Returning the tube to its correct placement level will require deflation of the tube's cuff and careful withdrawal, while one EMT ventilates and another auscultates the chest.
    (d) immediately pull the endotracheal tube completely out of the patient's airway and return to bag-valve-mask ventilation. Then notify the intubating EMT.
    (e) Either answer (a) or (d).

7. While ventilating the intubated patient, if the endotracheal tube appears to begin sliding out of the patient's airway (or you suddenly notice there is more of the tube visible), you should
    (a) push it back in, and resume ventilation of the patient. Do not interrupt ventilations or the activities of others.
    (b) leave it where it is; there is no need for concern. The endotracheal tube has a cuff at its distal end which will hold the tube's opening in the correct place, even though the exposed section of the tube appears longer. Do not interrupt ventilations or the activities of others.
    (c) immediately notify the intubating EMT. Checking the tube's placement will require one EMT to auscultate the epigastric area and chest, while another EMT ventilates the patient. If the tube has come out of the trachea and/or entered the patient's esophagus, it will have to be removed or the patient could die.
    (d) immediately pull the endotracheal tube completely out of the patient's airway and return to bag-valve-mask ventilation. Then notify the intubating EMT.
    (e) Either answer (a) or (d).

8. When ventilating an intubated patient that has her/his own respiratory effort, you should
    (a) time your ventilations to coincide with the patient's natural inhalations, as long as the patient is breathing at an appropriate rate.
    (b) assist the patient to attain a more rapid respiratory rate if she/he is breathing too slowly (or requires hyperventilation). Do this by ventilating with the patient's own inhalations, gently interposing extra ventilations between them.

(c) continue to observe that the tube placement level does not change and monitor that the patient continues to breathe on her/his own. Simply hold the bag-valve device steady, supporting its weight. A breathing patient does not need to be artificially ventilated.
(d) Either answer (a) or (b).
(e) None of the above. A patient who is intubated will not have her own respiratory effort. This is a trick question.

9. When ventilating an intubated patient, if you notice an increase in the resistance of the patient's lungs (if the bag-valve device becomes more difficult to squeeze), it may be a sign that

   (a) the patient is waking up. As long as the patient is restrained, disregard the increased resistance and squeeze more forcefully to continue ventilations.
   (b) a hole has developed in one or both lungs, leaking air into the chest cavity and compressing the lung(s). Immediately notify the intubating EMT. This is a serious development.
   (c) the esophagus needs to be decompressed. Notify the intubating EMT only if she/he is not busy with other activities (gastric distention in an intubated patient is not a concern).
   (d) Either answer (a) or (c).
   (e) None of the above. Increased lung resistance is a natural side effect of endotracheal ventilation and should be disregarded. Squeeze more forcefully to continue ventilations, without interrupting other providers' activities.

10. When ventilating an intubated patient, if you notice **any** change in the resistance of the patient's lungs (if the bag-valve device becomes more **or** less difficult to squeeze), it may be a sign that

    (a) the patient is about to vomit. Immediately discontinue ventilations and gather suctioning equipment.
    (b) the esophagus needs to be decompressed. Notify the intubating EMT only if she/he is not busy with other activities (gastric distention in an intubated patient is not a concern).
    (c) the endotracheal tube has slipped out of the trachea and/or entered the esophagus. Immediately notify the intubating EMT. This could be a fatal development.
    (d) Either answer (a) or (b).
    (e) None of the above. Changes in lung resistance (increased, decreased, whatever) are a natural side effect of endotracheal ventilation and should be disregarded. Continue ventilations without interrupting other providers' activities.

11. When ventilating an intubated cardiac arrest patient that is about to be defibrillated, you should
    (a) continue ventilations without worry. The rubber bag of the bag-valve device is designed to "ground" you and protect you from electrical shock. Additionally, it is vitally important that a cardiac arrest patient's ventilations not be interrupted, for any reason.
    (b) immediately drop the bag-valve device and get away from the patient. Do not disconnect it from the secured endotracheal tube, because doing so would delay your return to ventilating after the defibrillation.
    (c) carefully disconnect the bag-valve device from the endotracheal tube and then move away from the patient.
    (d) carefully disconnect the bag-valve device from the endotracheal tube and then hold the endotracheal tube in place. Make sure that you are not in contact with the patient's lips or body during defibrillation. The plastic endotracheal tube is designed to "ground" you and protect you from electrical shock.
    (e) remind the defibrillating EMT to deflate the tube's cuff and remove the endotracheal tube before defibrillation.

12. While ventilating an intubated patient, you also need to observe for signs of mental status changes in the patient. If the patient begins to move, you should
    (a) immediately notify the paramedic you are assisting. She/he will want to administer a sedative to the patient to prevent the patient from attempting to remove the endotracheal tube.
    (b) immediately notify the EMT you are assisting. If the patient's hands are free, they will need to be restrained.
    (c) stop ventilations and observe for a return of the patient's respiratory effort. If the patient has resumed breathing, discontinue ventilations and simply support the weight of the bag-valve device until the endotracheal tube can be removed and a nonrebreather mask applied.
    (d) Both answers (a) and (b).
    (e) Both answers (a) and (c).

13. While ventilating an intubated patient who has an oral airway inserted as a bite block, if you notice the patient beginning to gag, chew, or attempting to cough, you should

   (a) partially withdraw the oral airway, removing its tip from the posterior oropharynx. Keep a portion of the airway between the patient's teeth to continue to act as a bite block. Continue ventilations.
   (b) hold the oral airway in place (fully inserted), but stop ventilations and observe for a return of the patient's respiratory effort. If the patient has resumed breathing, discontinue ventilations and simply continue holding the airway in place, while supporting the weight of the bag-valve device.
   (c) hold the oral airway in place (fully inserted), and continue ventilations. It may be helpful to tape the oral airway in place.
   (d) remove the oral airway completely, before it stimulates the patient to vomit.
   (e) None of the above. Oral airways are not inserted after a patient is intubated, for any reason (endotracheal tubes are hard enough to be their own bite block).

14. Which of the following statements regarding assisting with medication delivery via the endotracheal tube is true?

   (a) Only paramedics may administer medications via the endotracheal tube, and EMTs may not assist with this. If asked to assist, respectfully (but firmly) decline.
   (b) After the medication is injected down the endotracheal tube, the assisting EMT should wait at least 15 seconds before resuming ventilation (to give the medication opportunity to be absorbed). When resumed, ventilations should be very slow to allow the medication to continue to be absorbed.
   (c) After the medication is injected down the endotracheal tube, the assisting EMT may be asked to hyperventilate the patient. This will increase the rate of medication absorption.
   (d) Any of the above, depending on local protocols.
   (e) None of the above. Medication does not get injected into the airway!

ASSISTING WITH ECG APPLICATION AND USE

15. The electrocardiogram (ECG) provides graphic information about the

   (a) electrical activity of the heart.
   (b) electrical activity of the brain.
   (c) force and effectiveness of cardiac contraction.
   (d) Answers (a) and (c) only.
   (e) Answers (a), (b), and (c).

16. EMTs who wish to assist with ECG application and use should learn all of the following, except
    (a) how to turn the machine on and off.
    (b) how to record an ECG strip.
    (c) how to defibrillate a patient using transcranial ECG paddle placement.
    (d) how to change the ECG batteries.
    (e) how to change the ECG paper.

17. Types of electrodes used for the prehospital ECG include
    (a) small electrodes for monitoring only, and large electrodes that can monitor and deliver an electrical shock (defibrillate).
    (b) large electrodes for monitoring only, and small electrodes that can monitor and deliver an electrical shock (defibrillate).
    (c) dry (unlubricated) electrodes for monitoring only, and pre-lubricated electrodes that can monitor and deliver an electrical shock (defibrillate).
    (d) Both answers (a) and (c).
    (e) Any of the above, depending on the electrode brand.

18. Which of the following statements regarding application of ECG electrodes is false?
    (a) The best quality of ECG monitoring is achieved by electrodes placed on dry, bare skin.
    (b) It may be necessary to shave off the patient's hair in the areas where the electrodes will be placed.
    (c) If the patient has very oily skin, it may be necessary to wash the areas where the electrodes will be placed.
    (d) If the patient continues to be very sweaty (after initially wiping the skin dry), consider applying an antiperspirant to the areas where the electrodes will be placed.
    (e) None of the above are false.

19. Monitoring electrode placement may differ from system to system. The most common placement site for the electrode attached to the white (negative) ECG cable is
    (a) on the right arm or beneath the right clavicle.
    (b) on the left arm or beneath the left clavicle.
    (c) on the right leg or at the lowest corner of the right chest.
    (d) on the left leg or at the lowest corner of the left chest.
    (e) Either answer (b) or (c).

20. The most common placement site for the electrode attached to the red (positive) ECG cable is

    (a) on the right arm or beneath the right clavicle.
    (b) on the left arm or beneath the left clavicle.
    (c) on the right leg or at the lowest corner of the right chest.
    (d) on the left leg or at the lowest corner of the left chest.
    (e) Either answer (b) or (c).

21. The most common placement site for the electrode attached to the black or green (grounding) ECG cable is

    (a) on the right arm or beneath the right clavicle.
    (b) on the left arm or beneath the left clavicle.
    (c) on the right leg or at the lowest corner of the right chest.
    (d) on the left leg or at the lowest corner of the left chest.
    (e) Either answer (b) or (c).

PULSE OXIMETER USE

22. A pulse oximeter is a small, photoelectric device that monitors

    (a) the percentage of oxygen saturating the patient's blood.
    (b) the patient's pulse rate.
    (c) the amount of blood circulating in the patient's body.
    (d) Both answers (a) and (b), depending on the pulse oximeter model.
    (e) Answers (a), (b), and (c), depending on the pulse oximeter model.

23. The equipment used for pulse oximetry includes

    (a) the portable pulse oximeter monitor.
    (b) a sensing probe (cable and clip).
    (c) a grounding cable and clip.
    (d) Answers (a) and/or (b) only.
    (e) Answers (a), (b), and/or (c).

24. The sensing probe's clip may be attached to the patient's

    (a) ear.
    (b) finger.
    (c) tongue.
    (d) Answers (a) and/or (b) only.
    (e) Answers (a), (b), and/or (c).

25. Indications for the use of a pulse oximeter include all of the following, except

(a) to assess the oxygen saturation of a patient complaining of breathing difficulty.
(b) to determine whether or not a patient with shortness of breath truly needs oxygen.
(c) to assess the effectiveness of artificial ventilations.
(d) to assess the effectiveness of oxygen administration.
(e) to assess the effectiveness of bronchodilator medication therapy.

26. The optimal (target) blood oxygen saturation percentage is

(a) 95 to 100 percent.
(b) 90 to 94 percent.
(c) 85 to 89 percent.
(d) 80 to 84 percent.
(e) 75 to 79 percent.

27. The primary benefit of pulse oximetry is that it

(a) saves oxygen, by identifying "shortness of breath" patients who do not need supplemental oxygenation.
(b) encourages EMTs to provide higher concentrations of oxygen delivery.
(c) identifies patients who are hyperventilating for psychiatric reasons (as opposed to physical reasons) and do not need oxygen.
(d) Both answers (a) and (b).
(e) Both answers (a) and (c).

28. Which of the following statements regarding pulse oximeter accuracy is false?

(a) A patient in shock will produce an inaccurate pulse oximeter reading.
(b) The hypothermic patient will produce an inaccurate pulse oximeter reading.
(c) Pulse oximetry is 100 percent accurate when used to determine the oxygen need of patients who are chronic cigarette smokers.
(d) Excessive patient movement or the presence of nail polish can produce an inaccurate pulse oximeter reading.
(e) Patients with carbon monoxide poisoning will produce a falsely high pulse oximeter reading.

29. When using the pulse oximeter, check the patient's oxygen saturation reading every

    (a) minute.
    (b) 5 minutes.
    (c) 10 minutes.
    (d) 15 minutes.
    (e) 20 minutes.

ASSISTING WITH IV THERAPY

30. The medical abbreviation **IV** stands for the medical term

    (a) intravenous.
    (b) injection-venous.
    (c) innervenous.
    (d) intervessel.
    (e) intervascular.

31. There are two basic types of IV fluid administration sets (administration tubing). The primary difference between these sets is the number of drops required to deliver 1 cc (cubic centimeter) or ml (milliliter) of fluid. The IV tubing type that delivers 1 cc with every 60 drops is called the

    (a) mini-drip (or micro-drip) administration set.
    (b) tiny drop administration set.
    (c) infant drip (or pedi-drip) administration set.
    (d) small drip administration set.
    (e) Either answer (b) or (c).

32. The IV tubing type that delivers 1 cc with every 10 or 15 drops is called the

    (a) macro-drip (or maxi-drip) administration set.
    (b) big drop administration set.
    (c) infant drip (or pedi-drip) administration set.
    (d) large drip administration set.
    (e) Either answer (b) or (c).

33. The biggest difference in the physical appearance of these two IV tubing types consists of the different drip chamber configurations. The drip chamber of the _____ IV administration set contains a special tiny metal barrel, from which the drops emerge.

    (a) 10 drops/1 cc
    (b) 15 drops/1 cc
    (c) 60 drops/1 cc
    (d) Either answer (a) or (b).
    (e) Either answer (b) or (c).

34. Which of the following statements regarding an IV extension set is false?

(a) Attaching an extension set makes it easier to disrobe the patient without disturbing the IV site.
(b) IV extension tubing comes in two sizes: a 60 drop/1 cc size and a 10 or 15 drop/ 1 cc size.
(c) Attaching an extension set makes it easier to carry or move a patient without disturbing the IV site.
(d) Extension tubing should not be used with a 10 or 15 drop/1 cc administration set.
(e) None of the above are false.

35. When assisting with IV therapy, EMT-B (non-IV-certified) responsibilities include all of the following, except

(a) inspecting the IV fluid to make sure it is clear and free of contaminants.
(b) squeezing the IV fluid bag to check for any leaks.
(c) deciding which kind of IV fluid to set up.
(d) correctly identifying the requested IV administration set.
(e) maintaining connection site sterility during assembly.

36. Before connecting the administration set to the IV fluid container, the EMT must

(a) assemble the tubing's flow regulator.
(b) attach a flow regulator to the tubing.
(c) disconnect the flow regulator from the tubing.
(d) close the tubing's flow regulator.
(e) open the tubing's flow regulator.

37. Which of the following statements regarding IV assembly sterility factors is true?

(a) Although it would be best to keep the attaching parts sterile, sterility cannot be maintained in the prehospital setting.
(b) After removal of the tubing spike's protective cover, if the spike contacts an unsterile surface, cleanse it with an alcohol wipe and proceed with assembly.
(c) Sterility is not an important factor when assembling an emergency IV. Antibiotics will be administered at the hospital and will correct any IV-contaminant-caused infection.
(d) All of the above are true.
(e) None of the above are true.

38. The administration set's drip chamber should be

(a) completely filled with fluid to prevent air from entering the IV tubing.
(b) filled with enough fluid to cover the bottom of the drip port.

(c) filled only about one-third full of fluid (leaving two-thirds of the chamber filled with air).
(d) should be completely filled only for the 60 drops/1 cc administration set.
(e) should be completely filled only for the 10 to 15 drops/1 cc administration set.

39. Which of the following statements regarding "flushing" air from the IV tubing is true?

(a) To flush air from the tubing, the cap at the patient-connection-end of the tubing must be removed and discarded.
(b) All of the air bubbles (large and small) must be flushed from the IV tubing.
(c) IV fluid should not be wasted. Only the largest air bubbles must be flushed from the tubing. Small (2 to 3 cc) air bubbles will be absorbed and will not endanger the patient.
(d) Both answers (a) and (b) are true.
(e) Both answers (a) and (c) are true.

40. When the drips stop dripping in the drip chamber, it means that the IV fluid is no longer flowing through the tubing (into the patient). The EMT must investigate the cause of this. Which of the following is not a potential cause for the drips to stop dripping?

(a) A closed flow regulator or a closed tubing clamp.
(b) IV tubing that has become kinked or folded.
(c) IV tubing that has become caught under the patient's body or a piece of equipment.
(d) IV tubing that has become disconnected from the patient's IV catheter.
(e) The constricting band used to engorge the vein for IV catheter insertion has been left on the patient.

41. If the IV fluid stops flowing through the patient's IV catheter,

(a) a blood clot may form inside the catheter, rendering the IV site useless.
(b) the EMT should pull the catheter out of the patient (1 or 2 centimeters) and squeeze the bag with great force to get the IV running again.
(c) the EMT should inject 30 to 50 cc of air through the medication administration port to clear the IV of debris and get it running again.
(d) Answers (b) and (c) only.
(e) Answers (a), (b), and (c).

42. A "runaway IV"

(a) is an IV that is flowing too fast (faster than what the patient's condition requires).
(b) is when the IV needle and/or catheter has punctured the vein, and fluid is flowing into the tissues around the IV site instead of into the vein.
(c) may cause a fluid overload that may create serious problems for the patient.
(d) Both answers (a) and (c).
(e) Both answers (b) and (c).

43. An "infiltrated IV"

(a) is an IV that is flowing too fast (faster than what the patient's condition requires).
(b) is when the IV needle and/or catheter has punctured the vein, and fluid is flowing into the tissues around the IV site instead of into the vein.
(c) may cause a fluid overload that may create serious problems for the patient.
(d) Both answers (a) and (c).
(e) Both answers (b) and (c).

INFECTIOUS DISEASES

44. Of the following list of diseases, which diseases are **communicable**?

1. AIDS (acquired immune deficiency syndrome)
2. Bacterial meningitis
3. Chicken pox (varicella)
4. German measles (rubella)
5. Hepatitis
6. Measles (rubeola)
7. Mumps
8. Pneumonia (bacterial)
9. Pneumonia (viral)
10. Staphylococcal skin infections ("staff" infections)
11. Tuberculosis (TB)
12. Whooping cough (pertussis)

(a) 1, 2, 3, 4, 5, 6, 7, 8, 9, 10, 11, and 12 (all of them).
(b) 1, 4, 5, 7, 8, 10, 11, and 12 only.
(c) 1, 3, 4, 5, 8, 9, 11, and 12 only.
(d) 1, 2, 4, 5, 9, 10, and 11 only.
(e) 1, 5, and 11 only.

45. Of the diseases listed in question number 44, which are of the greatest concern (present the most significant threat) to health care providers?

    (a) 1, 2, 3, 4, 5, 6, 7, 8, 9, 10, 11, and 12 (all of them).
    (b) 1, 4, 5, 7, 8, 10, 11, and 12 only.
    (c) 1, 3, 4, 5, 8, 9, 11, and 12 only.
    (d) 1, 2, 4, 5, 9, 10, and 11 only.
    (e) 1, 5, and 11 only.

46. The infectious disease that **kills** the most health care providers in the United States (approximately ***200 every year***), is

    (a) AIDS.
    (b) bacterial meningitis.
    (c) hepatitis.
    (d) staphylococcal skin infections ("staff" infections)
    (e) tuberculosis (TB).

47. Infectious diseases can be transmitted by

    (a) bloodborne pathogens.
    (b) airborne pathogens.
    (c) any body surface (or clothing) contact with an infected person.
    (d) Answers (a) and (b) only.
    (e) Answers (a), (b), and (c).

48. Body substance isolation (BSI) infection control precautions consist of

    (a) wearing protective equipment (contact barriers).
    (b) following mandated procedures for infection control.
    (c) obtaining vaccinations for specific diseases.
    (d) Answers (a) and (b) only.
    (e) Answers (a), (b), and (c).

49. Which of the following statements regarding BSI infection control precautions is true?

    (a) For every single patient an EMT encounters, every available BSI infection control precaution should be utilized.
    (b) Only moist (undried) body fluids present an infection risk. (Once infectious fluids have dried, they no longer retain any form of infectious pathogen.)
    (c) Any body fluid, whether dried or moist, should be considered to be "infectious" until proven otherwise.
    (d) Both answers (a) and (b) are true.
    (e) Both answers (a) and (c) are true.

50. The infection that causes an inflammation of the liver is

  (a) AIDS.
  (b) bacterial meningitis.
  (c) hepatitis.
  (d) staphylococcal skin infections ("staff" infections)
  (e) tuberculosis (TB).

51. The infectious disease AIDS is contracted by

  (a) blood transfusions of AIDS-infected blood.
  (b) blood contact (via open wounds or IV drug use) and unprotected sexual contact with an AIDS-infected person.
  (c) any body surface (or clothing) contact with an AIDS-infected person.
  (d) Answers (a) and (b) only.
  (e) Answers (a), (b), and (c).

52. AIDS is caused by the

  (a) homosexual infected virus (HIV).
  (b) human immunodeficiency virus (HIV).
  (c) heroin intravenous virus (HIV).
  (d) homosexual intravenous virus (HIV).
  (e) human intravenous virus (HIV).

53. Which of the following statements regarding hepatitis is true?

  (a) Hepatitis is contracted via any body surface (or clothing) contact with an infected person.
  (b) Hepatitis is contracted via blood, stool, or other body fluids (both dried and moist).
  (c) Hepatitis is contracted via moist blood, stool, or other body fluids. Once dried, the hepatitis virus is rendered inactive.
  (d) Both answers (a) and (b) are true.
  (e) Both answers (a) and (c) are true.

54. Which of the following statements regarding AIDS is true?

  (a) AIDS is contracted via any body surface (or clothing) contact with an infected person.
  (b) AIDS is contracted via unprotected sexual contact or contact with AIDS-infected blood (both dried and moist).
  (c) AIDS is contracted via unprotected sexual contact or contact with AIDS-infected blood (moist blood, only). Once dried, the AIDS virus is rendered inactive.
  (d) Both answers (a) and (b) are true.
  (e) Both answers (a) and (c) are true.

55. Which of the following statements regarding staphylococcal skin infections ("staff" infections) is true?

  (a) An EMT who has direct, unprotected contact with infected wounds may become infected with "staff."
  (b) An EMT who has direct, unprotected contact with infected sores may become infected with "staff."
  (c) Any direct, unprotected contact with "staff"-contaminated objects may infect an EMT.
  (d) Answers (a) and (b) only.
  (e) Answers (a), (b), and (c).

56. Which of the following statements regarding tuberculosis (TB) is true?

  (a) TB was eradicated in the late 1950s. Health care provider contraction of TB (from patients) is unheard of in today's society.
  (b) TB contraction by health care providers from patients is a rare event, especially since health care providers are tested routinely for the disease.
  (c) TB is highly contagious, and TB cases have become more and more frequent since the late 1980s. Any patient with a cough should be suspected of having TB, until proven otherwise.
  (d) Answers (a) and (b) only.
  (e) None of the above are true.

57. Human skin is

  (a) a highly effective barrier against pathogen-caused infections, unless it is broken by a cut or opening.
  (b) a very poor barrier against pathogen-caused infections. Any lethal pathogen can be absorbed though unbroken skin.
  (c) only an effective barrier to viral pathogens (such as AIDS and hepatitis).
  (d) Any of the above.
  (e) None of the above.

58. Which of the following statements regarding mucous membranes is true?

  (a) Mucous membranes are present only in the mouth.
  (b) Mucous membranes are present only in the nose.
  (c) Mucous membranes cannot be crossed by infectious pathogens (they are the most effective barrier a person has, by virtue of the thickness of their secretions).
  (d) Mucous membranes are present in the mouth, the nose, and the eyes. They present an easy access for any sort of infectious pathogen.
  (e) Both answers (a) and (c) are true.

59. Which of the following statements regarding direct mouth-to-mouth artificial respiration delivery is true?

   (a) No EMT should ever have to perform direct mouth-to-mouth artificial respirations.
   (b) Every EMT, no matter what her/his certification level, must be prepared to perform direct mouth-to-mouth artificial respirations.
   (c) Only basic EMTs must be prepared to perform direct mouth-to-mouth artificial respirations. (Intermediate EMTs and paramedics may perform orotracheal intubation; thus they can avoid mouth-to-mouth artificial respirations.)
   (d) All of the above are true.
   (e) None of the above are true.

60. Cross-infection of one patient's pathogens to another patient is

   (a) a complication that is literally impossible, unless the contaminating pathogen remains moist.
   (b) a serious concern that is best avoided by vigorous hand washing between every patient contact. BSI precautions, alone, will not always protect the next patient from cross-infection.
   (c) will happen, no matter what kind of precautions a health care provider takes. It is a risk that all patients must face when accessing emergency care treatment.
   (d) something that occurs often but is so easily remedied by administration of IV antibiotics that it is not a concern for health care providers in the emergency setting.
   (e) something that is a serious concern for in-hospital care providers but does not apply to prehospital care providers.

61. Supplies and equipment that are exposed to infectious pathogens

   (a) do not present a cross-contamination (or EMT-contamination) threat unless the surface substance is still moist.
   (b) should not be left on the scene, whether they are moistly contaminated or dryly contaminated.
   (c) should not be left in the ambulance, unless the contamination site is dry.
   (d) Answers (a) and (b) only (leaving any articles on the scene is considered to be in "poor taste").
   (e) Answers (a) and (c) only.

62. According to federal law, every employer of emergency health care providers must provide, free of charge to the employee,

(a) personal protective equipment that does not allow blood or other infectious body fluid to pass through it.
(b) the hepatitis B series of vaccinations.
(c) education and training in the avoidance of infectious contact and procedures for infection control.
(d) Answers (a) and (c) only (vaccinations are the responsibility of the employee).
(e) Answers (a), (b), and (c).

The answer key for Test Section Nine is on pages 379 through 381.

National Registry of Emergency Medical Technicians Skills Sheets

PATIENT ASSESSMENT/MANAGEMENT
TRAUMA

		Points Possible	Points Awarded
Takes or verbalizes body substance isolation precautions		1	
SCENE SIZE-UP			
Determines the scene is safe		1	
Determines the mechanism of injury		1	
Determines the number of patients		1	
Requests additional help if necessary		1	
Considers stabilization of spine		1	
INITIAL ASSESSMENT			
Verbalizes general impression of patient		1	
Determines responsiveness		1	
Determines chief complaint/apparent life threats		1	
Assess airway and breathing	Assessment	1	
	Initiates appropriate oxygen therapy	1	
	Assures adequate ventilation	1	
	Injury Management	1	
Assess Circulation	Assesses for and controls major bleeding	1	
	Assesses pulse	1	
	Assesses skin (color, temperature and condition)	1	
Identifies priority patients/makes transport decision		1	
FOCUSED HISTORY AND PHYSICAL EXAM/RAPID TRAUMA ASSESSMENT			
Selects appropriate assessment (focused or rapid assessment)		1	
Obtains or directs assistant to obtain baseline vital signs		1	
Obtains SAMPLE history		1	
DETAILED PHYSICAL EXAMINATION			
Assesses the head	Inspects and palpates the scalp and ears	1	
	Assesses the eyes	1	
	Assesses the facial area including oral and nasal area	1	
Assesses the neck	Inspects and palpates the neck	1	
	Assesses for JVD	1	
	Assesses for tracheal deviation	1	
Assesses the chest	Inspects	1	
	Palpates	1	
	Auscultates the chest	1	
Assesses the abdomen/pelvis	Assesses the abdomen	1	
	Assesses the pelvis	1	
	Verbalizes assessment of genitalia/perineum as needed	1	
Assesses the extremities	1 point for each extremity includes inspection, palpation, and assessment of pulses, sensory and motor activities	4	
Assesses the posterior	Assesses thorax	1	
	Assesses lumbar	1	
Manages secondary injuries and wounds appropriately **1 point for appropriate management of secondary injury/wound**		1	
Verbalizes reassessment of the vital signs		1	
	TOTAL:	40	

CRITICAL CRITERIA

___ Did not take or verbalize body substance isolation precautions
___ Did not assess for spinal protection
___ Did not provide for spinal protection when indicated
___ Did not provide high concentration of oxygen
___ Did not find or manage problems associated with airway, breathing, hemorrhage or shock (hypoperfusion)
___ Did not differentiate patient's needing transportation versus continued on scene assessment
___ Does other detailed physical examination before assessing airway, breathing and circulation
___ Did not transport patient within ten (10) minute time limit

PATIENT ASSESSMENT/MANAGEMENT MEDICAL

	Points Possible	Points Awarded
Takes or verbalizes body substance isolation precautions	1	
SCENE SIZE-UP		
Determines the scene is safe	1	
Determines the mechanism of injury/nature of illness	1	
Determines the number of patients	1	
Requests additional help if necessary	1	
Considers stabilization of spine	1	
INITIAL ASSESSMENT		
Verbalizes general impression of patient	1	
Determines responsiveness/level of consciousness	1	
Determines chief complaint/apparent life threats	1	
Assess airway and breathing — Assessment	1	
Initiates appropriate oxygen therapy	1	
Assures adequate ventilation	1	
Assess Circulation — Assesses/controls major bleeding	1	
Assesses pulse	1	
Assesses skin (color, temperature and condition)	1	
Identifies priority patients/makes transport decision	1	
FOCUSED HISTORY AND PHYSICAL EXAM/RAPID ASSESSMENT		
Signs and Symptoms (Assess history of present illness)	4	

Respiratory	Cardiac	Altered Mental Status	Allergic Reaction	Poisoning/ Overdose	Environmental Emergency	Obstetrics	Behavioral
•Onset? •Provokes? •Quality? •Radiates? •Severity? •Time? •Interventions?	•Onset? •Provokes? •Quality? •Radiates? •Severity? •Time? •Interventions?	•Description of the episode •Onset? •Duration? •Associated symptoms? •Evidence of trauma? •Interventions? •Seizures? •Fever?	•History of allergies? •What were you exposed to? •How were you exposed? •Effects? •Progressions? •Interventions?	•Substance? •When did you ingest/become exposed? •How much did you ingest? •Over what time period? •Interventions? •Estimated weight? •Effects?	•Source? •Environment? •Duration? •Loss of consciousness? •Effects - General or local?	•Are you pregnant? •How long have you been pregnant? •Pain or contractions? •Bleeding or discharge? •Do you feel the need to push? •Last menstrual period? •Crowning?	•How do you feel? •Determine suicidal tendencies •Is the patient a threat to self or others? •Is there a medical problem? •Interventions?

	Points Possible	Points Awarded
Allergies	1	
Medications	1	
Past medical history	1	
Last Meal	1	
Events leading to present illness (rule out trauma)	1	
Performs focused physical examination Assesses affected body part/system or, if indicated, completes rapid assessment	1	
VITALS (Obtains baseline vital signs)	1	
INTERVENTIONS Obtains medical direction or verbalizes standing order for medication interventions and verbalizes proper additional intervention/treatment	1	
TRANSPORT (Re-evaluates transport decision)	1	
Verbalizes the consideration for completing a detailed physical examination	1	
ONGOING ASSESSMENT (verbalized)		
Repeats initial assessment	1	
Repeats vital signs	1	
Repeats focused assessment regarding patient complaint or injuries	1	
Checks interventions	1	
CRITICAL CRITERIA TOTAL:	34	

___ Did not take or verbalize body substance isolation precautions if necessary
___ Did not determine scene safety
___ Did not obtain medical direction or verbalize standing orders for medication interventions
___ Did not provide high concentration of oxygen
___ Did not evaluate and find conditions of airway, breathing, circulation
___ Did not find or manage problems associated with airway, breathing, hemorrhage or shock (hypoperfusion)
___ Did not differentiate patient's needing transportation versus continued assessment at the scene
___ Does detailed or focused history/physical examination before assessing airway, breathing and circulation
___ Did not ask questions about the present illness
___ Administered a dangerous or inappropriate intervention

CARDIAC ARREST MANAGEMENT/AED

	Points Possible	Points Awarded
ASSESSMENT		
Takes or verbalizes body substances isolation precautions	1	
Briefly questions rescuer about arrest events	1	
Directs rescuer to stop CPR	1	
Verifies absence of spontaneous pulse *(skill station examiner states "no pulse")*	1	
Turns on defibrillator power	1	
Attaches automated defibrillator to patient	1	
Ensures all individuals are standing clear of the patient	1	
Initiates analysis of rhythm	1	
Delivers shock (up to three successive shocks)	1	
Verifies absence of spontaneous pulse *(skill station examiner states "no pulse")*	1	
TRANSITION		
Directs resumption of CPR	1	
Gathers additional information on arrest event	1	
Confirms effectiveness of CPR (ventilation and compressions)	1	
INTEGRATION		
Directs insertion of a simple airway adjunct (oropharyngeal/nasopharyngeal)	1	
Directs ventilation of patient	1	
Assures high concentration of oxygen connected to the ventilatory adjunct	1	
Assures CPR continues without unnecessary/prolonged interruption		
Re-evaluates patient/CPR in approximately one minute	1	
Repeats defibrillator sequence	1	
TRANSPORTATION		
Verbalizes transportation of patient	1	
TOTAL:	20	

CRITICAL CRITERIA

___ Did not take or verbalize body substance isolation precautions
___ Did not evaluate the need for immediate use of the AED
___ Did not direct initiation/resumption of ventilation/compressions at appropriate times
___ Did not assure all individuals were clear of patient before delivering each shock
___ Did not operate the AED properly (inability to deliver shock)

BAG-VALVE-MASK
APNEIC PATIENT

	Points Possible	Points Awarded
Takes or verbalizes body substance isolation precautions	1	
Voices opening the airway	1	
Voices inserting an airway adjunct	1	
Selects appropriate size mask	1	
Creates a proper mask-to-face seal	1	
Ventilates patient at no less than 800 ml volume *(The examiner must witness for at least 30 seconds)*	1	
Connects reservoir and oxygen	1	
Adjust liter flow to 15 liters/minute or greater	1	
The examiner indicates the arrival of second EMT. The second EMT is instructed to ventilate the patient while the candidate controls the mask and the airway.		
Voices re-opening the airway	1	
Creates a proper mask-to-face seal	1	
Instructs assistant to resume ventilation at proper volume per breath *(The examiner must witness for at least 30 seconds)*	1	
TOTAL:	11	

CRITICAL CRITERIA

___ Did not take or verbalize body substance isolation precautions
___ Did not immediately ventilate the patient
___ Interrupted ventilations for more than 20 seconds
___ Did not provide high concentration of oxygen
___ Did not provide or direct assistant to provide proper volume/breath
    (more than 2 ventilations per minute are below 800 ml)
___ Did not allow adequate exhalation

SPINAL IMMOBILIZATION
SUPINE PATIENT

	Points Possible	Points Awarded
Takes or verbalizes body substance isolation precautions	1	
Directs assistant to place/maintain head in neutral in-line position	1	
Directs assistant to maintain manual immobilization of the head	1	
Assesses motor, sensory, and distal circulation in extremities	1	
Applies appropriate size extrication collar	1	
Positions the immobilization device appropriately	1	
Directs movement of the patient onto device without compromising the integrity of the spine	1	
Applies padding to voids between the torso and the boards as necessary	1	
Immobilizes the patient's torso to the device	1	
Evaluates the pads behind the patient's head as necessary	1	
Immobilizes the patient's head to the device	1	
Secures the patient's leg to the device	1	
Secures the patient's arms to the device	1	
Reassesses motor, sensory, and distal circulation in extremities	1	
TOTAL:	14	

CRITICAL CRITERIA

___ Did not immediately direct or take manual immobilization of the head
___ Releases or orders release of manual immobilization before it was maintained mechanically
___ Patient manipulated or moved excessively causing potential spinal compromise
___ Patient moves excessively up, down, left, or right on the device.
___ Head immobilization allows for excessive movement
___ Upon completion of immobilization, head is not in the neutral in-line position
___ Did not reassess motor, sensory, and distal circulation after immobilization to the device
___ Immobilizes head to the board before securing torso

SPINAL IMMOBILIZATION
SEATED PATIENT

	Points Possible	Points Awarded
Takes or verbalizes body substance isolation precautions	1	
Directs assistant to place/maintain head in neutral in-line position	1	
Directs assistant to maintain manual immobilization of the head	1	
Reassesses motor, sensory, and distal circulation in extremities	1	
Applies appropriate size extrication collar	1	
Positions the immobilization device behind the patient	1	
Secures the device to the patient's torso	1	
Evaluates torso fixation and adjusts as necessary	1	
Evaluates and pads behind the patient's head as necessary	1	
Secures the patient's head to the device	1	
Verbalizes moving the patient to a long board	1	
Reassesses motor, sensory, and distal circulation in extremities	1	
TOTAL:	12	

CRITICAL CRITERIA

___ Did not immediately direct or take manual immobilization of the head
___ Releases or orders release or manual immobilization before it was maintained mechanically
___ Patient manipulated or moved excessively causing potential spinal compromise
___ Device moves excessively up, down, left, or right on patient's torso.
___ Head immobilization allows for excessive movement
___ Torso fixation inhibits chest rise resulting in respiratory compromise
___ Upon completion of immobilization, head is not in the neutral position
___ Did not reassess motor, sensory, and distal circulation after voicing immobilization to the long board
___ Immobilized head to the board before securing the torso

IMMOBILIZATION SKILLS
LONG BONE

	Points Possible	Points Awarded
Takes or verbalizes body substance isolation precautions	1	
Directs application of manual stabilization	1	
Assesses motor, sensory, and distal circulation	1	
NOTE: The examiner acknowledges present and normal		
Measures splint	1	
Applies splint	1	
Immobilizes the joint above the injury site	1	
Immobilizes the joint below the injury site	1	
Secures the entire injured extremity	1	
Immobilizes hand/foot in the position of function	1	
Reassesses motor, sensory, and distal circulation	1	
NOTE: The examiner acknowledges present and normal		
TOTAL:	10	

CRITICAL CRITERIA

___ Grossly moves injured extremity
___ Did not immobilize adjacent joints
___ Did not assess motor, sensory, and distal circulation before and after splinting

IMMOBILIZATION SKILLS
JOINT INJURY

	Points Possible	Points Awarded
Takes or verbalizes body substance isolation precautions	1	
Directs application of manual stabilization of the injury	1	
Assesses motor, sensory, and distal circulation	1	
NOTE: The examiner acknowledges present and normal		
Selects proper splinting material	1	
Immobilizes the site of the injury	1	
Immobilizes bone above injured joint	1	
Immobilizes bone below injured joint	1	
Reassesses motor, sensory, and distal circulation	1	
NOTE: The examiner acknowledges present and normal		
TOTAL:	8	

CRITICAL CRITERIA

___ Did not support the joint so that the joint did not bear distal weight

___ Did not immobilize bone above and below injured joint

___ Did not reassess motor, sensory, and distal circulation before and after splinting

IMMOBILIZATION SKILLS
TRACTION SPLINTING

	Points Possible	Points Awarded
Takes or verbalizes body substance isolation precautions	1	
Directs application of manual stabilization of the injured leg	1	
Directs the application of manual traction	1	
Assesses motor, sensory, and distal circulation	1	
NOTE: The examiner acknowledges present and normal.		
Prepares/adjusts splint to the proper length	1	
Positions the splint at the injured leg	1	
Applies the proximal securing device (e.g., ischial strap)	1	
Applies the distal securing device (e.g., ankle hitch)	1	
Applies mechanical traction	1	
Positions/secures the support straps	1	
Re-evaluates the proximal/distal securing devices	1	
Reassesses motor, sensory, and distal circulation	1	
NOTE: The examiner acknowledges present and normal		
NOTE: The examiner must ask candidate how he/she would prepare the patient for transportation.		
Verbalizes securing the torso to the long board to immobilize the hip	1	
Verbalizes securing the splint to the long board to prevent movement of the splint	1	
TOTAL:	**14**	

CRITICAL CRITERIA:

___ Loss of traction at any point after it is assumed
___ Did not reassess motor, sensory, and distal circulation before and after splinting
___ The foot is excessively rotated or extended after splinting
___ Did not secure the ischial strap before taking traction
___ Final immobilization failed to support the femur or prevent rotation of the injured leg
___ Secures leg to splint before applying mechanical traction

NOTE: If the Sager splint or Kendricks Traction Device is used without elevating the patient's leg, application of manual traction is not necessary. The candidate should be awarded 1 point as if manual traction were applied.

NOTE: If the leg is elevated at all, manual traction must be applied before elevating the leg. The ankle hitch may be applied before elevating the leg and used to provide manual traction.

BLEEDING CONTROL/SHOCK MANAGEMENT

	Points Possible	Points Awarded
Takes or verbalizes body substance isolation precautions	1	
Applied direct pressure to the wound	1	
Elevates the extremity	1	
NOTE: The examiner must now inform the candidate that the wound continues to bleed.		
Applies an additional dressing to the wound	1	
NOTE: The examiner must now inform the candidate that the wound still continues to bleed. The second dressing does not control the bleeding.		
Locates and applies pressure to appropriate arterial pressure point	1	
NOTE: The examiner must now inform the candidate that the bleeding is controlled.		
Bandages the wound	1	
NOTE: The examiner must now inform the candidate that the patient is showing signs and symptoms indicative of hypoperfusion.		
Properly positions the patient	1	
Applies high concentration oxygen	1	
Initiates steps to prevent heat loss from the patient	1	
Indicates need for immediate transportation	1	
TOTAL:	10	

CRITICAL CRITERIA

___ Did not take or verbalize body substance isolation precautions
___ Did not apply high concentrations of oxygen
___ Applies tourniquet before attempting other methods of bleeding control
___ Did not control hemorrhage in a timely manner
___ Did not indicate a need for immediate transportation

AIRWAY, OXYGEN, AND VENTILATION SKILLS
UPPER AIRWAY ADJUNCTS AND SUCTION

OROPHARYNGEAL AIRWAY

	Points Possible	Points Awarded
Takes or verbalizes body substance isolation precautions	1	
Selects appropriate size airway	1	
Measures airway	1	
Inserts airway without pushing the tongue posteriorly	1	
NOTE: The examiner must advise the candidate that the patient is gagging and becoming conscious.		
Removes oropharyngeal airway	1	

SUCTION

NOTE: The examiner must advise the candidate to suction the patient's oropharynx/nasopharynx		
Turns on/prepares suction device	1	
Assures presence of mechanical suction	1	
Inserts suction tip without suction	1	
Applies suction to the oropharynx/nasopharynx	1	

NASOPHARYNGEAL AIRWAY

NOTE: The examiner must advise the candidate to insert a nasopharyngeal airway.		
Selects appropriate airway	1	
Measures airway	1	
Verbalizes lubrication of the nasal airway	1	
Fully inserts the airway with the bevel facing toward the septum	1	
TOTAL:	13	

CRITICAL CRITERIA

___ Did not take or verbalize body substance isolation precautions
___ Did not obtain a patent airway with the oropharyngeal airway
___ Did not obtain a patent airway with the nasopharyngeal airway
___ Did not demonstrate an acceptable suction technique
___ Inserts any adjunct in a manner dangerous to the patient

MOUTH-TO-MASK WITH SUPPLEMENTAL OXYGEN

	Points Possible	Points Awarded
Takes or verbalizes body substance isolation precautions	1	
Connects one-way valve to mask	1	
Opens patient's airway or confirms patient's airway is open (manually or with adjunct)	1	
Establishes and maintains a proper mask to face seal	1	
Ventilates the patient at the proper volume and rate (800–1200 ml per breath/10–20 breaths per minute)	1	
Connects mask to high concentration oxygen	1	
Adjusts flow rate to 15 liters/minute or greater	1	
Continues ventilation at proper volume and rate (800–1200 ml per breath/10–20 breaths per minute)	1	
NOTE: The examiner must witness ventilations for at least 30 seconds.		
TOTAL:	8	

CRITICAL CRITERIA

___ Did not take or verbalize body substance isolation precautions

___ Did not adjust liter flow to 15 L/min or greater

___ Did not provide proper volume per breath
   (more than 2 ventilations per minute are below 800 ml)

___ Did not ventilate the patient at 10-20 breaths per minute

___ Did not allow for complete exhalation

OXYGEN ADMINISTRATION

	Points Possible	Points Awarded
Takes or verbalizes body substance isolation precautions	1	
Assembles regulator to tank	1	
Opens tank	1	
Checks for leaks	1	
Checks tank pressure	1	
Attaches non-rebreather mask	1	
Prefills reservoir	1	
Adjusts liter flow to 12 liters/minute or greater	1	
Applies and adjusts mask to the patient's face	1	
NOTE: The examiner must advise the candidate that the patient is not tolerating the non-rebreather mask. Medical direction has ordered you to apply a nasal cannula to the patient.		
Attaches nasal cannula to oxygen	1	
Adjusts liter flow up to 6 liters/minute or less	1	
Applies nasal cannula to the patient	1	
NOTE: The examiner must advise the candidate to discontinue oxygen therapy.		
Removes the nasal cannula	1	
Shuts off the regulator	1	
Relieves the pressure within the regulator	1	
TOTAL:	**15**	

CRITICAL CRITERIA

___ Did not take or verbalize body substance isolation precautions
___ Did not assemble the tank and regulator without leaks
___ Did not prefill the reservoir bag
___ Did not adjust the device to the correct liter flow for the non-rebreather mask (12 L/min or greater)
___ Did not adjust the device to the correct liter flow for the nasal cannula (up to 6 L/min)

VENTILATORY MANAGEMENT
ENDOTRACHEAL INTUBATION

NOTE: If a candidate elects to initially ventilate with a BVM attached to a reservoir and oxygen, full credit must be awarded for steps denoted by "**" if the first ventilation is delivered within the initial 30 seconds

		Points Possible	Points Awarded
Takes or verbalizes body substance isolation precautions		1	
Opens airway manually		1	
Elevates tongue and inserts simple airway adjunct (oropharyngeal or nasopharyngeal airway)		1	
NOTE: The examiner now informs the candidate no gag reflect is present and the patient accepts the adjunct.			
**Ventilates the patient immediately using a BVM device unattached to oxygen		1	
**Hyperventilates the patient with room air		1	
Note: The examiner now informs the candidate that ventilation is being performed without difficulty.			
Attaches the oxygen reservoir to the BVM		1	
Attaches BVM to high-flow oxygen		1	
Ventilates the patient at the proper volume and rate (800–1200 ml per breath/10–20 breaths per minute)		1	
NOTE: After 30 seconds, the examiner auscultates and reports breath sounds are present and equal bilaterally and medical control has ordered intubation. The examiner must now take over ventilation.			
Directs assistant to hyperventilate patient		1	
Identifies/selects proper equipment for intubation		1	
Checks equipment	Checks for cuff leaks	1	
	Checks laryngoscope operation and bulb tightness	1	
NOTE: The examiner must remove the OPA and move out of the way when the candidate is prepared to intubate.			
Positions the head properly		1	
Inserts the laryngoscope blade while displacing the tongue		1	
Elevates the mandible with the laryngoscope		1	
Introduces the ET tube and advances it to the proper depth		1	
Inflates the cuff to the proper pressure		1	
Disconnects the syringe from the cuff inlet port		1	
Directs ventilation of the patient		1	
Confirms proper placement by auscultation bilaterally and over the epigastrium		1	
NOTE: The examiner must ask, "If you had proper placement, what would you expect to hear?"			
Secures the ET tube (*may be verbalized*)		1	
	TOTAL:	21	

CRITICAL CRITERIA

___ Did not take or verbalize body substance isolation precautions
___ Did not initiate ventilations within 30 seconds after applying gloves or interrupts ventilations for greater than 30 seconds at any time
___ Did not voice or provide high oxygen concentrations (15 L/min or greater)
___ Did not ventilate patient at a rate of at least 10/minute
___ Did not provide adequate volume per breath (maximum of 2 errors/minute permissible)
___ Did not hyperventilate the patient prior to intubation
___ Did not successfully intubate within 3 attempts
___ Used the patient's teeth as a fulcrum
___ Did not assure proper tube placement by auscultation bilaterally and over the epigastrium
___ If used, the stylette extended beyond the end of the ET tube
___ Inserts any adjunct in a manner that would be dangerous to the patient
___ Did not disconnect syringe from cuff inlet port

VENTILATORY MANAGEMENT
DUAL LUMEN AIRWAY DEVICE (PTL OR COMBI-TUBE) INSERTION
FOLLOWING AN UNSUCCESSFUL ENDOTRACHEAL INTUBATION ATTEMPT

	Points Possible	Points Awarded
Continues body substance isolation precautions	1	
Confirms the patient is being properly ventilated with high percentage oxygen	1	
Directs assistant to hyperventilate the patient	1	
Checks/prepares airway device	1	
Lubricates distal tip of the device (*may be verbalized*)	1	
Removes the oropharyngeal airway	1	
Positions the head properly	1	
Performs a tongue-jaw lift	1	
Inserts airway device to proper depth	1	

COMBI-TUBE	PTL		
Inflates pharyngeal cuff and removes syringe	Secures strap	1	
Inflates distal cuff and removes syringe	Blows into tube #1 to inflate both cuffs	1	

Ventilates through proper first lumen	1	
Confirms placement by observing chest rise and auscultating over the epigastrium and bilaterally over the chest	1	
NOTE: The examiner states: "You do not see rise and fall of the chest and hear sounds only over the epigastrium."		
Ventilates through the alternate lumen	1	
Confirms placement by observing chest rise and auscultating over the epigastrium and bilaterally over the chest	1	
NOTE: The examiner confirms adequate chest rise, bilateral breath sounds, and absent sounds over the epigastrium.		
Secures tube at appropriate step in sequence	1	
TOTAL:	**16**	

CRITICAL CRITERIA

___ Did not take or verbalize body substance isolation precautions.
___ Interrupts ventilation for greater than 30 seconds.
___ Did not direct hyperventilation of the patient prior to placement of the device.
___ Did not assure proper placement of the device.
___ Did not successfully ventilate patient.
___ Did not provide high flow oxygen (15 L/min or greater).
___ Inserts any adjunct in a manner that would be dangerous to the patient.

VENTILATORY MANAGEMENT
ESOPHAGEAL OBTURATOR AIRWAY INSERTION FOLLOWING AN UNSUCCESSFUL ENDOTRACHEAL INTUBATION ATTEMPT

	Points Possible	Points Awarded
Continues body substance isolation precautions	1	
Confirms the patient is being properly ventilated	1	
Directs assistant to hyperventilate the patient	1	
Identifies/selects proper equipment	1	
Assembles airway	1	
Tests cuff	1	
Inflates mask	1	
Lubricates tube (*may be verbalized*)	1	
Removes the oropharyngeal airway	1	
Positions head properly with neck in the neutral or slightly flexed position	1	
Grasps and elevates tongue and mandible	1	
Inserts and elevates tongue and mandible	1	
Inserts tube in the same direction as the curvature of the pharynx	1	
Advances tube until the mask is sealed against the face	1	
Ventilates the patient while maintaining a tight mask seal	1	
Confirms placement by observing chest rise and auscultating over the epigastrium and bilaterally over the chest	1	
NOTE: The examiner confirms adequate chest rise, bilateral breath sounds and absent sounds over the epigastrium.		
Inflates the cuff to the proper pressure	1	
Disconnects the syringe	1	
Continues ventilation of the patient	1	
TOTAL:	**18**	

CRITICAL CRITERIA

___ Did not take or verbalize body substance isolation precautions.
___ Interrupts ventilation for more than 30 seconds
___ Did not direct hyperventilation of the patient prior to placement of the device.
___ Did not assure proper placement of the device
___ Did not successfully ventilate the patient
___ Did not provide high flow oxygen (15 L/min or greater)
___ Inserts any adjunct in a manner that would be dangerous to the patient

1994 REVISED EMT-BASIC NATIONAL STANDARDS REVIEW SELF-TEST

TEST SECTION *ONE* ANSWER SHEET—page one of three pages

1. ⓐ ⓑ ⓒ ⓓ ⓔ
2. ⓐ ⓑ ⓒ ⓓ ⓔ
3. ⓐ ⓑ ⓒ ⓓ ⓔ
4. ⓐ ⓑ ⓒ ⓓ ⓔ
5. ⓐ ⓑ ⓒ ⓓ ⓔ
6. ⓐ ⓑ ⓒ ⓓ ⓔ
7. ⓐ ⓑ ⓒ ⓓ ⓔ
8. ⓐ ⓑ ⓒ ⓓ ⓔ
9. ⓐ ⓑ ⓒ ⓓ ⓔ
10. ⓐ ⓑ ⓒ ⓓ ⓔ
11. ⓐ ⓑ ⓒ ⓓ ⓔ
12. ⓐ ⓑ ⓒ ⓓ ⓔ
13. ⓐ ⓑ ⓒ ⓓ ⓔ
14. ⓐ ⓑ ⓒ ⓓ ⓔ
15. ⓐ ⓑ ⓒ ⓓ ⓔ
16. ⓐ ⓑ ⓒ ⓓ ⓔ
17. ⓐ ⓑ ⓒ ⓓ ⓔ
18. ⓐ ⓑ ⓒ ⓓ ⓔ
19. ⓐ ⓑ ⓒ ⓓ ⓔ
20. ⓐ ⓑ ⓒ ⓓ ⓔ
21. ⓐ ⓑ ⓒ ⓓ ⓔ
22. ⓐ ⓑ ⓒ ⓓ ⓔ
23. ⓐ ⓑ ⓒ ⓓ ⓔ
24. ⓐ ⓑ ⓒ ⓓ ⓔ
25. ⓐ ⓑ ⓒ ⓓ ⓔ
26. ⓐ ⓑ ⓒ ⓓ ⓔ
27. ⓐ ⓑ ⓒ ⓓ ⓔ
28. ⓐ ⓑ ⓒ ⓓ ⓔ
29. ⓐ ⓑ ⓒ ⓓ ⓔ
30. ⓐ ⓑ ⓒ ⓓ ⓔ
31. ⓐ ⓑ ⓒ ⓓ ⓔ
32. ⓐ ⓑ ⓒ ⓓ ⓔ
33. ⓐ ⓑ ⓒ ⓓ ⓔ
34. ⓐ ⓑ ⓒ ⓓ ⓔ
35. ⓐ ⓑ ⓒ ⓓ ⓔ
36. ⓐ ⓑ ⓒ ⓓ ⓔ
37. ⓐ ⓑ ⓒ ⓓ ⓔ
38. ⓐ ⓑ ⓒ ⓓ ⓔ
39. ⓐ ⓑ ⓒ ⓓ ⓔ
40. ⓐ ⓑ ⓒ ⓓ ⓔ
41. ⓐ ⓑ ⓒ ⓓ ⓔ
42. ⓐ ⓑ ⓒ ⓓ ⓔ
43. ⓐ ⓑ ⓒ ⓓ ⓔ
44. ⓐ ⓑ ⓒ ⓓ ⓔ
45. ⓐ ⓑ ⓒ ⓓ ⓔ
46. ⓐ ⓑ ⓒ ⓓ ⓔ
47. ⓐ ⓑ ⓒ ⓓ ⓔ
48. ⓐ ⓑ ⓒ ⓓ ⓔ
49. ⓐ ⓑ ⓒ ⓓ ⓔ
50. ⓐ ⓑ ⓒ ⓓ ⓔ
51. ⓐ ⓑ ⓒ ⓓ ⓔ
52. ⓐ ⓑ ⓒ ⓓ ⓔ
53. ⓐ ⓑ ⓒ ⓓ ⓔ
54. ⓐ ⓑ ⓒ ⓓ ⓔ
55. ⓐ ⓑ ⓒ ⓓ ⓔ
56. ⓐ ⓑ ⓒ ⓓ ⓔ
57. ⓐ ⓑ ⓒ ⓓ ⓔ
58. ⓐ ⓑ ⓒ ⓓ ⓔ
59. ⓐ ⓑ ⓒ ⓓ ⓔ
60. ⓐ ⓑ ⓒ ⓓ ⓔ
61. ⓐ ⓑ ⓒ ⓓ ⓔ
62. ⓐ ⓑ ⓒ ⓓ ⓔ
63. ⓐ ⓑ ⓒ ⓓ ⓔ
64. ⓐ ⓑ ⓒ ⓓ ⓔ
65. ⓐ ⓑ ⓒ ⓓ ⓔ
66. ⓐ ⓑ ⓒ ⓓ ⓔ
67. ⓐ ⓑ ⓒ ⓓ ⓔ
68. ⓐ ⓑ ⓒ ⓓ ⓔ
69. ⓐ ⓑ ⓒ ⓓ ⓔ
70. ⓐ ⓑ ⓒ ⓓ ⓔ
71. ⓐ ⓑ ⓒ ⓓ ⓔ
72. ⓐ ⓑ ⓒ ⓓ ⓔ
73. ⓐ ⓑ ⓒ ⓓ ⓔ
74. ⓐ ⓑ ⓒ ⓓ ⓔ
75. ⓐ ⓑ ⓒ ⓓ ⓔ
76. ⓐ ⓑ ⓒ ⓓ ⓔ
77. ⓐ ⓑ ⓒ ⓓ ⓔ
78. ⓐ ⓑ ⓒ ⓓ ⓔ
79. ⓐ ⓑ ⓒ ⓓ ⓔ
80. ⓐ ⓑ ⓒ ⓓ ⓔ
81. ⓐ ⓑ ⓒ ⓓ ⓔ
82. ⓐ ⓑ ⓒ ⓓ ⓔ
83. ⓐ ⓑ ⓒ ⓓ ⓔ
84. ⓐ ⓑ ⓒ ⓓ ⓔ
85. ⓐ ⓑ ⓒ ⓓ ⓔ
86. ⓐ ⓑ ⓒ ⓓ ⓔ
87. ⓐ ⓑ ⓒ ⓓ ⓔ
88. ⓐ ⓑ ⓒ ⓓ ⓔ
89. ⓐ ⓑ ⓒ ⓓ ⓔ
90. ⓐ ⓑ ⓒ ⓓ ⓔ
91. ⓐ ⓑ ⓒ ⓓ ⓔ
92. ⓐ ⓑ ⓒ ⓓ ⓔ
93. ⓐ ⓑ ⓒ ⓓ ⓔ
94. ⓐ ⓑ ⓒ ⓓ ⓔ
95. ⓐ ⓑ ⓒ ⓓ ⓔ
96. ⓐ ⓑ ⓒ ⓓ ⓔ
97. ⓐ ⓑ ⓒ ⓓ ⓔ
98. ⓐ ⓑ ⓒ ⓓ ⓔ
99. ⓐ ⓑ ⓒ ⓓ ⓔ

1994 REVISED EMT-BASIC NATIONAL STANDARDS REVIEW SELF-TEST

TEST SECTION *ONE* ANSWER SHEET—page two of three pages

#	a	b	c	d	e		#	a	b	c	d	e		#	a	b	c	d	e
100.	ⓐ	ⓑ	ⓒ	ⓓ	ⓔ		133.	ⓐ	ⓑ	ⓒ	ⓓ	ⓔ		166.	ⓐ	ⓑ	ⓒ	ⓓ	ⓔ
101.	ⓐ	ⓑ	ⓒ	ⓓ	ⓔ		134.	ⓐ	ⓑ	ⓒ	ⓓ	ⓔ		167.	ⓐ	ⓑ	ⓒ	ⓓ	ⓔ
102.	ⓐ	ⓑ	ⓒ	ⓓ	ⓔ		135.	ⓐ	ⓑ	ⓒ	ⓓ	ⓔ		168.	ⓐ	ⓑ	ⓒ	ⓓ	ⓔ
103.	ⓐ	ⓑ	ⓒ	ⓓ	ⓔ		136.	ⓐ	ⓑ	ⓒ	ⓓ	ⓔ		169.	ⓐ	ⓑ	ⓒ	ⓓ	ⓔ
104.	ⓐ	ⓑ	ⓒ	ⓓ	ⓔ		137.	ⓐ	ⓑ	ⓒ	ⓓ	ⓔ		170.	ⓐ	ⓑ	ⓒ	ⓓ	ⓔ
105.	ⓐ	ⓑ	ⓒ	ⓓ	ⓔ		138.	ⓐ	ⓑ	ⓒ	ⓓ	ⓔ		171.	ⓐ	ⓑ	ⓒ	ⓓ	ⓔ
106.	ⓐ	ⓑ	ⓒ	ⓓ	ⓔ		139.	ⓐ	ⓑ	ⓒ	ⓓ	ⓔ		172.	ⓐ	ⓑ	ⓒ	ⓓ	ⓔ
107.	ⓐ	ⓑ	ⓒ	ⓓ	ⓔ		140.	ⓐ	ⓑ	ⓒ	ⓓ	ⓔ		173.	ⓐ	ⓑ	ⓒ	ⓓ	ⓔ
108.	ⓐ	ⓑ	ⓒ	ⓓ	ⓔ		141.	ⓐ	ⓑ	ⓒ	ⓓ	ⓔ		174.	ⓐ	ⓑ	ⓒ	ⓓ	ⓔ
109.	ⓐ	ⓑ	ⓒ	ⓓ	ⓔ		142.	ⓐ	ⓑ	ⓒ	ⓓ	ⓔ		175.	ⓐ	ⓑ	ⓒ	ⓓ	ⓔ
110.	ⓐ	ⓑ	ⓒ	ⓓ	ⓔ		143.	ⓐ	ⓑ	ⓒ	ⓓ	ⓔ		176.	ⓐ	ⓑ	ⓒ	ⓓ	ⓔ
111.	ⓐ	ⓑ	ⓒ	ⓓ	ⓔ		144.	ⓐ	ⓑ	ⓒ	ⓓ	ⓔ		177.	ⓐ	ⓑ	ⓒ	ⓓ	ⓔ
112.	ⓐ	ⓑ	ⓒ	ⓓ	ⓔ		145.	ⓐ	ⓑ	ⓒ	ⓓ	ⓔ		178.	ⓐ	ⓑ	ⓒ	ⓓ	ⓔ
113.	ⓐ	ⓑ	ⓒ	ⓓ	ⓔ		146.	ⓐ	ⓑ	ⓒ	ⓓ	ⓔ		179.	ⓐ	ⓑ	ⓒ	ⓓ	ⓔ
114.	ⓐ	ⓑ	ⓒ	ⓓ	ⓔ		147.	ⓐ	ⓑ	ⓒ	ⓓ	ⓔ		180.	ⓐ	ⓑ	ⓒ	ⓓ	ⓔ
115.	ⓐ	ⓑ	ⓒ	ⓓ	ⓔ		148.	ⓐ	ⓑ	ⓒ	ⓓ	ⓔ		181.	ⓐ	ⓑ	ⓒ	ⓓ	ⓔ
116.	ⓐ	ⓑ	ⓒ	ⓓ	ⓔ		149.	ⓐ	ⓑ	ⓒ	ⓓ	ⓔ		182.	ⓐ	ⓑ	ⓒ	ⓓ	ⓔ
117.	ⓐ	ⓑ	ⓒ	ⓓ	ⓔ		150.	ⓐ	ⓑ	ⓒ	ⓓ	ⓔ		183.	ⓐ	ⓑ	ⓒ	ⓓ	ⓔ
118.	ⓐ	ⓑ	ⓒ	ⓓ	ⓔ		151.	ⓐ	ⓑ	ⓒ	ⓓ	ⓔ		184.	ⓐ	ⓑ	ⓒ	ⓓ	ⓔ
119.	ⓐ	ⓑ	ⓒ	ⓓ	ⓔ		152.	ⓐ	ⓑ	ⓒ	ⓓ	ⓔ		185.	ⓐ	ⓑ	ⓒ	ⓓ	ⓔ
120.	ⓐ	ⓑ	ⓒ	ⓓ	ⓔ		153.	ⓐ	ⓑ	ⓒ	ⓓ	ⓔ		186.	ⓐ	ⓑ	ⓒ	ⓓ	ⓔ
121.	ⓐ	ⓑ	ⓒ	ⓓ	ⓔ		154.	ⓐ	ⓑ	ⓒ	ⓓ	ⓔ		187.	ⓐ	ⓑ	ⓒ	ⓓ	ⓔ
122.	ⓐ	ⓑ	ⓒ	ⓓ	ⓔ		155.	ⓐ	ⓑ	ⓒ	ⓓ	ⓔ		188.	ⓐ	ⓑ	ⓒ	ⓓ	ⓔ
123.	ⓐ	ⓑ	ⓒ	ⓓ	ⓔ		156.	ⓐ	ⓑ	ⓒ	ⓓ	ⓔ		189.	ⓐ	ⓑ	ⓒ	ⓓ	ⓔ
124.	ⓐ	ⓑ	ⓒ	ⓓ	ⓔ		157.	ⓐ	ⓑ	ⓒ	ⓓ	ⓔ		190.	ⓐ	ⓑ	ⓒ	ⓓ	ⓔ
125.	ⓐ	ⓑ	ⓒ	ⓓ	ⓔ		158.	ⓐ	ⓑ	ⓒ	ⓓ	ⓔ		191.	ⓐ	ⓑ	ⓒ	ⓓ	ⓔ
126.	ⓐ	ⓑ	ⓒ	ⓓ	ⓔ		159.	ⓐ	ⓑ	ⓒ	ⓓ	ⓔ		192.	ⓐ	ⓑ	ⓒ	ⓓ	ⓔ
127.	ⓐ	ⓑ	ⓒ	ⓓ	ⓔ		160.	ⓐ	ⓑ	ⓒ	ⓓ	ⓔ		193.	ⓐ	ⓑ	ⓒ	ⓓ	ⓔ
128.	ⓐ	ⓑ	ⓒ	ⓓ	ⓔ		161.	ⓐ	ⓑ	ⓒ	ⓓ	ⓔ		194.	ⓐ	ⓑ	ⓒ	ⓓ	ⓔ
129.	ⓐ	ⓑ	ⓒ	ⓓ	ⓔ		162.	ⓐ	ⓑ	ⓒ	ⓓ	ⓔ		195.	ⓐ	ⓑ	ⓒ	ⓓ	ⓔ
130.	ⓐ	ⓑ	ⓒ	ⓓ	ⓔ		163.	ⓐ	ⓑ	ⓒ	ⓓ	ⓔ		196.	ⓐ	ⓑ	ⓒ	ⓓ	ⓔ
131.	ⓐ	ⓑ	ⓒ	ⓓ	ⓔ		164.	ⓐ	ⓑ	ⓒ	ⓓ	ⓔ		197.	ⓐ	ⓑ	ⓒ	ⓓ	ⓔ
132.	ⓐ	ⓑ	ⓒ	ⓓ	ⓔ		165.	ⓐ	ⓑ	ⓒ	ⓓ	ⓔ		198.	ⓐ	ⓑ	ⓒ	ⓓ	ⓔ

1994 REVISED EMT-BASIC NATIONAL STANDARDS REVIEW SELF-TEST

TEST SECTION *ONE* ANSWER SHEET—page three of three pages

199. ⓐ ⓑ ⓒ ⓓ ⓔ
200. ⓐ ⓑ ⓒ ⓓ ⓔ
201. ⓐ ⓑ ⓒ ⓓ ⓔ
202. ⓐ ⓑ ⓒ ⓓ ⓔ
203. ⓐ ⓑ ⓒ ⓓ ⓔ
204. ⓐ ⓑ ⓒ ⓓ ⓔ
205. ⓐ ⓑ ⓒ ⓓ ⓔ
206. ⓐ ⓑ ⓒ ⓓ ⓔ
207. ⓐ ⓑ ⓒ ⓓ ⓔ
208. ⓐ ⓑ ⓒ ⓓ ⓔ
209. ⓐ ⓑ ⓒ ⓓ ⓔ
210. ⓐ ⓑ ⓒ ⓓ ⓔ
211. ⓐ ⓑ ⓒ ⓓ ⓔ
212. ⓐ ⓑ ⓒ ⓓ ⓔ
213. ⓐ ⓑ ⓒ ⓓ ⓔ
214. ⓐ ⓑ ⓒ ⓓ ⓔ
215. ⓐ ⓑ ⓒ ⓓ ⓔ
216. ⓐ ⓑ ⓒ ⓓ ⓔ
217. ⓐ ⓑ ⓒ ⓓ ⓔ
218. ⓐ ⓑ ⓒ ⓓ ⓔ
219. ⓐ ⓑ ⓒ ⓓ ⓔ
220. ⓐ ⓑ ⓒ ⓓ ⓔ
221. ⓐ ⓑ ⓒ ⓓ ⓔ
222. ⓐ ⓑ ⓒ ⓓ ⓔ
223. ⓐ ⓑ ⓒ ⓓ ⓔ
224. ⓐ ⓑ ⓒ ⓓ ⓔ

225. ⓐ ⓑ ⓒ ⓓ ⓔ
226. ⓐ ⓑ ⓒ ⓓ ⓔ
227. ⓐ ⓑ ⓒ ⓓ ⓔ
228. ⓐ ⓑ ⓒ ⓓ ⓔ
229. ⓐ ⓑ ⓒ ⓓ ⓔ
230. ⓐ ⓑ ⓒ ⓓ ⓔ
231. ⓐ ⓑ ⓒ ⓓ ⓔ
232. ⓐ ⓑ ⓒ ⓓ ⓔ
233. ⓐ ⓑ ⓒ ⓓ ⓔ
234. ⓐ ⓑ ⓒ ⓓ ⓔ
235. ⓐ ⓑ ⓒ ⓓ ⓔ
236. ⓐ ⓑ ⓒ ⓓ ⓔ
237. ⓐ ⓑ ⓒ ⓓ ⓔ
238. ⓐ ⓑ ⓒ ⓓ ⓔ
239. ⓐ ⓑ ⓒ ⓓ ⓔ
240. ⓐ ⓑ ⓒ ⓓ ⓔ
241. ⓐ ⓑ ⓒ ⓓ ⓔ
242. ⓐ ⓑ ⓒ ⓓ ⓔ
243. ⓐ ⓑ ⓒ ⓓ ⓔ
244. ⓐ ⓑ ⓒ ⓓ ⓔ
245. ⓐ ⓑ ⓒ ⓓ ⓔ
246. ⓐ ⓑ ⓒ ⓓ ⓔ
247. ⓐ ⓑ ⓒ ⓓ ⓔ
248. ⓐ ⓑ ⓒ ⓓ ⓔ
249. ⓐ ⓑ ⓒ ⓓ ⓔ
250. ⓐ ⓑ ⓒ ⓓ ⓔ

251. ⓐ ⓑ ⓒ ⓓ ⓔ
252. ⓐ ⓑ ⓒ ⓓ ⓔ
253. ⓐ ⓑ ⓒ ⓓ ⓔ
254. ⓐ ⓑ ⓒ ⓓ ⓔ
255. ⓐ ⓑ ⓒ ⓓ ⓔ
256. ⓐ ⓑ ⓒ ⓓ ⓔ
257. ⓐ ⓑ ⓒ ⓓ ⓔ
258. ⓐ ⓑ ⓒ ⓓ ⓔ
259. ⓐ ⓑ ⓒ ⓓ ⓔ
260. ⓐ ⓑ ⓒ ⓓ ⓔ
261. ⓐ ⓑ ⓒ ⓓ ⓔ
262. ⓐ ⓑ ⓒ ⓓ ⓔ
263. ⓐ ⓑ ⓒ ⓓ ⓔ
264. ⓐ ⓑ ⓒ ⓓ ⓔ
265. ⓐ ⓑ ⓒ ⓓ ⓔ
266. ⓐ ⓑ ⓒ ⓓ ⓔ
267. ⓐ ⓑ ⓒ ⓓ ⓔ
268. ⓐ ⓑ ⓒ ⓓ ⓔ
269. ⓐ ⓑ ⓒ ⓓ ⓔ
270. ⓐ ⓑ ⓒ ⓓ ⓔ
271. ⓐ ⓑ ⓒ ⓓ ⓔ
272. ⓐ ⓑ ⓒ ⓓ ⓔ
273. ⓐ ⓑ ⓒ ⓓ ⓔ
274. ⓐ ⓑ ⓒ ⓓ ⓔ
275. ⓐ ⓑ ⓒ ⓓ ⓔ

1994 REVISED EMT-BASIC NATIONAL STANDARDS REVIEW SELF-TEST

TEST SECTION *TWO* ANSWER SHEET—page one of one page

1. a b c d e	32. a b c d e	63. a b c d e
2. a b c d e	33. a b c d e	64. a b c d e
3. a b c d e	34. a b c d e	65. a b c d e
4. a b c d e	35. a b c d e	66. a b c d e
5. a b c d e	36. a b c d e	67. a b c d e
6. a b c d e	37. a b c d e	68. a b c d e
7. a b c d e	38. a b c d e	69. a b c d e
8. a b c d e	39. a b c d e	70. a b c d e
9. a b c d e	40. a b c d e	71. a b c d e
10. a b c d e	41. a b c d e	72. a b c d e
11. a b c d e	42. a b c d e	73. a b c d e
12. a b c d e	43. a b c d e	74. a b c d e
13. a b c d e	44. a b c d e	75. a b c d e
14. a b c d e	45. a b c d e	76. a b c d e
15. a b c d e	46. a b c d e	77. a b c d e
16. a b c d e	47. a b c d e	78. a b c d e
17. a b c d e	48. a b c d e	79. a b c d e
18. a b c d e	49. a b c d e	80. a b c d e
19. a b c d e	50. a b c d e	81. a b c d e
20. a b c d e	51. a b c d e	82. a b c d e
21. a b c d e	52. a b c d e	83. a b c d e
22. a b c d e	53. a b c d e	84. a b c d e
23. a b c d e	54. a b c d e	85. a b c d e
24. a b c d e	55. a b c d e	86. a b c d e
25. a b c d e	56. a b c d e	87. a b c d e
26. a b c d e	57. a b c d e	88. a b c d e
27. a b c d e	58. a b c d e	89. a b c d e
28. a b c d e	59. a b c d e	90. a b c d e
29. a b c d e	60. a b c d e	91. a b c d e
30. a b c d e	61. a b c d e	92. a b c d e
31. a b c d e	62. a b c d e	93. a b c d e

1994 REVISED EMT-BASIC NATIONAL STANDARDS REVIEW SELF-TEST

TEST SECTION *THREE* ANSWER SHEET—page one of two pages

1. ⓐ ⓑ ⓒ ⓓ ⓔ	34. ⓐ ⓑ ⓒ ⓓ ⓔ	67. ⓐ ⓑ ⓒ ⓓ ⓔ
2. ⓐ ⓑ ⓒ ⓓ ⓔ	35. ⓐ ⓑ ⓒ ⓓ ⓔ	68. ⓐ ⓑ ⓒ ⓓ ⓔ
3. ⓐ ⓑ ⓒ ⓓ ⓔ	36. ⓐ ⓑ ⓒ ⓓ ⓔ	69. ⓐ ⓑ ⓒ ⓓ ⓔ
4. ⓐ ⓑ ⓒ ⓓ ⓔ	37. ⓐ ⓑ ⓒ ⓓ ⓔ	70. ⓐ ⓑ ⓒ ⓓ ⓔ
5. ⓐ ⓑ ⓒ ⓓ ⓔ	38. ⓐ ⓑ ⓒ ⓓ ⓔ	71. ⓐ ⓑ ⓒ ⓓ ⓔ
6. ⓐ ⓑ ⓒ ⓓ ⓔ	39. ⓐ ⓑ ⓒ ⓓ ⓔ	72. ⓐ ⓑ ⓒ ⓓ ⓔ
7. ⓐ ⓑ ⓒ ⓓ ⓔ	40. ⓐ ⓑ ⓒ ⓓ ⓔ	73. ⓐ ⓑ ⓒ ⓓ ⓔ
8. ⓐ ⓑ ⓒ ⓓ ⓔ	41. ⓐ ⓑ ⓒ ⓓ ⓔ	74. ⓐ ⓑ ⓒ ⓓ ⓔ
9. ⓐ ⓑ ⓒ ⓓ ⓔ	42. ⓐ ⓑ ⓒ ⓓ ⓔ	75. ⓐ ⓑ ⓒ ⓓ ⓔ
10. ⓐ ⓑ ⓒ ⓓ ⓔ	43. ⓐ ⓑ ⓒ ⓓ ⓔ	76. ⓐ ⓑ ⓒ ⓓ ⓔ
11. ⓐ ⓑ ⓒ ⓓ ⓔ	44. ⓐ ⓑ ⓒ ⓓ ⓔ	77. ⓐ ⓑ ⓒ ⓓ ⓔ
12. ⓐ ⓑ ⓒ ⓓ ⓔ	45. ⓐ ⓑ ⓒ ⓓ ⓔ	78. ⓐ ⓑ ⓒ ⓓ ⓔ
13. ⓐ ⓑ ⓒ ⓓ ⓔ	46. ⓐ ⓑ ⓒ ⓓ ⓔ	79. ⓐ ⓑ ⓒ ⓓ ⓔ
14. ⓐ ⓑ ⓒ ⓓ ⓔ	47. ⓐ ⓑ ⓒ ⓓ ⓔ	80. ⓐ ⓑ ⓒ ⓓ ⓔ
15. ⓐ ⓑ ⓒ ⓓ ⓔ	48. ⓐ ⓑ ⓒ ⓓ ⓔ	81. ⓐ ⓑ ⓒ ⓓ ⓔ
16. ⓐ ⓑ ⓒ ⓓ ⓔ	49. ⓐ ⓑ ⓒ ⓓ ⓔ	82. ⓐ ⓑ ⓒ ⓓ ⓔ
17. ⓐ ⓑ ⓒ ⓓ ⓔ	50. ⓐ ⓑ ⓒ ⓓ ⓔ	83. ⓐ ⓑ ⓒ ⓓ ⓔ
18. ⓐ ⓑ ⓒ ⓓ ⓔ	51. ⓐ ⓑ ⓒ ⓓ ⓔ	84. ⓐ ⓑ ⓒ ⓓ ⓔ
19. ⓐ ⓑ ⓒ ⓓ ⓔ	52. ⓐ ⓑ ⓒ ⓓ ⓔ	85. ⓐ ⓑ ⓒ ⓓ ⓔ
20. ⓐ ⓑ ⓒ ⓓ ⓔ	53. ⓐ ⓑ ⓒ ⓓ ⓔ	86. ⓐ ⓑ ⓒ ⓓ ⓔ
21. ⓐ ⓑ ⓒ ⓓ ⓔ	54. ⓐ ⓑ ⓒ ⓓ ⓔ	87. ⓐ ⓑ ⓒ ⓓ ⓔ
22. ⓐ ⓑ ⓒ ⓓ ⓔ	55. ⓐ ⓑ ⓒ ⓓ ⓔ	88. ⓐ ⓑ ⓒ ⓓ ⓔ
23. ⓐ ⓑ ⓒ ⓓ ⓔ	56. ⓐ ⓑ ⓒ ⓓ ⓔ	89. ⓐ ⓑ ⓒ ⓓ ⓔ
24. ⓐ ⓑ ⓒ ⓓ ⓔ	57. ⓐ ⓑ ⓒ ⓓ ⓔ	90. ⓐ ⓑ ⓒ ⓓ ⓔ
25. ⓐ ⓑ ⓒ ⓓ ⓔ	58. ⓐ ⓑ ⓒ ⓓ ⓔ	91. ⓐ ⓑ ⓒ ⓓ ⓔ
26. ⓐ ⓑ ⓒ ⓓ ⓔ	59. ⓐ ⓑ ⓒ ⓓ ⓔ	92. ⓐ ⓑ ⓒ ⓓ ⓔ
27. ⓐ ⓑ ⓒ ⓓ ⓔ	60. ⓐ ⓑ ⓒ ⓓ ⓔ	93. ⓐ ⓑ ⓒ ⓓ ⓔ
28. ⓐ ⓑ ⓒ ⓓ ⓔ	61. ⓐ ⓑ ⓒ ⓓ ⓔ	94. ⓐ ⓑ ⓒ ⓓ ⓔ
29. ⓐ ⓑ ⓒ ⓓ ⓔ	62. ⓐ ⓑ ⓒ ⓓ ⓔ	95. ⓐ ⓑ ⓒ ⓓ ⓔ
30. ⓐ ⓑ ⓒ ⓓ ⓔ	63. ⓐ ⓑ ⓒ ⓓ ⓔ	96. ⓐ ⓑ ⓒ ⓓ ⓔ
31. ⓐ ⓑ ⓒ ⓓ ⓔ	64. ⓐ ⓑ ⓒ ⓓ ⓔ	97. ⓐ ⓑ ⓒ ⓓ ⓔ
32. ⓐ ⓑ ⓒ ⓓ ⓔ	65. ⓐ ⓑ ⓒ ⓓ ⓔ	98. ⓐ ⓑ ⓒ ⓓ ⓔ
33. ⓐ ⓑ ⓒ ⓓ ⓔ	66. ⓐ ⓑ ⓒ ⓓ ⓔ	99. ⓐ ⓑ ⓒ ⓓ ⓔ

1994 REVISED EMT-BASIC NATIONAL STANDARDS REVIEW SELF-TEST

TEST SECTION *THREE* ANSWER SHEET—page two of two pages

[Answer sheet bubbles for questions 100–189, each with options (a) (b) (c) (d) (e)]

1994 REVISED EMT-BASIC NATIONAL STANDARDS REVIEW SELF-TEST

TEST SECTION *FOUR* ANSWER SHEET—page one of four pages

1. ⓐ ⓑ ⓒ ⓓ ⓔ
2. ⓐ ⓑ ⓒ ⓓ ⓔ
3. ⓐ ⓑ ⓒ ⓓ ⓔ
4. ⓐ ⓑ ⓒ ⓓ ⓔ
5. ⓐ ⓑ ⓒ ⓓ ⓔ
6. ⓐ ⓑ ⓒ ⓓ ⓔ
7. ⓐ ⓑ ⓒ ⓓ ⓔ
8. ⓐ ⓑ ⓒ ⓓ ⓔ
9. ⓐ ⓑ ⓒ ⓓ ⓔ
10. ⓐ ⓑ ⓒ ⓓ ⓔ
11. ⓐ ⓑ ⓒ ⓓ ⓔ
12. ⓐ ⓑ ⓒ ⓓ ⓔ
13. ⓐ ⓑ ⓒ ⓓ ⓔ
14. ⓐ ⓑ ⓒ ⓓ ⓔ
15. ⓐ ⓑ ⓒ ⓓ ⓔ
16. ⓐ ⓑ ⓒ ⓓ ⓔ
17. ⓐ ⓑ ⓒ ⓓ ⓔ
18. ⓐ ⓑ ⓒ ⓓ ⓔ
19. ⓐ ⓑ ⓒ ⓓ ⓔ
20. ⓐ ⓑ ⓒ ⓓ ⓔ
21. ⓐ ⓑ ⓒ ⓓ ⓔ
22. ⓐ ⓑ ⓒ ⓓ ⓔ
23. ⓐ ⓑ ⓒ ⓓ ⓔ
24. ⓐ ⓑ ⓒ ⓓ ⓔ
25. ⓐ ⓑ ⓒ ⓓ ⓔ
26. ⓐ ⓑ ⓒ ⓓ ⓔ
27. ⓐ ⓑ ⓒ ⓓ ⓔ
28. ⓐ ⓑ ⓒ ⓓ ⓔ
29. ⓐ ⓑ ⓒ ⓓ ⓔ
30. ⓐ ⓑ ⓒ ⓓ ⓔ
31. ⓐ ⓑ ⓒ ⓓ ⓔ
32. ⓐ ⓑ ⓒ ⓓ ⓔ
33. ⓐ ⓑ ⓒ ⓓ ⓔ
34. ⓐ ⓑ ⓒ ⓓ ⓔ
35. ⓐ ⓑ ⓒ ⓓ ⓔ
36. ⓐ ⓑ ⓒ ⓓ ⓔ
37. ⓐ ⓑ ⓒ ⓓ ⓔ
38. ⓐ ⓑ ⓒ ⓓ ⓔ
39. ⓐ ⓑ ⓒ ⓓ ⓔ
40. ⓐ ⓑ ⓒ ⓓ ⓔ
41. ⓐ ⓑ ⓒ ⓓ ⓔ
42. ⓐ ⓑ ⓒ ⓓ ⓔ
43. ⓐ ⓑ ⓒ ⓓ ⓔ
44. ⓐ ⓑ ⓒ ⓓ ⓔ
45. ⓐ ⓑ ⓒ ⓓ ⓔ
46. ⓐ ⓑ ⓒ ⓓ ⓔ
47. ⓐ ⓑ ⓒ ⓓ ⓔ
48. ⓐ ⓑ ⓒ ⓓ ⓔ
49. ⓐ ⓑ ⓒ ⓓ ⓔ
50. ⓐ ⓑ ⓒ ⓓ ⓔ
51. ⓐ ⓑ ⓒ ⓓ ⓔ
52. ⓐ ⓑ ⓒ ⓓ ⓔ
53. ⓐ ⓑ ⓒ ⓓ ⓔ
54. ⓐ ⓑ ⓒ ⓓ ⓔ
55. ⓐ ⓑ ⓒ ⓓ ⓔ
56. ⓐ ⓑ ⓒ ⓓ ⓔ
57. ⓐ ⓑ ⓒ ⓓ ⓔ
58. ⓐ ⓑ ⓒ ⓓ ⓔ
59. ⓐ ⓑ ⓒ ⓓ ⓔ
60. ⓐ ⓑ ⓒ ⓓ ⓔ
61. ⓐ ⓑ ⓒ ⓓ ⓔ
62. ⓐ ⓑ ⓒ ⓓ ⓔ
63. ⓐ ⓑ ⓒ ⓓ ⓔ
64. ⓐ ⓑ ⓒ ⓓ ⓔ
65. ⓐ ⓑ ⓒ ⓓ ⓔ
66. ⓐ ⓑ ⓒ ⓓ ⓔ
67. ⓐ ⓑ ⓒ ⓓ ⓔ
68. ⓐ ⓑ ⓒ ⓓ ⓔ
69. ⓐ ⓑ ⓒ ⓓ ⓔ
70. ⓐ ⓑ ⓒ ⓓ ⓔ
71. ⓐ ⓑ ⓒ ⓓ ⓔ
72. ⓐ ⓑ ⓒ ⓓ ⓔ
73. ⓐ ⓑ ⓒ ⓓ ⓔ
74. ⓐ ⓑ ⓒ ⓓ ⓔ
75. ⓐ ⓑ ⓒ ⓓ ⓔ
76. ⓐ ⓑ ⓒ ⓓ ⓔ
77. ⓐ ⓑ ⓒ ⓓ ⓔ
78. ⓐ ⓑ ⓒ ⓓ ⓔ
79. ⓐ ⓑ ⓒ ⓓ ⓔ
80. ⓐ ⓑ ⓒ ⓓ ⓔ
81. ⓐ ⓑ ⓒ ⓓ ⓔ
82. ⓐ ⓑ ⓒ ⓓ ⓔ
83. ⓐ ⓑ ⓒ ⓓ ⓔ
84. ⓐ ⓑ ⓒ ⓓ ⓔ
85. ⓐ ⓑ ⓒ ⓓ ⓔ
86. ⓐ ⓑ ⓒ ⓓ ⓔ
87. ⓐ ⓑ ⓒ ⓓ ⓔ
88. ⓐ ⓑ ⓒ ⓓ ⓔ
89. ⓐ ⓑ ⓒ ⓓ ⓔ
90. ⓐ ⓑ ⓒ ⓓ ⓔ
91. ⓐ ⓑ ⓒ ⓓ ⓔ
92. ⓐ ⓑ ⓒ ⓓ ⓔ
93. ⓐ ⓑ ⓒ ⓓ ⓔ
94. ⓐ ⓑ ⓒ ⓓ ⓔ
95. ⓐ ⓑ ⓒ ⓓ ⓔ
96. ⓐ ⓑ ⓒ ⓓ ⓔ
97. ⓐ ⓑ ⓒ ⓓ ⓔ
98. ⓐ ⓑ ⓒ ⓓ ⓔ
99. ⓐ ⓑ ⓒ ⓓ ⓔ

TEST SECTION FOUR ANSWER SHEET

1994 REVISED EMT-BASIC NATIONAL STANDARDS REVIEW SELF-TEST

TEST SECTION *FOUR* ANSWER SHEET—page two of four pages

1994 REVISED EMT-BASIC NATIONAL STANDARDS REVIEW SELF-TEST

TEST SECTION *FOUR* ANSWER SHEET—page three of four pages

199. ⓐ ⓑ ⓒ ⓓ ⓔ	232. ⓐ ⓑ ⓒ ⓓ ⓔ	265. ⓐ ⓑ ⓒ ⓓ ⓔ
200. ⓐ ⓑ ⓒ ⓓ ⓔ	233. ⓐ ⓑ ⓒ ⓓ ⓔ	266. ⓐ ⓑ ⓒ ⓓ ⓔ
201. ⓐ ⓑ ⓒ ⓓ ⓔ	234. ⓐ ⓑ ⓒ ⓓ ⓔ	267. ⓐ ⓑ ⓒ ⓓ ⓔ
202. ⓐ ⓑ ⓒ ⓓ ⓔ	235. ⓐ ⓑ ⓒ ⓓ ⓔ	268. ⓐ ⓑ ⓒ ⓓ ⓔ
203. ⓐ ⓑ ⓒ ⓓ ⓔ	236. ⓐ ⓑ ⓒ ⓓ ⓔ	269. ⓐ ⓑ ⓒ ⓓ ⓔ
204. ⓐ ⓑ ⓒ ⓓ ⓔ	237. ⓐ ⓑ ⓒ ⓓ ⓔ	270. ⓐ ⓑ ⓒ ⓓ ⓔ
205. ⓐ ⓑ ⓒ ⓓ ⓔ	238. ⓐ ⓑ ⓒ ⓓ ⓔ	271. ⓐ ⓑ ⓒ ⓓ ⓔ
206. ⓐ ⓑ ⓒ ⓓ ⓔ	239. ⓐ ⓑ ⓒ ⓓ ⓔ	272. ⓐ ⓑ ⓒ ⓓ ⓔ
207. ⓐ ⓑ ⓒ ⓓ ⓔ	240. ⓐ ⓑ ⓒ ⓓ ⓔ	273. ⓐ ⓑ ⓒ ⓓ ⓔ
208. ⓐ ⓑ ⓒ ⓓ ⓔ	241. ⓐ ⓑ ⓒ ⓓ ⓔ	274. ⓐ ⓑ ⓒ ⓓ ⓔ
209. ⓐ ⓑ ⓒ ⓓ ⓔ	242. ⓐ ⓑ ⓒ ⓓ ⓔ	275. ⓐ ⓑ ⓒ ⓓ ⓔ
210. ⓐ ⓑ ⓒ ⓓ ⓔ	243. ⓐ ⓑ ⓒ ⓓ ⓔ	276. ⓐ ⓑ ⓒ ⓓ ⓔ
211. ⓐ ⓑ ⓒ ⓓ ⓔ	244. ⓐ ⓑ ⓒ ⓓ ⓔ	277. ⓐ ⓑ ⓒ ⓓ ⓔ
212. ⓐ ⓑ ⓒ ⓓ ⓔ	245. ⓐ ⓑ ⓒ ⓓ ⓔ	278. ⓐ ⓑ ⓒ ⓓ ⓔ
213. ⓐ ⓑ ⓒ ⓓ ⓔ	246. ⓐ ⓑ ⓒ ⓓ ⓔ	279. ⓐ ⓑ ⓒ ⓓ ⓔ
214. ⓐ ⓑ ⓒ ⓓ ⓔ	247. ⓐ ⓑ ⓒ ⓓ ⓔ	280. ⓐ ⓑ ⓒ ⓓ ⓔ
215. ⓐ ⓑ ⓒ ⓓ ⓔ	248. ⓐ ⓑ ⓒ ⓓ ⓔ	281. ⓐ ⓑ ⓒ ⓓ ⓔ
216. ⓐ ⓑ ⓒ ⓓ ⓔ	249. ⓐ ⓑ ⓒ ⓓ ⓔ	282. ⓐ ⓑ ⓒ ⓓ ⓔ
217. ⓐ ⓑ ⓒ ⓓ ⓔ	250. ⓐ ⓑ ⓒ ⓓ ⓔ	283. ⓐ ⓑ ⓒ ⓓ ⓔ
218. ⓐ ⓑ ⓒ ⓓ ⓔ	251. ⓐ ⓑ ⓒ ⓓ ⓔ	284. ⓐ ⓑ ⓒ ⓓ ⓔ
219. ⓐ ⓑ ⓒ ⓓ ⓔ	252. ⓐ ⓑ ⓒ ⓓ ⓔ	285. ⓐ ⓑ ⓒ ⓓ ⓔ
220. ⓐ ⓑ ⓒ ⓓ ⓔ	253. ⓐ ⓑ ⓒ ⓓ ⓔ	286. ⓐ ⓑ ⓒ ⓓ ⓔ
221. ⓐ ⓑ ⓒ ⓓ ⓔ	254. ⓐ ⓑ ⓒ ⓓ ⓔ	287. ⓐ ⓑ ⓒ ⓓ ⓔ
222. ⓐ ⓑ ⓒ ⓓ ⓔ	255. ⓐ ⓑ ⓒ ⓓ ⓔ	288. ⓐ ⓑ ⓒ ⓓ ⓔ
223. ⓐ ⓑ ⓒ ⓓ ⓔ	256. ⓐ ⓑ ⓒ ⓓ ⓔ	289. ⓐ ⓑ ⓒ ⓓ ⓔ
224. ⓐ ⓑ ⓒ ⓓ ⓔ	257. ⓐ ⓑ ⓒ ⓓ ⓔ	290. ⓐ ⓑ ⓒ ⓓ ⓔ
225. ⓐ ⓑ ⓒ ⓓ ⓔ	258. ⓐ ⓑ ⓒ ⓓ ⓔ	291. ⓐ ⓑ ⓒ ⓓ ⓔ
226. ⓐ ⓑ ⓒ ⓓ ⓔ	259. ⓐ ⓑ ⓒ ⓓ ⓔ	292. ⓐ ⓑ ⓒ ⓓ ⓔ
227. ⓐ ⓑ ⓒ ⓓ ⓔ	260. ⓐ ⓑ ⓒ ⓓ ⓔ	293. ⓐ ⓑ ⓒ ⓓ ⓔ
228. ⓐ ⓑ ⓒ ⓓ ⓔ	261. ⓐ ⓑ ⓒ ⓓ ⓔ	294. ⓐ ⓑ ⓒ ⓓ ⓔ
229. ⓐ ⓑ ⓒ ⓓ ⓔ	262. ⓐ ⓑ ⓒ ⓓ ⓔ	295. ⓐ ⓑ ⓒ ⓓ ⓔ
230. ⓐ ⓑ ⓒ ⓓ ⓔ	263. ⓐ ⓑ ⓒ ⓓ ⓔ	296. ⓐ ⓑ ⓒ ⓓ ⓔ
231. ⓐ ⓑ ⓒ ⓓ ⓔ	264. ⓐ ⓑ ⓒ ⓓ ⓔ	297. ⓐ ⓑ ⓒ ⓓ ⓔ

TEST SECTION FOUR ANSWER SHEET

1994 REVISED EMT-BASIC NATIONAL STANDARDS REVIEW SELF-TEST

TEST SECTION *FOUR* ANSWER SHEET—page four of four pages

298. ⓐ ⓑ ⓒ ⓓ ⓔ
299. ⓐ ⓑ ⓒ ⓓ ⓔ
300. ⓐ ⓑ ⓒ ⓓ ⓔ
301. ⓐ ⓑ ⓒ ⓓ ⓔ
302. ⓐ ⓑ ⓒ ⓓ ⓔ
303. ⓐ ⓑ ⓒ ⓓ ⓔ
304. ⓐ ⓑ ⓒ ⓓ ⓔ
305. ⓐ ⓑ ⓒ ⓓ ⓔ
306. ⓐ ⓑ ⓒ ⓓ ⓔ
307. ⓐ ⓑ ⓒ ⓓ ⓔ
308. ⓐ ⓑ ⓒ ⓓ ⓔ

309. ⓐ ⓑ ⓒ ⓓ ⓔ
310. ⓐ ⓑ ⓒ ⓓ ⓔ
311. ⓐ ⓑ ⓒ ⓓ ⓔ
312. ⓐ ⓑ ⓒ ⓓ ⓔ
313. ⓐ ⓑ ⓒ ⓓ ⓔ
314. ⓐ ⓑ ⓒ ⓓ ⓔ
315. ⓐ ⓑ ⓒ ⓓ ⓔ
316. ⓐ ⓑ ⓒ ⓓ ⓔ
317. ⓐ ⓑ ⓒ ⓓ ⓔ
318. ⓐ ⓑ ⓒ ⓓ ⓔ
319. ⓐ ⓑ ⓒ ⓓ ⓔ

320. ⓐ ⓑ ⓒ ⓓ ⓔ
321. ⓐ ⓑ ⓒ ⓓ ⓔ
322. ⓐ ⓑ ⓒ ⓓ ⓔ
323. ⓐ ⓑ ⓒ ⓓ ⓔ
324. ⓐ ⓑ ⓒ ⓓ ⓔ
325. ⓐ ⓑ ⓒ ⓓ ⓔ
326. ⓐ ⓑ ⓒ ⓓ ⓔ
327. ⓐ ⓑ ⓒ ⓓ ⓔ
328. ⓐ ⓑ ⓒ ⓓ ⓔ
329. ⓐ ⓑ ⓒ ⓓ ⓔ
330. ⓐ ⓑ ⓒ ⓓ ⓔ

1994 REVISED EMT-BASIC NATIONAL STANDARDS REVIEW SELF-TEST

TEST SECTION *FIVE* ANSWER SHEET—page one of two pages

1. ⓐ ⓑ ⓒ ⓓ ⓔ	34. ⓐ ⓑ ⓒ ⓓ ⓔ	67. ⓐ ⓑ ⓒ ⓓ ⓔ
2. ⓐ ⓑ ⓒ ⓓ ⓔ	35. ⓐ ⓑ ⓒ ⓓ ⓔ	68. ⓐ ⓑ ⓒ ⓓ ⓔ
3. ⓐ ⓑ ⓒ ⓓ ⓔ	36. ⓐ ⓑ ⓒ ⓓ ⓔ	69. ⓐ ⓑ ⓒ ⓓ ⓔ
4. ⓐ ⓑ ⓒ ⓓ ⓔ	37. ⓐ ⓑ ⓒ ⓓ ⓔ	70. ⓐ ⓑ ⓒ ⓓ ⓔ
5. ⓐ ⓑ ⓒ ⓓ ⓔ	38. ⓐ ⓑ ⓒ ⓓ ⓔ	71. ⓐ ⓑ ⓒ ⓓ ⓔ
6. ⓐ ⓑ ⓒ ⓓ ⓔ	39. ⓐ ⓑ ⓒ ⓓ ⓔ	72. ⓐ ⓑ ⓒ ⓓ ⓔ
7. ⓐ ⓑ ⓒ ⓓ ⓔ	40. ⓐ ⓑ ⓒ ⓓ ⓔ	73. ⓐ ⓑ ⓒ ⓓ ⓔ
8. ⓐ ⓑ ⓒ ⓓ ⓔ	41. ⓐ ⓑ ⓒ ⓓ ⓔ	74. ⓐ ⓑ ⓒ ⓓ ⓔ
9. ⓐ ⓑ ⓒ ⓓ ⓔ	42. ⓐ ⓑ ⓒ ⓓ ⓔ	75. ⓐ ⓑ ⓒ ⓓ ⓔ
10. ⓐ ⓑ ⓒ ⓓ ⓔ	43. ⓐ ⓑ ⓒ ⓓ ⓔ	76. ⓐ ⓑ ⓒ ⓓ ⓔ
11. ⓐ ⓑ ⓒ ⓓ ⓔ	44. ⓐ ⓑ ⓒ ⓓ ⓔ	77. ⓐ ⓑ ⓒ ⓓ ⓔ
12. ⓐ ⓑ ⓒ ⓓ ⓔ	45. ⓐ ⓑ ⓒ ⓓ ⓔ	78. ⓐ ⓑ ⓒ ⓓ ⓔ
13. ⓐ ⓑ ⓒ ⓓ ⓔ	46. ⓐ ⓑ ⓒ ⓓ ⓔ	79. ⓐ ⓑ ⓒ ⓓ ⓔ
14. ⓐ ⓑ ⓒ ⓓ ⓔ	47. ⓐ ⓑ ⓒ ⓓ ⓔ	80. ⓐ ⓑ ⓒ ⓓ ⓔ
15. ⓐ ⓑ ⓒ ⓓ ⓔ	48. ⓐ ⓑ ⓒ ⓓ ⓔ	81. ⓐ ⓑ ⓒ ⓓ ⓔ
16. ⓐ ⓑ ⓒ ⓓ ⓔ	49. ⓐ ⓑ ⓒ ⓓ ⓔ	82. ⓐ ⓑ ⓒ ⓓ ⓔ
17. ⓐ ⓑ ⓒ ⓓ ⓔ	50. ⓐ ⓑ ⓒ ⓓ ⓔ	83. ⓐ ⓑ ⓒ ⓓ ⓔ
18. ⓐ ⓑ ⓒ ⓓ ⓔ	51. ⓐ ⓑ ⓒ ⓓ ⓔ	84. ⓐ ⓑ ⓒ ⓓ ⓔ
19. ⓐ ⓑ ⓒ ⓓ ⓔ	52. ⓐ ⓑ ⓒ ⓓ ⓔ	85. ⓐ ⓑ ⓒ ⓓ ⓔ
20. ⓐ ⓑ ⓒ ⓓ ⓔ	53. ⓐ ⓑ ⓒ ⓓ ⓔ	86. ⓐ ⓑ ⓒ ⓓ ⓔ
21. ⓐ ⓑ ⓒ ⓓ ⓔ	54. ⓐ ⓑ ⓒ ⓓ ⓔ	87. ⓐ ⓑ ⓒ ⓓ ⓔ
22. ⓐ ⓑ ⓒ ⓓ ⓔ	55. ⓐ ⓑ ⓒ ⓓ ⓔ	88. ⓐ ⓑ ⓒ ⓓ ⓔ
23. ⓐ ⓑ ⓒ ⓓ ⓔ	56. ⓐ ⓑ ⓒ ⓓ ⓔ	89. ⓐ ⓑ ⓒ ⓓ ⓔ
24. ⓐ ⓑ ⓒ ⓓ ⓔ	57. ⓐ ⓑ ⓒ ⓓ ⓔ	90. ⓐ ⓑ ⓒ ⓓ ⓔ
25. ⓐ ⓑ ⓒ ⓓ ⓔ	58. ⓐ ⓑ ⓒ ⓓ ⓔ	91. ⓐ ⓑ ⓒ ⓓ ⓔ
26. ⓐ ⓑ ⓒ ⓓ ⓔ	59. ⓐ ⓑ ⓒ ⓓ ⓔ	92. ⓐ ⓑ ⓒ ⓓ ⓔ
27. ⓐ ⓑ ⓒ ⓓ ⓔ	60. ⓐ ⓑ ⓒ ⓓ ⓔ	93. ⓐ ⓑ ⓒ ⓓ ⓔ
28. ⓐ ⓑ ⓒ ⓓ ⓔ	61. ⓐ ⓑ ⓒ ⓓ ⓔ	94. ⓐ ⓑ ⓒ ⓓ ⓔ
29. ⓐ ⓑ ⓒ ⓓ ⓔ	62. ⓐ ⓑ ⓒ ⓓ ⓔ	95. ⓐ ⓑ ⓒ ⓓ ⓔ
30. ⓐ ⓑ ⓒ ⓓ ⓔ	63. ⓐ ⓑ ⓒ ⓓ ⓔ	96. ⓐ ⓑ ⓒ ⓓ ⓔ
31. ⓐ ⓑ ⓒ ⓓ ⓔ	64. ⓐ ⓑ ⓒ ⓓ ⓔ	97. ⓐ ⓑ ⓒ ⓓ ⓔ
32. ⓐ ⓑ ⓒ ⓓ ⓔ	65. ⓐ ⓑ ⓒ ⓓ ⓔ	98. ⓐ ⓑ ⓒ ⓓ ⓔ
33. ⓐ ⓑ ⓒ ⓓ ⓔ	66. ⓐ ⓑ ⓒ ⓓ ⓔ	99. ⓐ ⓑ ⓒ ⓓ ⓔ

1994 REVISED EMT-BASIC NATIONAL STANDARDS REVIEW SELF-TEST

TEST SECTION *FIVE* ANSWER SHEET—page two of two pages

100. ⓐ ⓑ ⓒ ⓓ ⓔ	114. ⓐ ⓑ ⓒ ⓓ ⓔ	128. ⓐ ⓑ ⓒ ⓓ ⓔ
101. ⓐ ⓑ ⓒ ⓓ ⓔ	115. ⓐ ⓑ ⓒ ⓓ ⓔ	129. ⓐ ⓑ ⓒ ⓓ ⓔ
102. ⓐ ⓑ ⓒ ⓓ ⓔ	116. ⓐ ⓑ ⓒ ⓓ ⓔ	130. ⓐ ⓑ ⓒ ⓓ ⓔ
103. ⓐ ⓑ ⓒ ⓓ ⓔ	117. ⓐ ⓑ ⓒ ⓓ ⓔ	131. ⓐ ⓑ ⓒ ⓓ ⓔ
104. ⓐ ⓑ ⓒ ⓓ ⓔ	118. ⓐ ⓑ ⓒ ⓓ ⓔ	132. ⓐ ⓑ ⓒ ⓓ ⓔ
105. ⓐ ⓑ ⓒ ⓓ ⓔ	119. ⓐ ⓑ ⓒ ⓓ ⓔ	133. ⓐ ⓑ ⓒ ⓓ ⓔ
106. ⓐ ⓑ ⓒ ⓓ ⓔ	120. ⓐ ⓑ ⓒ ⓓ ⓔ	134. ⓐ ⓑ ⓒ ⓓ ⓔ
107. ⓐ ⓑ ⓒ ⓓ ⓔ	121. ⓐ ⓑ ⓒ ⓓ ⓔ	136. ⓐ ⓑ ⓒ ⓓ ⓔ
108. ⓐ ⓑ ⓒ ⓓ ⓔ	122. ⓐ ⓑ ⓒ ⓓ ⓔ	137. ⓐ ⓑ ⓒ ⓓ ⓔ
109. ⓐ ⓑ ⓒ ⓓ ⓔ	123. ⓐ ⓑ ⓒ ⓓ ⓔ	138. ⓐ ⓑ ⓒ ⓓ ⓔ
110. ⓐ ⓑ ⓒ ⓓ ⓔ	124. ⓐ ⓑ ⓒ ⓓ ⓔ	139. ⓐ ⓑ ⓒ ⓓ ⓔ
111. ⓐ ⓑ ⓒ ⓓ ⓔ	125. ⓐ ⓑ ⓒ ⓓ ⓔ	140. ⓐ ⓑ ⓒ ⓓ ⓔ
112. ⓐ ⓑ ⓒ ⓓ ⓔ	126. ⓐ ⓑ ⓒ ⓓ ⓔ	141. ⓐ ⓑ ⓒ ⓓ ⓔ
113. ⓐ ⓑ ⓒ ⓓ ⓔ	127. ⓐ ⓑ ⓒ ⓓ ⓔ	142. ⓐ ⓑ ⓒ ⓓ ⓔ

1994 REVISED EMT-BASIC NATIONAL STANDARDS REVIEW SELF-TEST

TEST SECTION SIX ANSWER SHEET—page one of one page

1. ⓐ ⓑ ⓒ ⓓ ⓔ	16. ⓐ ⓑ ⓒ ⓓ ⓔ	31. ⓐ ⓑ ⓒ ⓓ ⓔ
2. ⓐ ⓑ ⓒ ⓓ ⓔ	17. ⓐ ⓑ ⓒ ⓓ ⓔ	32. ⓐ ⓑ ⓒ ⓓ ⓔ
3. ⓐ ⓑ ⓒ ⓓ ⓔ	18. ⓐ ⓑ ⓒ ⓓ ⓔ	33. ⓐ ⓑ ⓒ ⓓ ⓔ
4. ⓐ ⓑ ⓒ ⓓ ⓔ	19. ⓐ ⓑ ⓒ ⓓ ⓔ	34. ⓐ ⓑ ⓒ ⓓ ⓔ
5. ⓐ ⓑ ⓒ ⓓ ⓔ	20. ⓐ ⓑ ⓒ ⓓ ⓔ	35. ⓐ ⓑ ⓒ ⓓ ⓔ
6. ⓐ ⓑ ⓒ ⓓ ⓔ	21. ⓐ ⓑ ⓒ ⓓ ⓔ	36. ⓐ ⓑ ⓒ ⓓ ⓔ
7. ⓐ ⓑ ⓒ ⓓ ⓔ	22. ⓐ ⓑ ⓒ ⓓ ⓔ	37. ⓐ ⓑ ⓒ ⓓ ⓔ
8. ⓐ ⓑ ⓒ ⓓ ⓔ	23. ⓐ ⓑ ⓒ ⓓ ⓔ	38. ⓐ ⓑ ⓒ ⓓ ⓔ
9. ⓐ ⓑ ⓒ ⓓ ⓔ	24. ⓐ ⓑ ⓒ ⓓ ⓔ	39. ⓐ ⓑ ⓒ ⓓ ⓔ
10. ⓐ ⓑ ⓒ ⓓ ⓔ	25. ⓐ ⓑ ⓒ ⓓ ⓔ	40. ⓐ ⓑ ⓒ ⓓ ⓔ
11. ⓐ ⓑ ⓒ ⓓ ⓔ	26. ⓐ ⓑ ⓒ ⓓ ⓔ	41. ⓐ ⓑ ⓒ ⓓ ⓔ
12. ⓐ ⓑ ⓒ ⓓ ⓔ	27. ⓐ ⓑ ⓒ ⓓ ⓔ	42. ⓐ ⓑ ⓒ ⓓ ⓔ
13. ⓐ ⓑ ⓒ ⓓ ⓔ	28. ⓐ ⓑ ⓒ ⓓ ⓔ	43. ⓐ ⓑ ⓒ ⓓ ⓔ
14. ⓐ ⓑ ⓒ ⓓ ⓔ	29. ⓐ ⓑ ⓒ ⓓ ⓔ	
15. ⓐ ⓑ ⓒ ⓓ ⓔ	30. ⓐ ⓑ ⓒ ⓓ ⓔ	

1994 REVISED EMT-BASIC NATIONAL STANDARDS REVIEW SELF-TEST

TEST SECTION *SEVEN* ANSWER SHEET—page one of one page

1. ⓐ ⓑ ⓒ ⓓ ⓔ	10. ⓐ ⓑ ⓒ ⓓ ⓔ	19. ⓐ ⓑ ⓒ ⓓ ⓔ
2. ⓐ ⓑ ⓒ ⓓ ⓔ	11. ⓐ ⓑ ⓒ ⓓ ⓔ	20. ⓐ ⓑ ⓒ ⓓ ⓔ
3. ⓐ ⓑ ⓒ ⓓ ⓔ	12. ⓐ ⓑ ⓒ ⓓ ⓔ	21. ⓐ ⓑ ⓒ ⓓ ⓔ
4. ⓐ ⓑ ⓒ ⓓ ⓔ	13. ⓐ ⓑ ⓒ ⓓ ⓔ	22. ⓐ ⓑ ⓒ ⓓ ⓔ
5. ⓐ ⓑ ⓒ ⓓ ⓔ	14. ⓐ ⓑ ⓒ ⓓ ⓔ	23. ⓐ ⓑ ⓒ ⓓ ⓔ
6. ⓐ ⓑ ⓒ ⓓ ⓔ	15. ⓐ ⓑ ⓒ ⓓ ⓔ	24. ⓐ ⓑ ⓒ ⓓ ⓔ
7. ⓐ ⓑ ⓒ ⓓ ⓔ	16. ⓐ ⓑ ⓒ ⓓ ⓔ	25. ⓐ ⓑ ⓒ ⓓ ⓔ
8. ⓐ ⓑ ⓒ ⓓ ⓔ	17. ⓐ ⓑ ⓒ ⓓ ⓔ	26. ⓐ ⓑ ⓒ ⓓ ⓔ
9. ⓐ ⓑ ⓒ ⓓ ⓔ	18. ⓐ ⓑ ⓒ ⓓ ⓔ	27. ⓐ ⓑ ⓒ ⓓ ⓔ

1994 REVISED EMT-BASIC NATIONAL STANDARDS REVIEW SELF-TEST

TEST SECTION *EIGHT* ANSWER SHEET—page one of one page

1. ⓐ ⓑ ⓒ ⓓ ⓔ	27. ⓐ ⓑ ⓒ ⓓ ⓔ	53. ⓐ ⓑ ⓒ ⓓ ⓔ
2. ⓐ ⓑ ⓒ ⓓ ⓔ	28. ⓐ ⓑ ⓒ ⓓ ⓔ	54. ⓐ ⓑ ⓒ ⓓ ⓔ
3. ⓐ ⓑ ⓒ ⓓ ⓔ	29. ⓐ ⓑ ⓒ ⓓ ⓔ	55. ⓐ ⓑ ⓒ ⓓ ⓔ
4. ⓐ ⓑ ⓒ ⓓ ⓔ	30. ⓐ ⓑ ⓒ ⓓ ⓔ	56. ⓐ ⓑ ⓒ ⓓ ⓔ
5. ⓐ ⓑ ⓒ ⓓ ⓔ	31. ⓐ ⓑ ⓒ ⓓ ⓔ	57. ⓐ ⓑ ⓒ ⓓ ⓔ
6. ⓐ ⓑ ⓒ ⓓ ⓔ	32. ⓐ ⓑ ⓒ ⓓ ⓔ	58. ⓐ ⓑ ⓒ ⓓ ⓔ
7. ⓐ ⓑ ⓒ ⓓ ⓔ	33. ⓐ ⓑ ⓒ ⓓ ⓔ	59. ⓐ ⓑ ⓒ ⓓ ⓔ
8. ⓐ ⓑ ⓒ ⓓ ⓔ	34. ⓐ ⓑ ⓒ ⓓ ⓔ	60. ⓐ ⓑ ⓒ ⓓ ⓔ
9. ⓐ ⓑ ⓒ ⓓ ⓔ	35. ⓐ ⓑ ⓒ ⓓ ⓔ	61. ⓐ ⓑ ⓒ ⓓ ⓔ
10. ⓐ ⓑ ⓒ ⓓ ⓔ	36. ⓐ ⓑ ⓒ ⓓ ⓔ	62. ⓐ ⓑ ⓒ ⓓ ⓔ
11. ⓐ ⓑ ⓒ ⓓ ⓔ	37. ⓐ ⓑ ⓒ ⓓ ⓔ	63. ⓐ ⓑ ⓒ ⓓ ⓔ
12. ⓐ ⓑ ⓒ ⓓ ⓔ	38. ⓐ ⓑ ⓒ ⓓ ⓔ	64. ⓐ ⓑ ⓒ ⓓ ⓔ
13. ⓐ ⓑ ⓒ ⓓ ⓔ	39. ⓐ ⓑ ⓒ ⓓ ⓔ	65. ⓐ ⓑ ⓒ ⓓ ⓔ
14. ⓐ ⓑ ⓒ ⓓ ⓔ	40. ⓐ ⓑ ⓒ ⓓ ⓔ	66. ⓐ ⓑ ⓒ ⓓ ⓔ
15. ⓐ ⓑ ⓒ ⓓ ⓔ	41. ⓐ ⓑ ⓒ ⓓ ⓔ	67. ⓐ ⓑ ⓒ ⓓ ⓔ
16. ⓐ ⓑ ⓒ ⓓ ⓔ	42. ⓐ ⓑ ⓒ ⓓ ⓔ	68. ⓐ ⓑ ⓒ ⓓ ⓔ
17. ⓐ ⓑ ⓒ ⓓ ⓔ	43. ⓐ ⓑ ⓒ ⓓ ⓔ	69. ⓐ ⓑ ⓒ ⓓ ⓔ
18. ⓐ ⓑ ⓒ ⓓ ⓔ	44. ⓐ ⓑ ⓒ ⓓ ⓔ	70. ⓐ ⓑ ⓒ ⓓ ⓔ
19. ⓐ ⓑ ⓒ ⓓ ⓔ	45. ⓐ ⓑ ⓒ ⓓ ⓔ	71. ⓐ ⓑ ⓒ ⓓ ⓔ
20. ⓐ ⓑ ⓒ ⓓ ⓔ	46. ⓐ ⓑ ⓒ ⓓ ⓔ	72. ⓐ ⓑ ⓒ ⓓ ⓔ
21. ⓐ ⓑ ⓒ ⓓ ⓔ	47. ⓐ ⓑ ⓒ ⓓ ⓔ	73. ⓐ ⓑ ⓒ ⓓ ⓔ
22. ⓐ ⓑ ⓒ ⓓ ⓔ	48. ⓐ ⓑ ⓒ ⓓ ⓔ	74. ⓐ ⓑ ⓒ ⓓ ⓔ
23. ⓐ ⓑ ⓒ ⓓ ⓔ	49. ⓐ ⓑ ⓒ ⓓ ⓔ	75. ⓐ ⓑ ⓒ ⓓ ⓔ
24. ⓐ ⓑ ⓒ ⓓ ⓔ	50. ⓐ ⓑ ⓒ ⓓ ⓔ	76. ⓐ ⓑ ⓒ ⓓ ⓔ
25. ⓐ ⓑ ⓒ ⓓ ⓔ	51. ⓐ ⓑ ⓒ ⓓ ⓔ	77. ⓐ ⓑ ⓒ ⓓ ⓔ
26. ⓐ ⓑ ⓒ ⓓ ⓔ	52. ⓐ ⓑ ⓒ ⓓ ⓔ	78. ⓐ ⓑ ⓒ ⓓ ⓔ

1994 REVISED EMT-BASIC NATIONAL STANDARDS REVIEW SELF-TEST

TEST SECTION *NINE* ANSWER SHEET—page one of one page

(Answer sheet with questions 1–62, each with options a, b, c, d, e)

1994 Revised EMT-Basic National Standards Review Self-Test
ANSWER SECTION ONE

The page numbers following each answer indicate that subject's reference page within Brady's **Emergency Care**, 7th ed., 1994. If you do not have access to Brady's text, utilize the index of the text you do have to obtain information for review of each question's subject.

Following some answers is "g/d." This indicates that you should consult the glossary of your EMT text and/or a medical dictionary. Occasionally, some information contained in the DOT guidelines is not presented in many textbooks.

QUESTION	ANSWER	PAGE KEY	SUBJECT
1.	(e)	pages 9–12	EMT roles and responsibilities
2.	(d)	pages 9–12	EMT professional attributes
3.	(a)	pages 9–12	quality improvement
4.	(b)	pages 9–12	medical director
5.	(e)	pages 9–12	quality improvement
6.	(d)	pages 9–12	on-line medical direction
7.	(c)	pages 9–12	off-line medical direction
8.	(a)	pages 1–20	EMS stress
9.	(e)	pages 17–20	signs and symptoms of stress
10.	(b)	pages 17–20	dealing with stress
11.	(b)	pages 17–20	Critical Incident Stress Debriefing
12.	(e)	pages 17–20	stages of death and dying
13.	(b)	pages 17–20	stages of death and dying
14.	(c)	pages 17–20	stages of death and dying
15.	(c)	page 20	pathogens
16.	(e)	page 20	infectious disease transmission
17.	(a)	page 21	personal protective equipment
18.	(b)	page 22	immunizations
19.	(b)	pages 22–25	hazardous material incidents
20.	(e)	pages 22–25	hazardous rescue operations
21.	(d)	pages 22–25	violent crime scenes
22.	(d)	page 29	EMT scope of practice
23.	(d)	g/d	battery
24.	(e)	pages 30–31	expressed consent
25.	(e)	pages 30–31	implied consent
26.	(d)	pages 30–31	consent of minor children and mentally incompetent adults
27.	(a)	pages 30–31	refusal of care
28.	(a)	pages 30–31	implied consent
29.	(b)	pages 30–31	refusal of care

QUESTION	ANSWER	PAGE KEY	SUBJECT
30.	(b)	pages 30–31	protection from liability
31.	(c)	pages 31–34	Do Not Resuscitate orders
32.	(e)	pages 31–34	Do Not Resuscitate orders
33.	(e)	pages 34–35	negligence
34.	(a)	pages 34–35	abandonment
35.	(c)	pages 34–35	Good Samaritan laws
36.	(a)	pages 34–35	patient confidentiality
37.	(e)	pages 34–35	patient confidentiality exceptions
38.	(e)	page 35	medical identification devices
39.	(a)	pages 37–38	crime scenes and evidence preservation
40.	(b)	pages 37–38	mandatory report situations
41.	(a)	page 43	anatomy
42.	(b)	page 43	physiology
43.	(e)	pages 43–46	anatomical position
44.	(e)	pages 43–46	lateral
45.	(c)	pages 43–46	midline
46.	(e)	pages 43–46	lateral
47.	(a)	g/d	unilateral
48.	(b)	pages 43–46	bilateral
49.	(d)	pages 43–46, g/d	lateral rotation
50.	(b)	g/d	extension
51.	(e)	pages 43–46, g/d	medial rotation
52.	(c)	g/d	flexion
53.	(b)	pages 43–46	mid-clavicular line
54.	(c)	pages 43–46	mid-axillary line
55.	(a)	g/d	apex
56.	(d)	pages 43–46	inferior
57.	(a)	pages 43–46	superior
58.	(b)	pages 43–46	medial
59.	(e)	pages 43–46	distal
60.	(b)	pages 43–46	anterior
61.	(e)	pages 43–46	distal
62.	(d)	pages 43–46	posterior
63.	(c)	pages 43–46	anterior
64.	(e)	pages 43–46	supine
65.	(a)	pages 43–46	prone
66.	(b)	pages 43–46	lateral recumbent
67.	(c)	g/d	abduction
68.	(a)	g/d	adduction
69.	(a)	pages 43–46	dorsal
70.	(b)	pages 43–46	ventral
71.	(d)	pages 43–46	palmar
72.	(c)	pages 43–46	plantar
73.	(e)	pages 46–49	musculoskeletal system
74.	(b)	pages 46–49	skull
75.	(b)	pages 46–49	orbit
76.	(c)	pages 46–49	nasal bone
77.	(d)	pages 46–49	maxilla
78.	(e)	pages 46–49	zygoma (zygomatic bone)

TEST SECTION ONE ANSWER KEY

QUESTION	ANSWER	PAGE KEY	SUBJECT
79.	(a)	pages 46–49	mandible
80.	(e)	pages 46–49	spine
81.	(b)	pages 46–49	sacral spine (sacrum)
82.	(a)	pages 46–49	thoracic spine
83.	(d)	pages 46–49	cervical spine
84.	(e)	pages 46–49	coccyx
85.	(c)	pages 46–49	lumbar spine
86.	(c)	pages 46–49	thoracic cavity (thorax)
87.	(c)	pages 46–49	7 vertebra in the cervical spine
88.	(a)	pages 46–49	12 vertebra in the thoracic spine
89.	(d)	pages 46–49	5 vertebra in the lumbar spine
90.	(d)	pages 46–49	5 fused vertebra in the sacrum
91.	(e)	pages 46–49	4 fused vertebra in the coccyx
92.	(b)	pages 46–49	12 pairs of ribs
93.	(b)	pages 46–49	2 pairs of "floating" ribs
94.	(c)	pages 46–49	sternum
95.	(d)	pages 46–49	manubrium
96.	(a)	pages 46–49	xyphoid process
97.	(b)	pages 46–49	hip
98.	(a)	pages 46–49	ilium
99.	(c)	pages 46–49	pubis
100.	(d)	pages 46–49	acetabulum
101.	(c)	pages 46–49	femur
102.	(e)	pages 46–49	patella
103.	(a)	pages 46–49	tibia
104.	(b)	pages 46–49	fibula
105.	(a)	pages 46–49	medial malleolus
106.	(b)	pages 46–49	lateral malleolus
107.	(c)	pages 46–49	phalanges
108.	(a)	pages 46–49	tarsals and metatarsals
109.	(d)	pages 46–49	calcaneus
110.	(c)	pages 46–49	phalanges
111.	(b)	pages 46–49	carpals and metacarpals
112.	(d)	pages 46–49	clavicle
113.	(c)	pages 46–49	scapula
114.	(b)	pages 46–49	acromion
115.	(b)	pages 46–49	humerus
116.	(c)	pages 46–49	radius
117.	(a)	pages 46–49	ulna
118.	(b)	pages 46–49	ball-and-socket joint
119.	(a)	pages 46–49	hinge joint
120.	(b)	pages 46–49	voluntary muscle
121.	(a)	pages 46–49	involuntary muscle
122.	(d)	pages 46–49	cardiac muscle
123.	(c)	pages 46–49	voluntary muscle
124.	(a)	pages 46–49	involuntary muscle
125.	(b)	pages 46–49	cardiac muscle
126.	(b)	pages 50–52	the respiratory system
127.	(e)	pages 50–52	oropharynx

QUESTION	ANSWER	PAGE KEY	SUBJECT
128.	(b)	pages 50–52	nasopharynx
129.	(d)	pages 50–52	epiglottis
130.	(e)	pages 50–52	trachea
131.	(a)	pages 50–52	cricoid cartilage
132.	(b)	pages 50–52	larynx
133.	(b)	pages 50–52	right or left bronchi
134.	(c)	pages 50–52	alveoli
135.	(d)	pages 50–52	mechanics of inspiration
136.	(b)	pages 50–52	mechanics of expiration
137.	(a)	pages 50–52	active phase of respiration
138.	(b)	pages 50–52	passive phase of respiration
139.	(d)	pages 50–52	respiratory gas exchange
140.	(b)	pages 75–76	normal adult respiratory rate
141.	(e)	pages 75–76	normal infant respiratory rate
142.	(c)	pages 75–76	normal child respiratory rate
143.	(e)	pages 75–76	components of respiratory assessment
144.	(b)	pages 50–52	pediatric airway anatomy considerations
145.	(d)	pages 50–52	pediatric airway anatomy considerations
146.	(d)	pages 52–56	right-sided heart circulation
147.	(d)	pages 52–56	right atrium
148.	(e)	pages 52–56	left atrium
149.	(b)	pages 52–56	right ventricle
150.	(a)	pages 52–56	left ventricle
151.	(c)	pages 52–56	cardiac valves
152.	(a)	pages 52–56	arteries
153.	(b)	pages 52–56	veins
154.	(d)	pages 52–56	pulmonary arteries
155.	(e)	pages 52–56	pulmonary veins
156.	(c)	pages 52–56	aorta
157.	(d)	pages 52–56	superior and inferior vena cava
158.	(d)	pages 52–56	coronary arteries
159.	(c)	pages 52–56	carotid arteries
160.	(a)	pages 52–56	femoral arteries
161.	(e)	pages 52–56	brachial arteries
162.	(b)	pages 52–56	radial arteries
163.	(e)	pages 52 56	brachial artery
164.	(b)	pages 52–56	posterior tibial artery
165.	(c)	pages 52–56	dorsalis pedis artery
166.	(d)	pages 52–56	capillaries
167.	(c)	pages 52–56	arteriole
168.	(c)	pages 52–56	venule
169.	(c)	pages 52–56	erythrocytes
170.	(a)	pages 52–56	leukocytes
171.	(b)	pages 52–56	platelets
172.	(d)	pages 52–56	plasma
173.	(c)	pages 52–56	pulse formation
174.	(b)	pages 52–56	pulse palpation
175.	(a)	pages 52–56	peripheral pulses
176.	(a)	pages 52–56	central pulses
177.	(c)	pages 52–56	systolic blood pressure

TEST SECTION ONE ANSWER KEY

QUESTION	ANSWER	PAGE KEY	SUBJECT
178.	(a)	pages 52–56	diastolic blood pressure
179.	(e)	pages 56–58	the nervous system
180.	(a)	pages 56–58	central nervous system
181.	(e)	pages 56–58	peripheral nervous system
182.	(c)	pages 56–58	spinal cord
183.	(b)	pages 56–58	sensory nerves
184.	(a)	pages 56–58	motor nerves
185.	(c)	pages 56–58	autonomic nervous system
186.	(c)	pages 58–59	functions of the skin
187.	(b)	pages 58–59	epidermis
188.	(c)	pages 58–59	dermis
189.	(c)	pages 58–59	dermis
190.	(d)	pages 58–59	subcutaneous skin layer
191.	(b)	page 59	hormones
192.	(e)	pages 60–66	diaphragm
193.	(c)	pages 60–66	right upper abdominal quadrant
194.	(b)	pages 60–66	left lower abdominal quadrant
195.	(d)	pages 60–66	left upper abdominal quadrant
196.	(e)	pages 60–66	right lower abdominal quadrant
197.	(a)	page 73	vital signs
198.	(a)	pages 75–77	respiratory rate measurement
199.	(c)	g/d	tachypnea
200.	(d)	g/d	bradypnea
201.	(e)	pages 298, 326, 327	dyspnea
202.	(b)	pages 298, 326, 327	apnea
203.	(c)	pages 75–77	counting respiratory rates
204.	(a)	pages 75–77	respiratory quality assessment
205.	(d)	pages 75–77	accessory muscle use assessment
206.	(b)	pages 75–77	snoring respirations
207.	(c)	pages 75–77	wheezing
208.	(a)	pages 75–77	gurgling respirations
209.	(d)	pages 75–77	crowing
210.	(e)	pages 75–77	respiratory rhythm
211.	(c)	pages 74–75	pulse rate assessment
212.	(d)	pages 74–75	carotid pulse
213.	(a)	pages 74–75	carotid pulse assessment
214.	(a)	pages 74–75	radial pulse
215.	(c)	pages 74–75	radial pulse assessment
216.	(d)	pages 74–75	pulse quality
217.	(d)	pages 74–75	irregular pulse rate assessment
218.	(a)	pages 74–75	absent radial pulse assessment
219.	(e)	pages 74–75	absent radial pulse assessment
220.	(c)	pages 74–75	normal adult pulse rate
221.	(b)	pages 74–75	athletic adult normal pulse rate
222.	(d)	pages 74–75	normal emergency situation pulse rates
223.	(b)	pages 74–75	serious injury or illness pulse rates
224.	(c)	pages 74–75	tachycardia
225.	(d)	pages 74–75	bradycardia
226.	(e)	pages 74–75	infant and child pulse rates
227.	(a)	page 77	skin and hemodynamic perfusion

QUESTION	ANSWER	PAGE KEY	SUBJECT
228.	(e)	page 77	skin color assessment
229.	(d)	page 77	cyanotic skin color (cyanosis)
230.	(e)	page 77	indications of cyanosis
231.	(e)	page 77	jaundice
232.	(a)	page 77	indications of jaundice
233.	(a)	page 77	indications of red, "flushed" skin
234.	(e)	page 77	indications of pale skin
235.	(e)	page 77	skin color assessment
236.	(d)	page 77	hot, moist skin indications
237.	(c)	page 77	hot, dry skin indications
238.	(a)	page 77	cool, moist ("clammy") skin indications
239.	(b)	page 77	cold, dry skin indications
240.	(b)	page 78	capillary refill
241.	(d)	page 78	pupil response to light
242.	(b)	page 78	pupil response to dark
243.	(b)	page 78	pupil response to fright
244.	(d)	page 78	pupil response to stroke or head injury
245.	(a)	pages 78–81	auscultation
246.	(c)	pages 78–81	palpation
247.	(d)	pages 78–81	sphygmomanometer
248.	(b)	pages 78–81	auscultation of blood pressure
249.	(c)	pages 78–81	palpation of blood pressure
250.	(a)	pages 78–81	auscultation of blood pressure
251.	(e)	pages 78–81	palpation of blood pressure
252.	(c)	pages 78–81	systolic blood pressure
253.	(a)	pages 78–81	diastolic blood pressure
254.	(c)	pages 78–81	palpated systolic blood pressure
255.	(e)	pages 78–81	palpated blood pressure
256.	(c)	page 79, g/d	hypotension
257.	(d)	page 79, g/d	hypotension
258.	(a)	page 79, g/d	hypertension
259.	(d)	page 79, g/d	hypertension
260.	(e)	page 82	stable vital sign assessment
261.	(e)	page 82	unstable vital sign assessment
262.	(e)	pages 82–83	definition of "sign"
263.	(d)	pages 82–83	definition of "symptom"
264.	(a)	pages 82–83	"S" of SAMPLE history
265.	(b)	pages 82–83	"A" of SAMPLE history
266.	(e)	pages 82–83	"M" of SAMPLE history
267.	(d)	pages 82–83	"P" of SAMPLE history
268.	(c)	pages 82–83	"L" of SAMPLE history
269.	(c)	pages 82–83	"E" of SAMPLE history
270.	(c)	pages 89–107	lifting and moving safety
271.	(d)	pages 89–107	pushing or pulling safety
272.	(d)	pages 89–107	emergency move
273.	(e)	pages 89–107	urgent move
274.	(b)	pages 89–107	emergency moves
275.	(e)	pages 89–107	patient positioning

1994 Revised EMT-Basic National Standards Review Self-Test
ANSWER SECTION TWO

The page numbers following each answer indicate that subject's reference page within Brady's **Emergency Care**, 7th ed., 1994. If you do not have access to Brady's text, utilize the index of the text you do have to obtain information for review of each question's subject.

Following some answers is "g/d." This indicates that you should consult the glossary of your EMT text and/or a medical dictionary. Occasionally, some information contained in the DOT guidelines is not presented in many textbooks.

QUESTION	ANSWER	PAGE KEY	SUBJECT
1.	(b)	pages 50–52	the respiratory system
2.	(e)	pages 50–52	oropharynx
3.	(b)	pages 50–52	nasopharynx
4.	(d)	pages 50–52	epiglottis
5.	(e)	pages 50–52	trachea
6.	(a)	pages 50–52	cricoid cartilage
7.	(b)	pages 50–52	larynx
8.	(b)	pages 50–52	right or left bronchi
9.	(c)	pages 50–52	alveoli
10.	(d)	pages 50–52	mechanics of inspiration
11.	(b)	pages 50–52	mechanics of expiration
12.	(a)	pages 50–52	active phase of respiration
13.	(b)	pages 50–52	passive phase of respiration
14.	(d)	pages 50–52	respiratory gas exchange
15.	(b)	pages 75–76	normal adult respiratory rate
16.	(e)	pages 75–76	normal infant respiratory rate
17.	(c)	pages 75–76	normal child respiratory rate
18.	(e)	pages 75–76	components of respiratory assessment
19.	(b)	pages 50–52	pediatric airway anatomy considerations
20.	(d)	pages 50–52	pediatric airway anatomy considerations
21.	(a)	pages 75–77	respiratory rate measurement
22.	(c)	g/d	tachypnea
23.	(d)	g/d	bradypnea
24.	(e)	pages 298, 326, 327	dyspnea
25.	(b)	pages 298, 326, 327	apnea
26.	(c)	pages 75–77	respiratory rate assessment
27.	(a)	pages 75–77	respiratory quality assessment
28.	(d)	pages 75–77	accessory muscle use assessment
29.	(b)	pages 75–77	snoring respirations
30.	(c)	pages 75–77	wheezing
31.	(a)	pages 75–77	gurgling respirations
32.	(d)	pages 75–77	crowing
33.	(e)	pages 75–77	respiratory rhythm assessment

QUESTION	ANSWER	PAGE KEY	SUBJECT
34.	(d)	page 116	cyanosis
35.	(e)	page 116	cyanosis indications
36.	(b)	pages 117–120	head-tilt chin-lift airway
37.	(c)	pages 117–120	jaw-thrust maneuver airway
38.	(e)	pages 120–125	oxygen administration/pocket face mask
39.	(a)	pages 120–125	pocket face mask positioning
40.	(c)	pages 120–125	adult ventilation/pocket face mask
41.	(b)	pages 120–125	pediatric ventilation/pocket face mask
42.	(b)	pages 120–125	bag-valve-mask (BVM) components
43.	(e)	pages 120–125	BVM components
44.	(d)	pages 120–125	BVM operation
45.	(c)	pages 120–125	adult ventilation/BVM
46.	(d)	pages 120–125	pediatric ventilation/BVM
47.	(d)	pages 120–125	oxygen percentage/BVM without oxygen reservoir
48.	(a)	pages 120–125	oxygen percentage/BVM with oxygen reservoir
49.	(b)	pages 120–125	preferred methods of ventilation
50.	(e)	pages 120–125	inadequate BVM ventilation assessment—no spinal injury
51.	(e)	pages 120–125	inadequate BVM ventilation assessment—with spinal injury
52.	(c)	pages 120–125	inadequate BVM ventilation assessment
53.	(c)	pages 120–125	adult ventilation/flow-restricted, oxygen-powered ventilation device
54.	(e)	pages 120–125	pediatric ventilation/flow-restricted, oxygen-powered ventilation device
55.	(d)	pages 125–129	oropharyngeal airways
56.	(e)	pages 125–129	nasopharyngeal airways
57.	(d)	pages 125–129	oral airway measurement
58.	(b)	pages 125–129	nasal airway measurement
59.	(b)	pages 125–129	adult oral airway insertion
60.	(b)	pages 125–129	pediatric oral airway insertion
61.	(d)	pages 125–129	nasal airway insertion
62.	(b)	pages 129–133	suction indications
63.	(a)	pages 129–133	"Yankauer" (rigid) suction catheter
64.	(c)	pages 129–133	soft suction catheter
65.	(a)	pages 129–133	"Yankauer" (rigid) suction catheter
66.	(e)	pages 129–133	soft suction catheter
67.	(a)	pages 129–133	suctioning techniques
68.	(d)	pages 133–134	atmospheric oxygen
69.	(e)	pages 133–134	hypoxia
70.	(c)	pages 133–134	CPR effectiveness
71.	(c)	pages 133–134	hazards of oxygen therapy
72.	(b)	page 135	oxygen tank capacity
73.	(a)	page 135	"D" size oxygen cylinder
74.	(b)	page 135	"E" size oxygen cylinder
75.	(c)	page 135	"M" size oxygen cylinder
76.	(d)	page 135	"G" size oxygen cylinder

QUESTION	ANSWER	PAGE KEY	SUBJECT
77.	(e)	page 135	"H" size oxygen cylinder
78.	(b)	pages 139–143	nonrebreather mask
79.	(b)	pages 139–143	nonrebreather mask oxygen flow rate
80.	(b)	pages 139–143	nonrebreather mask oxygen percentage
81.	(c)	pages 50, 134, 286, 289–290	normal respiratory stimulus
82.	(b)	pages 50, 134, 286, 289–290	hypoxic drive physiology
83.	(c)	pages 50, 134, 286, 289–290	hypoxic drive physiology
84.	(a)	pages 50, 134, 286, 289–290	hypoxic drive
85.	(a)	pages 50, 134, 286, 289–290	hypoxic drive physiology and prehospital oxygen administration
86.	(a)	pages 50, 134, 286, 289–290	hypoxic drive physiology and prehospital oxygen administration
87.	(d)	pages 139–143	The DOT considers the nasal cannula to be an inadequate oxygen delivery device for prehospital emergency care.
88.	(d)	pages 139–143	nasal cannula oxygen flow rate
89.	(c)	pages 139–143	nasal cannula oxygen percentage
90.	(b)	page 143	facial injury airway management
91.	(d)	page 143	airway obstructions management
92.	(d)	page 144	pediatric airway considerations
93.	(a)	page 788	laryngectomy patient airway management

1994 Revised EMT-Basic National Standards Review Self-Test
ANSWER SECTION THREE

The page numbers following each answer indicate that subject's reference page within Brady's ***Emergency Care***, 7th ed., 1994. If you do not have access to Brady's text, utilize the index of the text you do have to obtain information for review of each question's subject.

QUESTION	ANSWER	PAGE KEY	SUBJECT
1.	(e)	pages 151–160	scene size-up
2.	(a)	pages 151–160	scene safety
3.	(c)	pages 151–160	disease causes
4.	(e)	pages 151–160	disease spreading
5.	(a)	pages 151–160	personal protective equipment
6.	(d)	pages 151–160	mechanism of injury
7.	(e)	pages 151–160	sources of patient information
8.	(c)	pages 151–160	multiple-patient situations
9.	(a)	pages 164–176	steps of initial assessment
10.	(b)	page 82	"A" of SAMPLE mnemonic
11.	(a)	page 168	"A" of AVPU mnemonic
12.	(c)	page 168	"V" of AVPU mnemonic
13.	(d)	page 82	"P" of SAMPLE mnemonic
14.	(a)	page 168	"P" of AVPU mnemonic
15.	(d)	page 168	"U" of AVPU mnemonic
16.	(c)	pages 164–176	general impression
17.	(a)	pages 164–176	initial circulation assessment
18.	(e)	pages 164–176	skin color assessment
19.	(a)	pages 164–176	skin temperature
20.	(a)	pages 164–176	capillary refill
21.	(d)	pages 164–176	conscious patient airway assessment
22.	(a)	pages 164–176	breathing assessment and oxygenation
23.	(c)	pages 164–176	initial assessment encounter of life-threat
24.	(b)	pages 164–176	patients requiring ALS or rapid transport
25.	(b)	pages 182–201	Focused History and Physical Examination of trauma patients
26.	(c)	pages 182–201	significant mechanisms of injury
27.	(b)	pages 182–201	significant mechanisms of injury
28.	(a)	pages 182–201	significant pediatric mechanisms of injury
29.	(d)	pages 182–201	seat belt use
30.	(c)	pages 182–201	airbag use
31.	(c)	pages 182–201	airbag use assessment
32.	(e)	pages 182–201	Focused History and Physical Examination of trauma patients

TEST SECTION THREE ANSWER KEY

QUESTION	ANSWER	PAGE KEY	SUBJECT
33.	(e)	pages 182–201	"D" of DCAP-BTLS mnemonic
34.	(a)	pages 182–201	"C" of DCAP-BTLS mnemonic
35.	(c)	pages 182–201	"A" of DCAP-BTLS mnemonic
36.	(b)	pages 182–201	"P" of DCAP-BTLS mnemonic
37.	(d)	pages 182–201	"B" of DCAP-BTLS mnemonic
38.	(a)	pages 182–201	"T" of DCAP-BTLS mnemonic
39.	(d)	pages 182–201	"L" of DCAP-BTLS mnemonic
40.	(b)	pages 182–201	"S" of DCAP-BTLS mnemonic
41.	(d)	pages 182–201	focused examination for crepitation
42.	(b)	pages 182–201	focused neck assessment
43.	(c)	pages 182–201	focused chest assessment
44.	(d)	pages 182–201	focused chest auscultation locations
45.	(d)	pages 182–201	focused abdominal assessment
46.	(a)	pages 182–201	focused extremity assessment
47.	(a)	pages 75–77, 200	respiratory rate vital sign
48.	(c)	pages 75–77	accurate respiratory rate assessment
49.	(a)	pages 75–77	assessment of respiratory quality
50.	(d)	page s 75–77	adult accessory muscle use assessment
51.	(c)	pages 74–75	pulse rate assessment
52.	(d)	pages 74–75	pulse quality assessment
53.	(d)	pages 74–75	irregular pulse rate assessment
54.	(c)	pages 74–75	normal adult pulse rate
55.	(b)	pages 74–75	athletic adult normal pulse rate
56.	(d)	pages 74–75	normal emergency situation pulse rates
57.	(b)	pages 74–75	serious injury or illness pulse rates
58.	(e)	pages 74–75	infant and child pulse rates
59.	(d)	pages 78–82	seriously low blood pressure
60.	(a)	pages 78–82	seriously high blood pressure
61.	(a)	page 207	"S" of SAMPLE mnemonic
62.	(e)	page 207	"M" of SAMPLE mnemonic
63.	(c)	page 207	"L" of SAMPLE mnemonic
64.	(c)	page 207	"E" of SAMPLE mnemonic
65.	(c)	page 199	colostomy
66.	(b)	page 196	crepitation (or crepitus)
67.	(d)	page 199	distention
68.	(a)	page 197	paradoxical motion or movement
69.	(b)	page 199	priapism
70.	(b)	page 207	"O" of O-P-Q-R-S-T mnemonic
71.	(d)	page 207	"P" of O-P-Q-R-S-T mnemonic
72.	(e)	page 207	"Q" of O-P-Q-R-S-T mnemonic
73.	(a)	page 207	"R" of O-P-Q-R-S-T mnemonic
74.	(a)	page 207	"S" of O-P-Q-R-S-T mnemonic
75.	(c)	page 207	"T" of O-P-Q-R-S-T mnemonic
76.	(b)	page 207	SAMPLE history
77.	(a)	pages 206–212	Focused Rapid Physical Exam of a responsive (conscious) medical patient.
78.	(b)	pages 206–212	Focused Rapid Physical Exam of an unresponsive (unconscious) medical patient

QUESTION	ANSWER	PAGE KEY	SUBJECT
79.	(e)	page 212	medical ID information devices
80.	(e)	page 213	"Vial of Life" identification stickers
81.	(e)	pages 222–227	the Detailed Physical Exam
82.	(b)	pages 222–227	scalp and cranium Detailed Physical Exam
83.	(c)	pages 222–227	Detailed Physical Exam of the ears
84.	(e)	pages 222–227	Detailed Physical Exam of the eyes
85.	(a)	pages 222–227	Detailed Physical Exam of the nose
86.	(e)	pages 222–227	Detailed Physical Exam of the mouth
87.	(b)	pages 231–237	the Ongoing Assessment
88.	(a)	page 232	trending
89.	(e)	pages 231–237	steps of the Ongoing Assessment
90.	(e)	pages 231–237	initial and repeated patient assessment
91.	(b)	page 242	base station
92.	(d)	page 242	mobile two-way radio
93.	(a)	page 242	portable radio
94.	(c)	page 242	repeater
95.	(e)	page 242	cellular telephones
96.	(a)	page 243	the Federal Communications Commission
97.	(e)	pages 243–246	medical direction communication
98.	(b)	pages 243–246	radio transmission content
99.	(d)	pages 243–246	EMT/physician radio communications
100.	(c)	pages 243–246	radio communication principles
101.	(b)	pages 243–246	radio communication principles
102.	(b)	pages 243–246	radio communication principles
103.	(a)	pages 243–246	radio communication principles
104.	(a)	pages 243–246	order of radioed patient medical report
105.	(c)	pages 243–246	repeat radio contact reports
106.	(c)	pages 243–246	ambulance dispatch notification
107.	(d)	pages 243–246	reporting to emergency department staff
108.	(e)	pages 246–248	interpersonal patient communications
109.	(b)	pages 246–248	interpersonal patient communications
110.	(c)	pages 251–262	written prehospital care report
111.	(c)	pages 251–262	written prehospital care report
112.	(b)	pages 251–262	objective information
113.	(c)	pages 251–262	subjective information
114.	(c)	pages 251–262	subjective information
115.	(d)	pages 251–262	pertinent negative information
116.	(b)	pages 251–262	objective information
117.	(a)	pages 251–262	narrative section of prehospital documents
118.	(a)	pages 251–262	written prehospital documentation
119.	(c)	pages 251–262	use of medical abbreviations
120.	(d)	pages 251–262	written prehospital documentation
121.	(d)	pages 251–262	written prehospital documentation
122.	(d)	pages 251–262	errors of omission
123.	(c)	pages 251–262	errors of commission
124.	(c)	pages 251–262	charting errors of omission or commission
125.	(e)	pages 251–262	falsification of information implications
126.	(e)	pages 251–262	patient refusal procedure

TEST SECTION THREE ANSWER KEY

QUESTION	ANSWER	PAGE KEY	SUBJECT
127.	(e)	pages 251–262	patient refusal procedure
128.	(a)	pages 251–262	error correction of written reports
129.	(d)	pages 251–262	error correction of written reports
130.	(a)	pages 251–262	multiple casualty incident reporting

The following 59 questions are an elective group of Medical Abbreviations and Symbols Questions. These symbols and abbreviations do not necessarily represent DOT-required knowledge for the EMT-Basic.* Page numbers keyed to Brady's **Emergency Care**, 7th ed., are not provided for these questions. Instead, refer to the Common Medical Abbreviations and Symbols available in the appendix to this text (pages 383 through 387).

QUESTION	ANSWER	SUBJECT
131.	(a)	before ($\bar{a}$)
132.	(e)	without ($\bar{s}$)
133.	(d)	with ($\bar{c}$)
134.	(b)	after ($\bar{p}$)
135.	(c)	every ($\bar{q}$)
136.	(c)	abdomen or abdominal (abd)
137.	(e)	acute myocardial infarction (AMI)
138.	(b)	"two times a day," bid or b.i.d. (from the Latin **bis in die**)
139.	(a)	"every day," qd or q.d. (from the Latin **quaque die**)
140.	(d)	"four times a day," qid or q.i.d. (from the Latin **quarter in die**)
141.	(c)	"at bedtime," hs or h.s. (from the Latin **hora somni**)
142.	(e)	"three times a day," tid or t.i.d. (from the Latin **ter in die**)
143.	(d)	breath sounds or blood sugar (BS)
144.	(a)	bowel movement (BM)
145.	(b)	bag-valve-mask (BVM)
146.	(d)	cancer (CA)
147.	(e)	congestive heart failure (CHF)
148.	(e)	closed head injury (CHI)
149.	(c)	central nervous system (CNS)
150.	(c)	chronic obstructive pulmonary disease (COPD)
151.	(b)	cerebrovascular accident (CVA)
152.	(b)	gastrointestinal (GI)
153.	(d)	gunshot wound (GSW)
154.	(a)	genitourinary (GU)
155.	(d)	headache (HA)
156.	(c)	history (Hx)
157.	(b)	jugular vein distention (JVD)
158.	(a)	long backboard (LBB)
159.	(e)	left lower (abdominal) quadrant (LLQ)
160.	(a)	last menstrual period (LMP)
161.	(b)	liters per minute (lpm)
162.	(d)	left upper (abdominal) quadrant (LUQ)
163.	(a)	level of consciousness (LOC)
164.	(c)	nasal cannula (nc)

* All DOT-required medical terminology will be presented in appropriate test sections of this text. The DOT does not list specific, "standard" medical abbreviations or symbols.

165.	(e)	nonrebreather mask (NRB)
166.	(b)	nitroglycerine (NTG)
167.	(c)	nausea and vomiting (n/v)
168.	(e)	nausea, vomiting, and diarrhea (n/v/d)
169.	(a)	pulmonary embolism (PE)
170.	(d)	pelvic inflammatory disease (PID)
171.	(c)	peripheral nervous system (PNS)
172.	(e)	prior to our arrival (PTOA)
173.	(a)	rule out (R/O)
174.	(b)	right lower (abdominal) quadrant (RLQ)
175.	(e)	right upper (abdominal) quadrant (RUQ)
176.	(a)	shortness of breath (SOB)
177.	(c)	transient ischemic attack (TIA)
178.	(b)	upper respiratory infection (URI)
179.	(c)	urinary tract infection (UTI)
180.	(e)	within normal limits (WNL)
181.	(d)	years old (y/o)
182.	(c)	approximately (∿∿)
183.	(a)	change (△)
184.	(b)	greater than (>)
185.	(a)	less than (<)
186.	(c)	female symbol (♀)
187.	(b)	male symbol (♂)
188.	(c)	above or increased (↑)
189.	(d)	below or decreased (↓)

1994 Revised EMT-Basic National Standards Review Self-Test
ANSWER SECTION FOUR

The page numbers following each answer indicate that subject's reference page within Brady's ***Emergency Care***, 7th ed., 1994. If you do not have access to Brady's text, utilize the index of the text you do have to obtain information for review of each question's subject.

Following some answers is "g/d." This indicates that you should consult the glossary of your EMT text and/or a medical dictionary. Occasionally, some information contained in the DOT guidelines is not presented in many textbooks.

QUESTION	ANSWER	PAGE KEY	SUBJECT
1.	(c)	page 271	pharmacology
2.	(d)	page 271	EMT-B medication administration
3.	(d)	page 271	EMT-B assist with patient's medications
4.	(a)	page 274	generic drug names
5.	(c)	page 274	trade, proprietary, or brand drug names
6.	(d)	page 274	drug indications
7.	(a)	page 274	drug contraindications
8.	(c)	page 274	drug side effects
9.	(c)	page 274	suspension medication forms
10.	(d)	page 274	sublingual spray, compressed powder, or tablet medication forms
11.	(b)	page 274	injectable liquid medication forms
12.	(a)	page 274	gel medication forms
13.	(c)	page 274	gas medication forms
14.	(e)	page 274	a metered dose of fine powder for inhalation medication forms
15.	(e)	page 274	sublingual medication administration
16.	(b)	page 283	signs of adequate artificial ventilation
17.	(e)	pages 281–282	signs of difficulty breathing
18.	(a)	pages 281–282	signs of difficulty breathing
19.	(b)	page 284	the tripod position for difficulty breathing
20.	(b)	page 284	barrel chest appearance
21.	(e)	page 284	stridor
22.	(b)	page 284	audible wheezing
23.	(c)	pages 286–288	treatment of the dyspneic patient without a prescribed inhaler
24.	(c)	pages 286–288	treatment of the dyspneic patient who has a prescribed inhaler
25.	(b)	page 288	generic inhaler names
26.	(e)	page 288	trade names for inhalers

QUESTION	ANSWER	PAGE KEY	SUBJECT
27.	(e)	pages 286–288	criteria for assisted inhaler administration
28.	(d)	pages 286–288	contraindications for assisted inhaler administration
29.	(d)	pages 286–288	inhaler dosage
30.	(c)	pages 286–288	assisted inhaler administration
31.	(a)	pages 286–288	assisted inhaler administration steps
32.	(c)	page 288	a spacer device
33.	(d)	page 286	bronchoconstriction
34.	(a)	page 286	bronchodilation
35.	(b)	pages 286–288	beta agonist bronchodilator medications
36.	(e)	pages 286–288	side effects of inhaler medications
37.	(e)	pages 286–288	care after assisted medication inhalation
38.	(d)	pages 289–290	chronic obstructive pulmonary disease (COPD)
39.	(c)	pages 289–290	asthma
40.	(c)	pages 289–290	blood oxygen level is the normal body breathing stimulus
41.	(b)	pages 289–290	chronically increased carbon dioxide levels in COPD patients
42.	(b)	pages 289–290	blood carbon dioxide level is the normal breathing stimulus in COPD patients
43.	(a)	pages 289–290	hypoxic drive
44.	(a)	pages 289–290	COPD once considered a contraindication to high-flow oxygen administration
45.	(a)	pages 289–290	COPD no longer a contraindication to high-flow oxygen administration
46.	(c)	pages 289–290	asthma
47.	(d)	pages 289–290	Pediatric cases of emphysema and chronic bronchitis are rare.
48.	(b)	pages 289–290	chronic bronchitis
49.	(a)	pages 289–290	emphysema
50.	(d)	pages 289–290	COPD
51.	(c)	pages 289–290	asthma
52.	(e)	pages 289–290	Specific respiratory disease diagnosis is unnecessary to prehospital care.
53.	(d)	pages 52–55	blood flow through the heart
54.	(c)	pages 52–55	blood flow through the heart
55.	(a)	pages 52–55	blood flow through the heart
56.	(b)	pages 52–55	blood flow through the heart
57.	(e)	pages 52–55	cardiac valves
58.	(e)	pages 52–55	the cardiac conductive system
59.	(c)	page 308	ACLS (advanced cardiac life support)
60.	(e)	page 300	CHF (congestive heart failure)
61.	(b)	page 298	CAD (coronary artery disease)
62.	(d)	page 324	atherosclerosis
63.	(a)	page 325	arteriosclerosis
64.	(c)	page 325	aneurysm
65.	(e)	page 325	thrombus
66.	(c)	page 325	embolism
67.	(a)	page 325	occlusion

TEST SECTION FOUR ANSWER KEY

QUESTION	ANSWER	PAGE KEY	SUBJECT
68.	(e)	pages 297–298	cardiac compromise
69.	(e)	pages 297–298	cardiac compromise signs and symptoms
70.	(e)	pages 297–298	cardiac compromise signs and symptoms
71.	(d)	pages 297–298	cardiac compromise signs and symptoms
72.	(c)	page 299	angina pectoris (pain in the chest)
73.	(e)	page 299	causes of angina
74.	(d)	page 299	angina
75.	(d)	page 299	nitroglycerin effects
76.	(d)	page 299	nitroglycerin forms of administration
77.	(e)	pages 299–300	causes of AMI (acute myocardial infarction)
78.	(e)	page 300	sudden death
79.	(e)	page 300	causes of cardiac arrest
80.	(c)	page 300	thrombolytic medications
81.	(c)	pages 300, 326	edema
82.	(b)	page 326	pedal edema
83.	(c)	page 326	ascites
84.	(a)	page 326	pulmonary edema
85.	(e)	page 326	edema and congestive heart failure (CHF)
86.	(a)	page 326	causes of CHF
87.	(c)	page 326	diuretic
88.	(b)	page 301	cardiac compromise position of comfort
89.	(c)	page 301	cardiac compromise and oxygenation
90.	(b)	pages 301–304	nitroglycerin administration indications
91.	(e)	pages 301–304	nitroglycerin contraindications
92.	(d)	pages 301–304	nitroglycerin re administration
93.	(d)	page 304	nitroglycerin side effects
94.	(a)	page 304	blood pressure check after nitroglycerin
95.	(a)	pages 306–308	cardiac arrest survival factors
96.	(a)	pages 308–324	automated external defibrillator (AED) facts and operation
97.	(d)	pages 308–324	AED facts and operation
98.	(d)	pages 308–324	AED facts and operation
99.	(d)	pages 308–324	AED facts and operation
100.	(c)	pages 308–324	AED facts and operation
101.	(a)	pages 308–324	AED facts and operation
102.	(e)	pages 308–324	AED facts and operation
103.	(b)	pages 308–324	AED facts and operation
104.	(b)	page 310	ventricular fibrillation
105.	(c)	page 310	asystole
106.	(a)	page 310	ventricular tachycardia
107.	(b)	page 310	ventricular fibrillation
108.	(c)	page 310	asystole
109.	(a)	page 310	ventricular tachycardia
110.	(c)	page 310	pulseless electrical activity (PEA)
111.	(b)	page 310	ventricular fibrillation
112.	(a)	page 310	ventricular tachycardia
113.	(e)	pages 308–324	indications for AED application
114.	(e)	pages 308–324	AED operation
115.	(b)	pages 308–324	AED operation

QUESTION	ANSWER	PAGE KEY	SUBJECT
116.	(e)	pages 308–324	transport after AED, without ALS
117.	(e)	pages 308–324	AED operation with only 2 responders
118.	(d)	pages 308–324	AED contraindications
119.	(b)	pages 308–324	AED voice recorders
120.	(c)	pages 308–324	AED voice recorder use
121.	(b)	pages 308–324	AED white cable pad
122.	(a)	pages 308–324	AED red cable pad
123.	(e)	pages 308–324	AEDs have only two cables/pads.
124.	(c)	pages 308–324	AED cable/pad placement phrase
125.	(a)	pages 308–324	AED operation steps
126.	(b)	pages 308–324	AED operation steps
127.	(d)	pages 308–324	AED operation steps
128.	(c)	pages 308–324	AED joules of energy, third shock
129.	(b)	pages 308–324	AED joules of energy, second shock
130.	(a)	pages 308–324	AED joules of energy, first shock
131.	(c)	pages 308–324	AED operation steps
132.	(c)	pages 308–324	AED use and ALS coordination
133.	(a)	pages 308–324	AED safety
134.	(e)	pages 308–324	AED use and patients with pacemakers
135.	(e)	pages 308–324	AED use and patients with automatic implantable cardioverter defibrillators (AICDs)
136.	(b)	page 332	hypoglycemia
137.	(a)	page 339	hyperglycemia
138.	(c)	page 337	idiopathic
139.	(b)	pages 332, 339	rapid onset of altered levels of consciousness
140.	(a)	pages 332, 339	diabetes
141.	(b)	pages 332, 339	diabetes pathophysiology
142.	(d)	page 332	hypoglycemia
143.	(d)	page 332	hypoglycemia-inducing situations
144.	(c)	page 332	hypoglycemia signs and symptoms
145.	(e)	page 332	likelihood of hypoglycemia
146.	(a)	page 333	medications prescribed for hypoglycemia
147.	(a)	page 333	insulin, location of storage
148.	(e)	pages 333–336	administration of oral glucose
149.	(c)	pages 333–336	administration of oral glucose
150.	(a)	pages 333–336	actions of oral glucose
151.	(d)	page 339	hyperglycemia
152.	(a)	page 337	seizures
153.	(d)	page 337	causes of seizures
154.	(c)	page 337	causes of seizures
155.	(a)	page 337	idiopathic seizures
156.	(d)	page 337	most common cause for adult seizures
157.	(b)	page 337	most common cause for pediatric seizures
158.	(b)	page 337	epilepsy
159.	(b)	page 338	treatment of a seizure patient
160.	(d)	page 338	treatment of a seizure patient
161.	(b)	page 338	status epilepticus
162.	(e)	page 340	aura
163.	(d)	pages 340–341	partial seizures

TEST SECTION FOUR ANSWER KEY

QUESTION	ANSWER	PAGE KEY	SUBJECT
164.	(e)	pages 340–341	generalized seizures
165.	(b)	page 341	cerebral-vascular accident (CVA)
166.	(e)	page 341	causes of CVA
167.	(e)	page 341	signs and symptoms of CVA
168.	(c)	page 341	signs and symptoms of CVA
169.	(c)	page 346	allergen
170.	(a)	page 346	allergic reaction
171.	(b)	page 346	anaphylaxis or anaphylactic shock
172.	(d)	page 352	epinephrine
173.	(a)	pages 346–348	allergic or anaphylactic reaction causes
174.	(a)	g/d	erythema
175.	(d)	page 348, g/d	urticaria or "hives"
176.	(e)	pages 346–348	allergic reactions or anaphylactic shock
177.	(c)	pages 349–353	assisted prescribed medication administration for anaphylaxis
178.	(e)	page 348	anaphylaxis skin signs and symptoms
179.	(c)	page 348	anaphylaxis respiratory signs and symptoms
180.	(d)	page 348	anaphylaxis cardiac signs and symptoms
181.	(a)	page 348	general anaphylaxis signs and symptoms
182.	(b)	pages 348–349	allergic reaction/anaphylaxis interview
183.	(d)	pages 348–349	allergic reaction/anaphylaxis oxygenation
184.	(e)	pages 349–353	assisted epinephrine injection indications
185.	(b)	pages 349–353	assisted epinephrine injection indications
186.	(a)	pages 349–353	assisted epinephrine injection indications
187.	(c)	pages 349–353	repeated assisted epinephrine injections
188.	(c)	page 353	pediatric assisted epinephrine injections
189.	(c)	pages 352–353	location of assisted epinephrine injections
190.	(b)	pages 352–353	side effects of epinephrine injections
191.	(e)	pages 352–353	repeated assisted epinephrine injections
192.	(c)	pages 361–362	poisoning or overdose interview
193.	(c)	page 364	activated charcoal names
194.	(e)	pages 362–365	activated charcoal contraindications
195.	(b)	pages 362–365	activated charcoal medication form
196.	(b)	pages 362–365	activated charcoal adult dose
197.	(c)	pages 362–365	activated charcoal pediatric dose
198.	(c)	pages 362–365	activated charcoal administration
199.	(d)	pages 362–365	activated charcoal actions
200.	(e)	pages 362–365	activated charcoal side effects
201.	(c)	pages 362–365	activated charcoal contraindications
202.	(a)	page 384	hypothermia
203.	(c)	page 391	hyperthermia
204.	(a)	pages 383–384	heat loss by radiation
205.	(d)	pages 383–384	heat loss by evaporation
206.	(e)	pages 383–384	heat loss by breathing (respiration)
207.	(c)	pages 383–384	heat loss by conduction
208.	(b)	pages 383–384	heat loss by convection
209.	(c)	g/d	normal body temperature
210.	(c)	g/d	normal body temperature
211.	(b)	page 384	hypothermia risk factors

QUESTION	ANSWER	PAGE KEY	SUBJECT
212.	(a)	pages 384–385	hypothermia risk factors
213.	(b)	pages 384–385	hypothermia pediatric risk factors
214.	(e)	pages 384–385	hypothermia risk factors
215.	(e)	pages 384–385	hypothermia risk factors
216.	(e)	pages 384–385	hypothermia risk factors
217.	(e)	pages 384–385	hypothermia risk factors
218.	(d)	page 386	skin temperature assessment
219.	(c)	page 386	hypothermia signs and symptoms
220.	(e)	page 386	hypothermia signs and symptoms
221.	(d)	pages 386–387	treatment of hypothermia
222.	(a)	page 387	severe hypothermia pulse assessment
223.	(c)	pages 386–387	passive rewarming techniques
224.	(e)	pages 386–387	active rewarming techniques
225.	(a)	pages 386–387	active rewarming techniques
226.	(e)	pages 386–387	passive rewarming techniques
227.	(b)	page 388	early/superficial local cold injuries
228.	(a)	page 388	late/deep local cold injuries
229.	(c)	page 388	early/superficial local cold injuries signs and symptoms
230.	(a)	page 388	late/deep local cold injuries signs and symptoms
231.	(e)	pages 388–390	treatment (tx) of local cold injuries
232.	(e)	pages 388–390	tx of early/superficial local cold injuries
233.	(a)	pages 388–390	tx of late/deep local cold injuries
234.	(b)	pages 388–390	active, rapid rewarming
235.	(c)	pages 388–390	active, rapid rewarming
236.	(c)	pages 391–392	heat injuries and the elderly
237.	(d)	pages 391–392	heat injuries
238.	(b)	pages 391–392	heat injuries and infants/children
239.	(b)	pages 391–392	heat cramps or "moist, pale, normal to cool skin temperature"
240.	(b)	pages 391–392	heat exhaustion or "moist, pale, normal to cool skin temperature"
241.	(c)	pages 391–392	heat stroke or "hot, dry or moist skin"
242.	(d)	pages 391–392	heat exhaustion or "moist, pale, normal to cool skin temperature"
243.	(b)	pages 391–392	heat stroke or "hot, dry or moist skin"
244.	(e)	pages 391–392	heat exhaustion or "moist, pale, normal to cool skin temperature"
245.	(a)	pages 391–392	heat stroke or "hot, dry or moist skin"
246.	(e)	pages 393–397	near-drowning
247.	(e)	pages 393–397	drowning and near-drowning
248.	(e)	pages 393–397	treatment of drowning and near-drowning
249.	(d)	pages 393–397	drowning and near-drowning
250.	(c)	pages 393–397	treatment of drowning and near-drowning
251.	(b)	pages 393–397	drowning and near-drowning
252.	(e)	pages 397–401	bites and stings
253.	(c)	pages 397–401	insect stinger care
254.	(a)	pages 397–401	treatment of bites and stings

QUESTION	ANSWER	PAGE KEY	SUBJECT
255.	(e)	pages 409–416	behavioral emergencies
256.	(b)	pages 409–416	nonpsychiatric abnormal behavior
257.	(a)	pages 409–416	behavioral emergencies
258.	(c)	pages 409–416	risk factors for suicide
259.	(c)	pages 409–416	behavioral emergency safety
260.	(a)	pages 409–416	behavioral emergency medico-legal considerations
261.	(c)	pages 409–416	use of force
262.	(b)	pages 409–416	calming the behavioral emergency patient
263.	(c)	pages 409–416	calming the behavioral emergency patient
264.	(c)	pages 409–416	patient restraint
265.	(d)	pages 409–416	patient communication
266.	(b)	page 422	fetus
267.	(e)	page 422	uterus
268.	(a)	page 422	the birth canal
269.	(c)	page 422	placenta
270.	(d)	page 422	umbilical cord
271.	(a)	page 422	amniotic sac ("bag of waters")
272.	(e)	page 422	vagina
273.	(b)	page 434	perineum
274.	(d)	page 423	crowning
275.	(b)	page 423	beginning of labor
276.	(c)	page 423	end of labor
277.	(c)	pages 423–430	presenting part
278.	(b)	pages 423–430	crowning
279.	(d)	pages 423–430	bloody show
280.	(d)	pages 439–440	miscarriage
281.	(e)	pages 439–440	abortion
282.	(d)	pages 439–440	miscarriage
283.	(e)	page 439	seizures in pregnancy
284.	(a)	page 439	seizures in pregnancy
285.	(e)	pages 438–442	vaginal bleeding
286.	(d)	pages 438–442	vaginal bleeding
287.	(c)	pages 438–442	trauma and pregnancy
288.	(b)	page 424	contraction frequency
289.	(a)	pages 423–426	signs, symptoms, and patient history factors not related to assessing the likelihood of imminent delivery
290.	(c)	pages 423–426	signs, symptoms, and patient history factors indicating imminent delivery is not likely
291.	(b)	pages 423–426	signs, symptoms, and patient history factors indicating imminent delivery is highly likely
292.	(e)	pages 426–430	assisted delivery on scene
293.	(d)	pages 426–430	prevention of explosive delivery
294.	(c)	pages 426–430	breaking the amniotic sac
295.	(a)	pages 426–430	an umbilical cord around the infant's neck
296.	(c)	pages 426–430	infant suctioning

QUESTION	ANSWER	PAGE KEY	SUBJECT
297.	(d)	pages 430–435	care upon infant delivery
298.	(d)	pages 430–435	clamping the umbilical cord
299.	(b)	pages 430–435	cutting the umbilical cord
300.	(d)	pages 430–435	bleeding from the umbilical cord
301.	(b)	pages 433–434	delivery of the placenta
302.	(a)	pages 433–434	care of the placenta
303.	(a)	pages 433–434	maternal care after delivery
304.	(b)	pages 433–434	postdelivery vaginal bleeding
305.	(d)	pages 430–433	initial care of the newborn
306.	(b)	pages 430–433	the inverted pyramid of newborn resuscitation
307.	(d)	pages 430–433	time factor of spontaneous breathing in a newborn (within 30 seconds after birth)
308.	(d)	pages 430–433	newborn respiratory rates
309.	(c)	pages 430–433	newborn ventilatory rate
310.	(a)	pages 430–433	reassessment of newborn respirations
311.	(c)	pages 430–433	newborn heart rate (bradycardia)
312.	(d)	pages 430–433	care for newborn bradycardia
313.	(e)	pages 430–433	cyanotic limbs in a newborn
314.	(e)	pages 430–433	central cyanosis in a newborn
315.	(c)	pages 435–439	prolapsed cord presentation
316.	(b)	pages 435–439	treatment of a prolapsed cord presentation
317.	(c)	pages 435–439	breech birth presentation
318.	(d)	pages 435–439	limb presentation
319.	(b)	pages 435–439	multiple births
320.	(c)	pages 435–439	meconium
321.	(e)	pages 435–439	premature newborns
322.	(e)	page 442	sexual assault

The following 8 questions are an elective group of questions about gynecological and/or obstetrical conditions, emergencies, and/or medical terminology.

QUESTION	ANSWER	PAGE KEY	SUBJECT
323.	(e)	page 442	stillborn infant
324.	(b)	pages 438–439	placenta previa
325.	(a)	pages 438–439	abruptio placentae
326.	(a)	pages 439–442	trauma and pregnancy
327.	(e)	page 426	supine hypotensive syndrome signs and symptoms
328.	(a)	page 426	supine hypotensive syndrome transport position
329.	(b)	page 426	supine hypotensive syndrome
330.	(c)	page 443	cephalic presentation

1994 Revised EMT-Basic National Standards Review Self-Test
ANSWER SECTION FIVE

The page numbers following each answer indicate that subject's reference page within Brady's **Emergency Care**, 7th ed., 1994. If you do not have access to Brady's text, utilize the index of the text you do have to obtain information for review of each question's subject.

QUESTION	ANSWER	PAGE KEY	SUBJECT
1.	(d)	pages 52–56	right-sided heart circulation
2.	(d)	pages 52–56	right atrium
3.	(e)	pages 52–56	left atrium
4.	(b)	pages 52–56	right ventricle
5.	(a)	pages 52–56	left ventricle
6.	(c)	pages 52–56	cardiac valves
7.	(a)	pages 52–56, 449	arteries
8.	(b)	pages 52–56, 450	veins
9.	(d)	pages 52–56	pulmonary arteries
10.	(e)	pages 52–56	pulmonary veins
11.	(c)	pages 52–56	aorta
12.	(d)	pages 52–56	superior and inferior vena cava
13.	(d)	pages 52–56	coronary arteries
14.	(c)	pages 52–56	carotid arteries
15.	(a)	pages 52–56	femoral arteries
16.	(e)	pages 52–56	brachial arteries
17.	(b)	pages 52–56	radial arteries
18.	(e)	pages 52–56	brachial artery
19.	(b)	pages 52–56	posterior tibial artery
20.	(c)	pages 52–56	dorsalis pedis artery
21.	(d)	pages 52–56, 450	capillaries
22.	(c)	pages 52–56	arteriole
23.	(c)	pages 52–56	venule
24.	(c)	pages 52–56	erythrocytes
25.	(a)	pages 52–56	leukocytes
26.	(b)	pages 52–56	platelets
27.	(d)	pages 52–56	plasma
28.	(c)	pages 52–56	pulse formation
29.	(b)	pages 52–56	pulse palpation
30.	(a)	pages 52–56	peripheral pulses
31.	(a)	pages 52–56	central pulses
32.	(e)	page 450	perfusion
33.	(b)	page 450	hemorrhage
34.	(c)	pages 450–451	arterial bleeding
35.	(d)	pages 450–451	capillary and venous bleeding

QUESTION	ANSWER	PAGE KEY	SUBJECT
36.	(c)	pages 450–451	arterial bleeding
37.	(b)	pages 450–451	venous bleeding
38.	(a)	pages 450–451	capillary bleeding
39.	(c)	pages 450–451	arterial bleeding
40.	(b)	pages 450–451	venous bleeding
41.	(c)	page 451	serious blood loss from the adult
42.	(c)	page 451	serious blood loss from the child
43.	(b)	page 451	serious blood loss from the infant
44.	(a)	pages 451–452	blood loss severity determination
45.	(b)	page 451	hypoperfusion
46.	(c)	pages 451–459	bleeding control methods
47.	(a)	pages 451–459	pressure points
48.	(e)	pages 451–459	tourniquet use
49.	(c)	pages 451–459	tourniquet use
50.	(a)	page 459	nose bleeding
51.	(b)	page 459	epistaxis
52.	(d)	page 459	bleeding from the ears or nose
53.	(a)	page 459	nosebleed care
54.	(c)	pages 459–460	internal bleeding
55.	(e)	pages 459–460	internal bleeding mechanism of injury
56.	(b)	pages 459–460	internal bleeding signs and symptoms
57.	(c)	pages 460–463	hypovolemic signs and symptoms
58.	(d)	pages 460–463	late signs and symptoms of shock
59.	(a)	pages 460–463	early signs and symptoms of shock
60.	(c)	pages 460–463	late signs and symptoms of shock
61.	(b)	pages 460–463	hypoperfusion syndrome
62.	(e)	pages 460–463	hypovolemic or hemorrhagic shock
63.	(e)	pages 460–463	cause of shock
64.	(d)	pages 460–463	infants and children in shock
65.	(e)	pages 463–465	emergency medical treatment of shock
66.	(c)	pages 472–473	functions of the skin
67.	(b)	pages 472–473	epidermis
68.	(c)	pages 472–473	dermis
69.	(c)	pages 472–473	dermis
70.	(d)	pages 472–473	subcutaneous skin layer
71.	(a)	pages 473–477	closed injuries
72.	(c)	pages 473–477	crush injuries
73.	(b)	pages 473–477	open injuries
74.	(b)	pages 473–477	open injuries
75.	(b)	pages 473–477	open injuries
76.	(d)	pages 473–477	hematoma
77.	(c)	pages 473–477	contusion
78.	(e)	pages 473–477	laceration
79.	(a)	pages 473–477	abrasion
80.	(b)	pages 473–477	avulsion
81.	(b)	pages 473–477	avulsion
82.	(c)	pages 485–488	treatment of open chest injuries
83.	(b)	pages 488–491, 507	treatment of open abdominal injuries

TEST SECTION FIVE ANSWER KEY

QUESTION	ANSWER	PAGE KEY	SUBJECT
84.	(d)	page 501	occlusive dressing
85.	(b)	pages 488–491	evisceration
86.	(a)	pages 488–491	treatment of evisceration
87.	(c)	pages 479–481	impaled object treatment
88.	(e)	pages 481–483	treatment of avulsions
89.	(a)	pages 481–483	treatment of full avulsions or amputations
90.	(d)	page 483	treatment of large, open neck wounds
91.	(a)	page 492	first degree or superficial burn
92.	(c)	page 492	third degree or full thickness burn
93.	(d)	page 492	burn skin color
94.	(b)	page 492	second degree or partial thickness burn
95.	(d)	page 492	burns and pain
96.	(c)	page 492	full thickness burn, loss of sensation
97.	(e)	page 494	Palmar Surface (Rule of Palm) method of measuring amount of burned surface area
98.	(c)	page 494	Rule of Nines, adult burn patient
99.	(e)	page 494	Rule of Nines, adult burn patient
100.	(b)	page 494	Rule of Nines, pediatric burn patient
101.	(a)	page 494	Rule of Nines, pediatric burn patient
102.	(d)	pages 492–495	critical burns
103.	(a)	pages 492–495	critical burns
104.	(d)	pages 492–494	circumferential burns
105.	(c)	pages 493–496	thermal burn treatment steps
106.	(b)	pages 493–496	thermal burn treatment
107.	(d)	pages 496–497	chemical burn treatment
108.	(a)	pages 497–499	electrical burn treatment
109.	(b)	page 499	dressings
110.	(a)	page 499	bandages
111.	(c)	pages 502–504	open wound care
112.	(c)	pages 516–518	mechanism of injury for bone damage
113.	(c)	pages 516–518	bone injury diagnosis
114.	(b)	pages 478, 519	emergency care of bone or joint injuries
115.	(c)	pages 519–522	general rules of splinting
116.	(e)	pages 518–522	improper splinting
117.	(a)	pages 522–527	traction splinting
118.	(d)	pages 522–527	traction splinting
119.	(a)	pages 566–567	mechanism of injury to the spine
120.	(c)	pages 566–567	mechanism of injury to the spine
121.	(e)	pages 566–569	spinal injury assessment
122.	(a)	pages 562–565	head (scalp, skull, and brain) injuries

The following 20 questions are an elective group of questions about traumatic conditions, emergencies, and/or medical terminology.

QUESTION	ANSWER	PAGE KEY	SUBJECT
123.	(b)	page 465	functions of blood
124.	(c)	pages 465–466	cardiogenic shock
125.	(b)	pages 465–466	septic shock

QUESTION	ANSWER	PAGE KEY	SUBJECT
126.	(a)	pages 465–466	systemic infections/septic shock
127.	(a)	pages 465–466	anaphylactic shock
128.	(d)	pages 465–466	neurogenic shock
129.	(d)	pages 465–466	neurogenic shock
130.	(b)	pages 462–466	compensated shock
131.	(a)	pages 462–466	decompensated shock
132.	(e)	pages 485–488, 504–506	pneumothorax
133.	(a)	pages 485–488, 504–506	sucking chest wound
134.	(c)	pages 485–488, 504–506	occlusive dressing of open chest wound
135.	(b)	pages 485–488, 504–506	occlusive dressing of open chest wound
136.	(b)	pages 485–488, 504–506	pneumothorax
137.	(d)	pages 485–488, 504–506	hemothorax
138.	(c)	pages 485–488, 504–506	tension pneumothorax
139.	(e)	pages 485–488, 504–506	hemopneumothorax
140.	(a)	pages 485–488, 504–506	traumatic asphyxia signs and symptoms
141.	(b)	pages 485–488, 504–506	cardiac tamponade
142.	(d)	pages 485–488, 504–506	cardiac tamponade signs and symptoms

1994 Revised EMT-Basic National Standards Review Self-Test
ANSWER SECTION SIX

The page numbers following each answer indicate that subject's reference page within Brady's **Emergency Care**, 7th ed., 1994. If you do not have access to Brady's text, utilize the index of the text you do have to obtain information for review of each question's subject.

QUESTION	ANSWER	PAGE KEY	SUBJECT
1.	(c)	pages 600–601	infant age range
2.	(b)	pages 600–601	toddler age range
3.	(a)	pages 600–601	preschooler age range
4.	(e)	pages 600–601	school-age age range
5.	(d)	pages 600–601	adolescent age range
6.	(d)	pages 600–601	infant concern characteristics
7.	(a)	pages 600–601	toddler concern characteristics
8.	(c)	pages 600–601	preschool and school-age concern characteristics
9.	(b)	pages 600–601	adolescent concern characteristics
10.	(c)	page 602	pediatric airway considerations
11.	(c)	pages 602–603	pediatric airway positioning
12.	(a)	pages 604–606	pediatric airway obstruction treatment
13.	(c)	pages 604–606	pediatric airway obstruction treatment
14.	(c)	pages 604–606	pediatric airway obstruction treatment
15.	(e)	pages 604–606	pediatric airway obstruction treatment
16.	(e)	pages 126–127, 604	pediatric oral airway adjunct use
17.	(d)	page 604	pediatric oxygen administration
18.	(e)	page 604	pediatric artificial ventilation rate
19.	(e)	page 609	pediatric respiratory assessment
20.	(c)	page 611	normal infant pulse rate
21.	(b)	page 611	normal preschooler pulse rate
22.	(b)	page 611	normal toddler respiratory rate
23.	(e)	pages 74–75	infant and child pulse rates
24.	(c)	page 610	pediatric blood pressure assessment
25.	(c)	page 610	detailed physical exam order
26.	(e)	pages 614–616	airway obstruction care
27.	(c)	pages 282–284, 288, 614	pediatric respiratory distress (EMT-assisted inhaler use)
28.	(b)	pages 120–125	pediatric ventilation/pocket face mask
29.	(e)	pages 120–125	pediatric ventilation/flow-restricted, oxygen-powered ventilation device
30.	(c)	page 353	pediatric assisted epinephrine injections
31.	(d)	pages 616–617	pediatric seizures
32.	(e)	page 618	treatment of pediatric poisoning

QUESTION	ANSWER	PAGE KEY	SUBJECT
33.	(d)	page 618	treatment of pediatric poisoning
34.	(e)	page 613	pediatric fevers
35.	(a)	pages 618–619	pediatric shock
36.	(c)	page 619	near-drowning transportation factors
37.	(e)	pages 619–620	sudden infant death syndrome
38.	(e)	pages 619–620	sudden infant death syndrome
39.	(a)	pages 620–621	pediatric trauma
40.	(d)	pages 620–621	pediatric trauma
41.	(d)	pages 622–625	child abuse and neglect
42.	(e)	pages 622–625	child abuse and neglect
43.	(b)	pages 622–625	child abuse and neglect

1994 Revised EMT-Basic National Standards Review Self-Test
ANSWER SECTION SEVEN

The page numbers following each answer indicate that subject's reference page within Brady's ***Emergency Care***, 7th ed., 1994. If you do not have access to Brady's text, utilize the index of the text you do have to obtain information for review of each question's subject.

QUESTION	ANSWER	PAGE KEY	SUBJECT
1.	(a)	pages 643–646	emergency vehicle operation with lights and sirens in use
2.	(e)	pages 643–646	emergency vehicle operation with lights and sirens in use
3.	(d)	pages 643–646	emergency vehicle operation without lights and sirens in use
4.	(b)	pages 643–646	use of sirens
5.	(e)	pages 643–646	use of lights and sirens
6.	(a)	pages 643–646	use of sirens
7.	(d)	pages 643–646	use of excessive speed
8.	(b)	pages 643–646	use of emergency escort
9.	(c)	page 646	most common emergency vehicle accident site
10.	(c)	pages 667–679	rescue and extrication duties
11.	(e)	pages 667–679	rescue and extrication duties
12.	(b)	pages 667–679	EMS and rescue priorities
13.	(a)	pages 667–679	EMS and rescue priorities
14.	(a)	page 679	simple access rescue techniques
15.	(a)	pages 647, 690	parking upwind of the hazardous materials scene
16.	(b)	pages 689–691	hazardous materials scene duties
17.	(d)	pages 689–691	hazardous materials identification
18.	(e)	pages 689–691	hazardous materials identification
19.	(d)	pages 693–696	multiple-casualty incident (MCI), or multiple-casualty situation (MCS)
20.	(e)	pages 693–696	incident management system
21.	(b)	pages 693–696	incident management system activation
22.	(c)	pages 693–696	triage
23.	(d)	pages 693–696	goal of triage
24.	(c)	pages 693–696	triage category, Priority 1
25.	(a)	pages 693–696	triage category, Priority 2
26.	(b)	pages 693–696	triage category, Priority 3
27.	(d)	pages 693–696	triage category, Priority 4 (Priority 0)

1994 Revised EMT-Basic National Standards Review Self-Test
ANSWER SECTION EIGHT

The page numbers following each answer indicate that subject's reference page within Brady's ***Emergency Care***, 7th ed., 1994. If you do not have access to Brady's text, utilize the index of the text you do have to obtain information for review of each question's subject.

QUESTION	ANSWER	PAGE KEY	SUBJECT
1.	(e)	page 710	oropharynx
2.	(b)	page 710	nasopharynx
3.	(d)	page 710	hypopharynx
4.	(d)	page 710	epiglottis
5.	(c)	page 710	valecula
6.	(e)	page 710	trachea
7.	(a)	page 710	cricoid cartilage
8.	(b)	page 710	larynx
9.	(b)	page 710	right and left bronchi
10.	(c)	page 710	alveoli
11.	(a)	page 712	cricoid cartilage—the narrowest area of the pediatric airway
12.	(b)	pages 713–723	endotracheal tube
13.	(c)	page 713	intubation
14.	(b)	page 713	orotracheal intubation
15.	(a)	pages 714–715	laryngoscope
16.	(c)	page 713	orotracheal intubation advantages
17.	(a)	pages 713–714	orotracheal intubation complications
18.	(e)	pages 713–714	orotracheal intubation complications
19.	(c)	pages 713–714	orotracheal intubation complications
20.	(d)	pages 714–715	laryngoscope blade sizes
21.	(b)	pages 714–715	use of the straight laryngoscope blade
22.	(a)	pages 714–715	use of the curved laryngoscope blade
23.	(c)	page 716	average male endotracheal tube
24.	(e)	page 716	average female endotracheal tube
25.	(c)	page 716	average adult endotracheal tube
26.	(c)	page 716	endotracheal tube 15 mm adapter
27.	(b)	page 716	Murphy's eye
28.	(c)	page 716	endotracheal tube inflatable cuff
29.	(b)	page 716	endotracheal tube inflatable cuff
30.	(a)	page 716	endotracheal tube pilot balloon
31.	(d)	page 716	endotracheal tube length
32.	(c)	page 717	average airway distances
33.	(b)	page 717	average airway distances
34.	(a)	page 717	average airway distances

TEST SECTION EIGHT ANSWER KEY

QUESTION	ANSWER	PAGE KEY	SUBJECT
35.	(d)	page 717	endotracheal tube stylet
36.	(d)	page 717	lubricants for intubation
37.	(e)	pages 717–718	orotracheal intubation indications
38.	(c)	pages 717–718	orotracheal intubation preparation
39.	(e)	pages 717–718	orotracheal intubation preparation
40.	(c)	page 718	orotracheal intubation head positioning
41.	(a)	page 718	orotracheal intubation head positioning for the trauma patient
42.	(c)	page 718	holding the laryngoscope
43.	(d)	pages 718–722	use of the laryngoscope
44.	(b)	pages 720–722	Sellick's maneuver
45.	(a)	page 722	visualization of the glottic opening
46.	(a)	page 722	insertion of the endotracheal tube
47.	(e)	page 722	preparing to check tube placement
48.	(d)	page 722	most accurate tube placement verification
49.	(a)	page 722	auscultation of epigastrium first
50.	(c)	page 723	right mainstem bronchus intubation
51.	(b)	page 723	gastric intubation
52.	(e)	pages 722–723	securing the endotracheal tube
53.	(e)	page 723	reassessing tube placement
54.	(e)	pages 723–724	indications for pediatric orotracheal intubation
55.	(b)	page 716	premature infant endotracheal tube size
56.	(c)	page 724	newborn and small infant endotracheal tube size
57.	(d)	page 724	large infant (up to 1 year old) endotracheal tube size
58.	(a)	page 724	mathematic formula for pediatric endotracheal tube size
59.	(e)	page 724	physical method of selecting pediatric endotracheal tube size
60.	(a)	page 724	uncuffed pediatric endotracheal tube
61.	(d)	page 724	pediatric laryngoscope blades
62.	(c)	pages 724–725	pediatric intubation head positioning
63.	(c)	pages 724–725	pediatric intubation head positioning for the trauma patient
64.	(e)	page 603	towel elevation of pediatric shoulders to improve alignment of the airway
65.	(d)	page 725	most accurate pediatric endotracheal tube placement verification
66.	(d)	page 725	poor chest rise with ventilation
67.	(c)	page 725	nasogastric tube purpose
68.	(d)	page 726	nasogastric tube indications
69.	(d)	page 726	nasogastric tube complications
70.	(a)	page 726	steps of nasogastric tube insertion
71.	(b)	page 726	orotracheal suctioning
72.	(e)	page 726	orotracheal suctioning indications

QUESTION	ANSWER	PAGE KEY	SUBJECT
73.	(c)	page 726	orotracheal suctioning requires sterile technique
74.	(d)	pages 726–729	orotracheal suctioning preparation
75.	(c)	pages 726–729	orotracheal suctioning techniques
76.	(a)	pages 726–729	orotracheal suctioning techniques
77.	(b)	pages 726–729	orotracheal suctioning techniques
78.	(d)	page 729	complications of orotracheal suctioning

1994 Revised EMT-Basic National Standards Review Self-Test
ANSWER SECTION NINE

APPENDICES A AND B OF BRADY'S *EMERGENCY CARE*, 7TH ED.

ALS-ASSIST SKILLS AND INFECTIOUS DISEASES

The page numbers following each answer indicate that subject's reference page within Brady's *Emergency Care*, 7th ed., 1994. If you do not have access to Brady's text, utilize the index of the text you do have to obtain information for review of each question's subject.

ASSISTING WITH ENDOTRACHEAL INTUBATION

QUESTION	ANSWER	PAGE KEY	SUBJECT
1.	(c)	page 739	hyperventilation before endotracheal intubation
2.	(c)	pages 739–741	endotracheal intubation head positioning
3.	(a)	pages 739–741	trauma patient endotracheal intubation head positioning
4.	(b)	pages 739–741	Sellick's maneuver
5.	(e)	pages 739–741	monitoring endotracheal tube depth
6.	(c)	pages 739–741	monitoring endotracheal tube depth
7.	(c)	pages 739–741	monitoring endotracheal tube depth
8.	(d)	pages 739–741	ventilation of the intubated patient
9.	(b)	pages 739–741	increased lung resistance with ventilations
10.	(c)	pages 739–741	changes in lung resistance with ventilations
11.	(c)	pages 739–741	ventilating and defibrillation
12.	(b)	pages 739–741	ventilating and changes in patient level of consciousness
13.	(a)	pages 739–741	oral airway bite blocks and ventilations
14.	(c)	pages 739–741	endotracheal tube medication administration

ASSISTING WITH ECG APPLICATION AND USE QUESTION

QUESTION	ANSWER	PAGE KEY	SUBJECT
15.	(a)	pages 741–742	the electrocardiogram (ECG)
16.	(c)	pages 741–742	EMT ECG assistance
17.	(a)	pages 741–742	ECG electrodes
18.	(e)	pages 741–742	ECG electrode application
19.	(a)	pages 741–742	monitoring electrode placement
20.	(d)	pages 741–742	monitoring electrode placement
21.	(e)	pages 741–742	monitoring electrode placement

PULSE OXIMETER USE

QUESTION	ANSWER	PAGE KEY	SUBJECT
22.	(d)	pages 742–743	the pulse oximeter
23.	(d)	pages 742–743	pulse oximetry equipment
24.	(d)	pages 742–743	sensing probe application
25.	(b)	pages 742–743	indications for pulse oximetry
26.	(a)	pages 742–743	target blood O2 saturation
27.	(b)	pages 742–743	primary benefit of pulse oximetry
28.	(c)	pages 742–743	causes of inaccurate pulse oximeter readings
29.	(b)	pages 742–743	pulse oximeter monitoring

ASSISTING WITH IV THERAPY

QUESTION	ANSWER	PAGE KEY	SUBJECT
30.	(a)	page 743	intravenous
31.	(a)	page 743	micro or mini drip administration set
32.	(a)	page 743	macro or maxi drip administration set
33.	(c)	page 743	micro/mini drip chamber barrel
34.	(b)	page 744	IV tubing extension set
35.	(c)	page 744	responsibilities of assembling the IV equipment
36.	(d)	page 744	the tubing flow regulator
37.	(e)	page 744	sterile assembly
38.	(c)	page 744	the drip chamber fluid level
39.	(c)	page 744	flushing the IV tubing
40.	(d)	page 745	IV flow obstructions
41.	(a)	page 745	blood clotting the IV catheter
42.	(d)	page 745	runaway IV
43.	(b)	page 745	infiltrated IV

INFECTIOUS DISEASES

QUESTION	ANSWER	PAGE KEY	SUBJECT
44.	(a)	page 748	communicable diseases
45.	(e)	page 747	diseases most dangerous to health care providers
46.	(c)	page 747	the most dangerous disease for health care providers
47.	(d)	pages 20–21, 747	infectious disease transmission
48.	(d)	pages 748–750	body substance isolation (BSI) precautions
49.	(c)	pages 20–21, 747–749	BSI precautions
50.	(c)	page 747	hepatitis
51.	(d)	pages 747–748	AIDS (acquired immune deficiency syndrome)
52.	(b)	pages 747–748	AIDS/HIV (human immunodeficiency virus)
53.	(b)	page 747	hepatitis
54.	(c)	page 747	AIDS
55.	(e)	page 748	staphylococcal skin infections ("staff")

TEST SECTION NINE ANSWER KEY

QUESTION	ANSWER	PAGE KEY	SUBJECT
56.	(c)	page 747	tuberculosis (TB)
57.	(a)	page 748	human skin as an infection barrier
58.	(d)	page 748	mucous membranes and infections
59.	(a)	page 749	contraindication of direct mouth-to-mouth respirations
60.	(b)	page 749	cross-infection of pathogens
61.	(b)	page 749	contaminated supplies and equipment
62.	(e)	pages 749–750	federal law and EMS employer's responsibilities

1994 REVISED EMT-BASIC NATIONAL STANDARDS REVIEW SELF-TEST

GUIDE TO COMMON MEDICAL ABBREVIATIONS AND SYMBOLS

Many of the following abbreviations were used in this text. For the purpose of self-improvement, the EMT should study the list here, which is more comprehensive. It contains abbreviations the professional EMT should be familiar with and use on a regular basis. When an abbreviation is based on the Latin or Greek form of a word, the Latin or Greek word is presented in parentheses to improve the EMT's understanding of the abbreviation's origin.

The appropriate use of upper- and lowercase letters is an important distinction in medical abbreviations. For example, "cc" is the abbreviation for cubic centimeter, whereas "CC" is the abbreviation for chief complaint; and "Ca" is the abbreviation for calcium, whereas "CA" is the abbreviation for cancer.

$\bar{a}$	before (***ante***)
AAOx3	alert and oriented to person/place/time
abd or abdo	abdomen
AMA	against medical advice
AMI	acute myocardial infarction/heart attack
ASA	acetylsalicylic acid/aspirin
ASHD	arteriosclerotic heart disease
BCP	birth control pills
bid (or b.i.d.)	twice a day (***bis in die***)
BM	bowel movement
BS	breath sounds ***or*** blood sugar
BVM	bag-valve-mask device
$\bar{c}$	with (***cum***)
CA	cancer
CAD	coronary artery disease
CAOx3	conscious, alert, oriented to person/place/time
cc	cubic centimeter
CC	chief complaint
CHF	congestive heart failure
CHI	closed head injury
cm	centimeter
CNS	central nervous system
c/o	complains of
CO	carbon monoxide

CO_2	carbon dioxide
conx	conscious
COPD/COLD	chronic obstructive pulmonary (lung) disease
cp	chest pain
CSF	cerebrospinal fluid
CVA	cerebrovascular accident/stroke
dc	discontinue
Dx	diagnosis/dislocation
ea	each
ED	Emergency Department
EMS	Emergency Medical Services
EMT	Emergency Medical Technician
EMT-B	Emergency Medical Technician-Basic level
EMT-I	Emergency Medical Technician-Intermediate
EMT-P	Emergency Medical Technician-Paramedic
ER	Emergency Room
et	and (*et*)
ETOH	alcohol (ethyl alcohol)
FROM	full range of motion
Fx	fracture
GI	gastrointestinal
Gm/gm	gram
GSW	gunshot wound
GU	genitourinary
GYN	gynecological
HA	headache
HEENT	head, ears, eyes, nose, throat
hs (or h.s.)	at bedtime (***hora somni***)
Hx	history
ICP	intercranial pressure
ICS	intercostal space
JVD	jugular vein distention
Kg/kg	kilogram

Ⓛ	left
lac	laceration
LBB	long backboard
LLQ	left lower quadrant
LMP	last menstrual period
lpm	liters per minute
LUQ	left upper quadrant
LOC	level of consciousness (**not** loss of consciousness!)
MAST	military anti-shock trousers
mg	milligram
MI	myocardial infarction/heart attack
MICU	mobile intensive care unit
ml	milliliter
mm	millimeter
MOI	mechanism of injury
N/A	not applicable
NPO	nothing by mouth (nothing **per os**)
nc	nasal cannula
NRB	nonrebreather mask
NTG	nitroglycerine
n/v	nausea and vomiting
n/v/d	nausea, vomiting, and diarrhea
OB	obstetrics
OBS	organic brain syndrome
OD	overdose/right eye (**occulus dexter**)
p̄	after (**post**)
PASG	pneumatic anti-shock garment
PE	pulmonary embolism
PEARL	pupils equal and reactive to light
PID	pelvic inflammatory disease
PNS	peripheral nervous system
po	by mouth (**per os**)
prn	as needed (**pro re nata**)
PTOA	prior to our arrival
PMH	past medical history

q̄ . . . . every (***quaque***)
qd (or q.d.) . . . . every day (***quaque die***)
qid (or q.i.d.) . . . . . . four times a day (quarter in die)

Ⓡ . . . . right
RBC . . . . red blood cell
R/O . . . . rule out
RLQ . . . . right lower quadrant
RUQ . . . . right upper quadrant
ROM . . . . range of motion
Rx . . . . recipe/prescription

s̄ . . . . without (the Latin ***sine*** or the French, ***sans***)
sc/sq . . . . subcutaneous
sl . . . . sublingual
SOB . . . . shortness of breath
s/s . . . . signs and symptoms
Sx . . . . symptoms

TIA . . . . transient ischemic attack/"mini-stroke"
tid (or t.i.d.) . . . . three times a day (***ter in die***)
trans . . . . transport
Tx . . . . treatment (***not*** transportation)

U/A . . . . upon arrival
UA . . . . urine analysis
unconx . . . . unconscious
URI . . . . upper respiratory infection
UTI . . . . urinary tract infection

WBC . . . . white blood cell
w/d . . . . warm and dry
w/d/pink . . . . warm, dry, and pink
WNL . . . . within normal limits

y/o . . . . years old

COMMON MEDICAL SYMBOLS

Symbol	Meaning	Symbol	Meaning
∿∿	approximately	⊕	positive for
△	change	⊖	negative for
>	greater than	Ⓗ	husband
<	less than	Ⓕ	father
↓	below or decreased	Ⓜ	mother
↑	above or increased	Ⓦ	wife
=	equal to	♀	female
2°	secondary to	♂	male
X	"times"/multiply by	⊙—	supine
			sitting
			standing